Advances in Trauma and Critical Care
Volume 9

Advances in Trauma and Critical Care
Volumes 1 through 6 (out of print)

Volume 7

What's New in Multiple System Organ Failure, by Arthur E. Baue and Eugen Faist
Advances in Oxygen Delivery, by Niels Lund
Inotropes in the Intensive Care Unit, by Thomas M. Scalea and Sharon M. Henry
Selective Decontamination in the Intensive Care Unit, by Jan A. Goris and Roelof van Dalen
Bacterial Translocation: Fact or Fancy, by Lena M. Napolitano and Christopher C. Baker
Monitoring and Treatment of Renal Failure, by Charles E. Lucas, Jonathon M. Saxe, Stephen T. Wysong, and Anna M. Ledgerwood
Chest Wall Injuries: New Trends in Analgesia, by Robert C. Mackersie
Emergency Department Thoracotomy for Trauma: A Reappraisal, by M. Margaret Knudson
Exsanguinating Craniofacial Trauma, by Richard B. Fratianne and Christine S. Cocanour
Perineal Injuries, by Ronald M. Stewart and Kenneth A. Kudsk
Imaging Techniques in Trauma, by Yoram Ben-Menachem
Tracheobronchial Injuries, by Philip D. Feliciano and Donald D. Trunkey

Volume 8

Blunt Pulmonary Injury, by Frederick A. Moore, James B. Haenel, and Ernest E. Moore
Hepatic Trauma, by James Jaggers and Philip D. Feliciano
Blood Transfusion Therapy in the Surgical Intensive Care Unit, by Roderick L. Johnson and Joyce Atlee Campbell
Penetrating Torso Trauma, by Ricardo Ferrada and Alberto Garcia
Injury Severity Scoring in Trauma Patients, by Robert Rutledge and Samir M. Fakhry
Blunt Traumatic Rupture of the Thoracic Aorta, by Aurelio Rodriguez and David Elliott
Head Injury From the General Surgeon's Perspective, by David H. Wisner
Peripheral Venous Injury, by James M. Edwards and Gregory L. Moneta
Nutritional Support of the Critically Ill and Injured Patient, by K. Dean Gubler and Gregory J. Jurkovich
Ethical Considerations in the Intensive Care Unit, by Glenn C. Graber
Current Management of Hand Injuries, by John H. Ganser and Alan E. Seyfer

Advances in Trauma and Critical Care

Editor-in-Chief
Kimball I. Maull, M.D.
Professor and Vice Chairman, Department of Surgery, Stritch School of Medicine; Director, Division of Trauma and Emergency Medical Services, Loyola University Medical Center, Maywood, Illinois

Associate Editors
Henry C. Cleveland, M.D.
Clinical Professor of Surgery, University of Colorado Health Sciences Center; President and CEO, ETHIX Sloans Lake, A Health Care Corporation, Denver, Colorado

David V. Feliciano, M.D.
Professor of Surgery, Emory University School of Medicine, Chief of Surgery, Grady Memorial Hospital, Atlanta, Georgia

Charles L. Rice, M.D.
Professor of Surgery, University of Illinois College of Medicine, Chicago, Illinois

Donald D. Trunkey, M.D.
Professor and Chairman, Department of Surgery, Oregon Health Sciences University School of Medicine, Portland, Oregon

Charles C. Wolferth, Jr., M.D.
Emilie & Roland T. deHellebrandth Professor of Surgery, University of Pennsylvania School of Medicine; Surgeon-in-Chief, Department of Surgery, The Graduate Hospital, Philadelphia, Pennsylvania

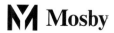

Volume 9 • 1994

St. Louis Baltimore Berlin Boston Carlsbad Chicago London Madrid
Naples New York Philadelphia Sydney Tokyo Toronto

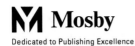
Mosby
Dedicated to Publishing Excellence

Vice President and Publisher, Continuity Publishing: Kenneth H. Killion
Director, Editorial Development: Gretchen C. Murphy
Developmental Editor: Bernadette Buchholz
Sr. Production Editor: Jill Waite
Project Supervisor: Maria Nevinger
Proofreading Supervisor: Barbara M. Kelly
Vice President, Professional Sales and Marketing: George M. Parker
Marketing and Circulation Manager: Barry J. Bowlus
Marketing Coordinator: Lynn Stevenson

Copyright © 1994 by Mosby-Year Book, Inc.

All rights reserved. No part of this publication may be reproduced, stored in a retrieval system, or transmitted, in any form or by any means, electronic, mechanical, photocopying, recording, or otherwise, without prior written permission from the publisher.

Permission to photocopy or reproduce solely for internal or personal use is permitted for libraries or other users registered with the Copyright Clearance Center, provided that the base fee of $4.00 per chapter plus $.10 per page is paid directly to the Copyright Clearance Center, 27 Congress Street, Salem, MA 01970. This consent does not extend to other kinds of copying, such as copying for general distribution, for advertising or promotional purposes, for creating new collected works, or for resale.

Printed in the United States of America
Composition by The Clarinda Company
Printing/binding by The Maple-Vail Book Manufacturing Group

Editorial Office:
Mosby–Year Book, Inc.
200 North LaSalle St.
Chicago, IL 60601

Mosby-Year Book, Inc.
11830 Westline Industrial Drive
St. Louis, Missouri 63146
International Standard Serial Number: 0886–7755
International Standard Book Number: 0–8151–6201–4

Contributors

Lawrence B. Bone, M.D.
Associate Professor of Orthopaedic Surgery, State University of New York at Buffalo; Director of Musculoskeletal Trauma Service, Erie County Medical Center, Buffalo, New York

Ulf Borg, B.S.
Research Associate, Co-Director, Extracorporeal Lung Assist Program, Department of Critical Care, University of Maryland School of Medicine, R. Adams Cowley Shock Trauma Center, Baltimore, Maryland

Christopher T. Born, M.D.
Associate Professor of Clinical Surgery, Department of Surgery, University of Medicine and Dentistry of New Jersey/Robert Wood Johnson Medical School-Camden, Cooper Hospital/University Medical Center, Camden, New Jersey

John B. Catalano, M.D.
Fellow in Orthopaedic Traumatology, Department of Surgery, University of Medicine and Dentistry of New Jersey/Robert Wood Johnson Medical School-Camden, Cooper Hospital/University Medical Center, Camden, New Jersey

David V. Feliciano, M.D.
Chief of Surgery, Grady Memorial Hospital; Professor of Surgery, Emory University School of Medicine, Atlanta, Georgia

John B. Fortune, M.D.
Associate Professor of Surgery, Department of Surgery, Albany Medical Center, Albany, New York

Larry M. Gentilello, M.D.
Assistant Professor of Surgery, Harborview Medical Center, University of Washington School of Medicine, Seattle, Washington

Nadar Habashi, M.D.
Intensivist, Assistant Professor of Medicine, Co-Director, Extracorporeal Lung Assist Program, Department of Critical Care, University of Maryland School of Medicine, R. Adams Cowley Shock Trauma Center, Baltimore, Maryland

David B. Hoyt, M.D.
Associate Professor of Surgery, Chief, Division of Trauma, University of California, San Diego School of Medicine, San Diego, California

Roger E. Huckfeldt, M.D.
Instructor, Trauma Fellow, Division of General Surgery, Oregon Health Sciences University, Portland, Oregon

Rao R. Ivatury, M.D.
Professor of Surgery, New York Medical College; Director, Trauma, Co-Director, Surgical Intensive Care Unit, Lincoln Medical & Mental Health Center, Bronx, New York

Lenworth M. Jacobs, M.D., M.P.H.
Professor of Surgery, University of Connecticut Health Center; Director, Trauma Program, Hartford Hospital, Hartford, Connecticut

David H. Kuehler, M.D.
Assistant Professor of Surgery, Department of Surgery, Albany Medical Center, Albany, New York

Wendy J. Marshall, M.D.
Associate Professor of Surgery, Stritch School of Medicine; Director, Trauma Services, Loyola University Medical Center, Maywood, Illinois

Reginald W. Martin, M.D.
Assistant Professor of Surgery, Department of Surgery, University of Mississippi Medical Center, Jackson, Mississippi

Richard J. Mullins, M.D.
Associate Professor, Director, Trauma Service, Division of General Surgery, Oregon Health Sciences University, Portland, Oregon

Stephane Panic, M.D.
Trauma/Surgical Critical Care Fellow, Hartford Hospital, Hartford, Connecticut

H. Neal Reynolds, M.D.
Intensivist, Assistant Professor of Medicine, Co-Director, Extracorporeal Lung Assist Program, Department of Critical Care, University of Maryland School of Medicine, R. Adams Cowley Shock Trauma Center, Baltimore, Maryland

Robert S. Rhodes, M.D.
James D. Hardy Professor and Chairman, Department of Surgery, University of Mississippi Medical Center, Jackson, Mississippi

J. David Richardson, M.D.
Professor and Vice Chairman, Department of Surgery, University of Louisville, Louisville, Kentucky

Michael Rohman, M.D.
Professor of Surgery, New York Medical College; Chief, Cardio-thoracic Surgery, Lincoln Medical & Mental Health Center, Bronx, New York

Alexander S. Rosemurgy, II, M.D.
Associate Professor of Surgery, Department of Surgery, University of South Florida, Tampa, Florida

Steven E. Ross, M.D.
Associate Professor of Surgery, Department of Surgery, University of Medicine and Dentistry of New Jersey/Robert Wood Johnson Medical School-Camden, Cooper Hospital/University Medical Center, Camden, New Jersey

Ronald J. Simon, M.D.
Assistant Professor of Surgery, New York Medical College; Attending Surgeon, Lincoln Medical & Mental Health Center, Bronx, New York

Richard K. Simons, M.B., B.Chir., F.R.C.S., F.R.C.S.(C)
Assistant Professor of Surgery, Department of Surgery, Division of Trauma, University of California, San Diego School of Medicine, San Diego, California

Philip M. Stegemann, M.D.
Clinical Assistant Professor of Orthopaedic Surgery, State University of New York at Buffalo, Erie County Medical Center, Buffalo, New York

John F. Sweeney, M.D.
Surgery—Immunology Research Fellow, Department of Surgery, University of South Florida, Tampa, Florida

Donald D. Trunkey, M.D.
Professor, Chairman, Department of Surgery, Division of General Surgery, Oregon Health Sciences University, Portland, Oregon

Contents

Contributors v

Prehospital Care: What Works, What Does Not
By Lenworth M. Jacobs and Stephane Panic **1**
   Prevention 1
   Prehospital Time Factor 2
   Basic Life Support vs. Advanced Life Support 3
   Airway Management 5
   Intravenous Line Placement in the Field 7
   Pneumatic Antishock Garment 8
   Immobilization 8
   Conclusions 10

Diagnosis, Temporary Stabilization, and Definitive Treatment of Injuries to the Cervical Spine
By John B. Catalano, Christopher T. Born, and Steven E. Ross . . **15**
   Clinical Risk Factors 16
   Initial Radiographic Evaluation 18
   Temporary Spinal Immobilization 20
   Specialty Beds for Immobilization of the Spine 21
   Traction, Collars, or the Halo for Cervical Immobilization in the Hospital 22
   Specific Injury Patterns and Treatment 22
      Fracture of the Occipital Condyles 22
      Occipital-atlantal Injuries 23
      Fractures of C1 24
      Atlantoaxial Rotation Injuries 25
      Odontoid Fractures 26
      Hangman's Fracture 27
      Injuries to the Lower Cervical Spine 28
      Penetrating Trauma to the Cervical Spine 33

Practical Approaches to Hypothermia
By Larry M. Gentilello **39**
   Definitions 39
   Hypothermia in the Trauma Victim 41
   Thermoregulation 43

Hypothermia and Oxygen Consumption. 45
Temperature and Metabolism 46
Induced Hypothermia 47
Detrimental Effects of Hypothermia 49
    Cardiovascular 49
    Respiratory System 51
    Central Nervous System 52
    Renal 53
    Gastrointestinal 53
    Endocrine 54
    Blood 54
Mechanisms of Heat Loss and Heat Transfer 55
    Conduction 55
    Convection 56
    Radiation 56
    Evaporation 57
Treatment 57
    Passive External Rewarming 57
    Active External Rewarming 58
    Active Core Rewarming 62
Summary 69

Protective Surgical Wear
By Reginald W. Martin and Robert S. Rhodes **81**

Pathogens 82
    Tuberculosis 82
    Hepatitis B Virus 82
    Human Immunodeficiency Virus 83
The Role and Development of Specific Attire 84
    Gloves 84
    Gowns 84
    Masks/Caps 85
    Eyewear 86
    Footwear and Accessory Recommendations 86
Conclusion 86

Minimally Invasive Surgery
By Wendy J. Marshall **89**

History 90
Technique 92
Complications 92
Gasless Laparoscopy 93

Pediatric Laparoscopy. 93
Thoracoscopy 94
Summary 96

New Directions and Applications for Extracorporeal Cardiopulmonary Support
By H. Neal Reynolds, Nadar Habashi, and Ulf Borg **99**

Historical Perspective 100
   Acute Respiratory Failure and Ventilatory Support 100
   Extracorporeal Life Support. 101
Nomenclature for Extracorporeal Life Support 104
Patient Selection Criteria and Applications 106
   Respiratory Failure Caused by Diffuse Acute Lung Disease . . 106
   Respiratory Failure Resulting From Status Asthmaticus 107
Nonpulmonary Indications for Extracorporeal Support 108
   Rewarming After Accidental Hypothermia 108
   Repair of Traumatic Rupture of the Aorta 109
   Failure of Cardiopulmonary Resuscitation 111
   Cardiac Failure and Cardiogenic Shock 112
   Bridge to Transplantation 112
Technique of Extracorporeal Support. 113
   Equipment 113
"Sweep Gas" 115
   Cannulation. 115
   Pressure Monitoring. 116
   Technical Variations. 117
Ventilator Management Before and During $ECCO_2R$/ECMO . . . 117
Anticoagulant Therapy 118
Complications of Extracorporeal Circulatory Support. 120
The Future of Extracorporeal Circulatory Support 122

Immunomodulation
By Richard K. Simons and David B. Hoyt **135**

Normal Host Defenses 135
   Barriers 135
   Humoral Mechanisms 136
   Cellular Mechanisms 137
   Mediators. 137
Immune Dysfunction After Trauma. 138
Mechanisms of Immunosuppression After Trauma 140
   Tissue Injury 140
   Gastrointestinal Tract and Bacterial Translocation 141

    Stress Hormones. 141
    Mediators. 141
    Suppressor Factors 142
    Suppressor Cells 142
    Hypoxia and Ischemia. 143
    Nutritional Deficiency 143
Sepsis and the Systemic Inflammatory Response 143
Immunomodulation. 144
    Preservation of Normal Defenses. 144
    Immunologic Stimulation. 146
    Sepsis and Immunologic Blockade 150
Summary 157

Treatment of the Pediatric Patient in an Adult Trauma Center
By John B. Fortune and David H. Kuehler **169**

Adult and Pediatric Trauma 170
    Demographics and Injury Types 170
Special Aspects of Pediatric Trauma 173
    Physiologic Differences of the Injured Child 173
    Airway. 174
    Breathing. 175
    Circulation 176
    Disability 178
    Abdominal Injuries 178
The Ideal Pediatric Trauma Center. 179
    Standards for Pediatric Trauma Centers 179
    The Problem With Pediatric Trauma Centers 179
Treatment of the Pediatric Patient in a Comprehensive Adult Trauma Center 181
    Commitment and Scope. 181
    Composition of the Pediatric Trauma Team 183
    Facilities 184
    Follow-up Care/Rehabilitation/Psychosocial Care 187
    Evaluation of a Pediatric Trauma Program in an Adult Trauma Center 188
Decision Tree for Triage of the Pediatric Patient. 192
Conclusion 196

Pelvic Fractures
By Roger E. Huckfeldt, Richard J. Mullins, and Donald D. Trunkey **199**

Incidence. 199

Anatomy 200
Classification 200
Concomitant Injuries 204
Hemorrhage 205
Soft-Tissue Injury/Open Pelvic Fracture 213
Rectal Injury 214
Vaginal Injuries 215
Urinary Tract Injury 216
Neurologic Injury 219
Complications 219
   Respiratory Failure 219
   Thrombosis 221
   Sepsis 222
Acetabular Fractures 222
Orthopaedic Considerations 223
Summary 223

Opportunistic *Candida* Infection Complicating Major Injury: A Consequence of Immune Suppression
By Alexander S. Rosemurgy, II, and John F. Sweeney **227**

Esophageal Injury
By Rao R. Ivatury, Michael Rohman, and Ronald J. Simon **245**
Surgical Anatomy 245
Etiology of Esophageal Injury 248
   Injury From an Intraluminal Force 249
   Injury from External Trauma 251
Diagnosis of Esophageal Injury 252
   Clinical Symptoms and Signs 253
   Radiography 254
Treatment of Esophageal Injury 259
   Injuries to the Cervical Esophagus 259
   Injuries to the Thoracic Esophagus 260
Results and Prognostic Considerations 268
Special Considerations 269
   Combined Tracheoesophageal Injuries 269
   Thoracoscopy in Esophageal Injuries 270
Summary 272

Early Fixation of Long-Bone Fractures
By Lawrence B. Bone and Philip M. Stegemann **275**
Historical Perspective 275

Early Fracture Fixation 276
Indications for Early Long-Bone Stabilization 279
Contraindications to Early Fracture Stabilization 284
Physiologic Response to Early Fracture Stabilization (the Wound and Its Local Consequences) 288
Conclusion 291

Variations on a Theme: Does Enteral Feeding Make a Difference?
By J. David Richardson **295**
The Case for Early Enteral Feeding 297
Bacterial Translocation 299
   Bacterial Translocation in Surgical Patients 300
Clinical Studies of Enteral Feeding 302
Critical Analysis of the Effect of Enteral Feeding on Sepsis. . . 307
What Are the Disadvantages of Nutritional Therapy? 310
The Cost of Nutritional Support: Parenteral vs. Enteral 312
Does the Method of Nutritional Support Affect Outcome? . . . 312
Who Should Receive Enteral Support? 313
Summary 314

A New Look at Penetrating Carotid Artery Injuries
By David V. Feliciano **319**
Cervical Hematoma With Compromise of the Airway. 319
Diagnostic Evaluation of Penetrating Wounds in Zone I 321
Treatment of a Penetrating Wound in Zone III 323
Occlusion of the Internal Artery in an Asymptomatic Patient . . . 328
Routine Repairs in Zone II Injuries 329
Treatment of the Carotid Artery Injury With Associated Stroke or Coma 332
Balloon Catheter Tamponade. 334
Carotid-Jugular Fistula 338
Blowout of the Carotid Artery in the Postoperative Period 340

Index 347

Mosby Document Express

Copies of the full text of journal articles referenced in this book are available by calling Mosby Document Express, toll-free, at 1-800-55-MOSBY.

With Mosby Document Express, you have convenient 24-hour-a-day access to literally every journal reference within this book. In fact, through Mosby Document Express, virtually any medical or scientific article can be located and delivered by FAX, overnight delivery service, international airmail, electronic transmission of bitmapped images (via Internet), or regular mail. The average cost of a complete delivered copy of an article, including copyright clearance charges and first-class mail delivery, is $12.

For inquiries and pricing information, please call the toll-free number shown above.

Prehospital Care: What Works, What Does Not

Lenworth M. Jacobs, M.D., M.P.H.

Professor of Surgery, University of Connecticut Health Center; Director, Trauma Program, Hartford Hospital, Hartford, Connecticut

Stephane Panic, M.D.

Trauma/Surgical Critical Care Fellow, Hartford Hospital, Hartford, Connecticut

Trauma is a disease that has been present since the beginning of civilization. Its causes have changed over time, but the importance and impact of trauma remain. It strikes swiftly and without warning, and most often involves the young and productive. The modern age of high-speed travel and permissive society has made trauma a national epidemic. It is the leading cause of death in the first 4 decades of life and is surpassed only by cancer and atherosclerosis as the cause of death in all age groups. About 50 million injuries occur annually, a fifth of which are disabling.[1]

It is estimated that more than 140,000 deaths occur each year as a result of trauma and that, for each death, there are at least two cases of permanent disability.[1] The consequences are devastating. In a period when the health care industry has come under increasing regulation and scrutiny in an attempt to control costs, it is critical that we identify factors that can enhance the efficient use of increasingly limited resources for victims of trauma.[2]

Prevention

Prevention is the most important tool in the control of trauma.[3] William Haddon was a leader in documenting the influence that alcohol ingestion has on fatal motor vehicle and pedestrian crashes. Three strategies for injury control are used to classify most injury countermeasures: (1) education/persuasion, (2) laws and administrative rules, and (3) engineering/technology. Education and persuasion strategies are designed to alter the behavior of those who may be exposed to certain hazards. An example is teaching high school students the perils of driving while intoxicated.

The second countermeasure, laws and administrative rules, also is designed to alter behavior, but not through an educational forum. The change in behavior is generated primarily by requirements and penalties imposed by laws or rules (i.e., mandatory seat belt and motorcycle helmet use, and speed limit laws).

The third strategy involves protecting the potential victim by adjusting the agents, vehicles, or environment through laws, administrative rules, or persuasion addressed to manufacturers. The law regulating the installation of automatic restraining devices and airbags in automobiles is an engineering/technology approach to injury prevention. Overall, research indicates that education is the least effective strategy and automatic protection is the most effective.[4]

When preventive measures fail, the prehospital system must be well organized to deal quickly and effectively with the challenges that trauma presents. Studies have shown that deaths from trauma have a trimodal distribution.[1, 5] The first peak occurs within seconds to minutes after injury (immediate death) and usually is caused by lacerations of the brain, brain stem, high spinal cord, heart, aorta, or other large vessel. The second peak occurs from minutes to a few hours after injury (early death) and generally results from major internal hemorrhage of the head, chest, or abdominal cavity, or from multiple lesser injuries causing significant blood loss. The third peak in the death rate occurs several days or weeks after the traumatic event (late death) and is almost always a consequence of sepsis or multiple organ failure.

More than half of all traumatic deaths are classified as immediate. Early and late deaths account for about 30% and 20%, respectively, of deaths resulting from injury.

Data indicate that well-organized trauma systems can decrease the incidence of morbidity and mortality related to trauma. A well-organized trauma system, however, must integrate the prehospital system with the receiving trauma center for maximum benefit.[6-11]

Prehospital Time Factor

The time that elapses before arrival at a hospital is of paramount importance in the care of trauma patients. The first systematic approach to early treatment of patients with injuries to multiple systems developed from experiences in military conflicts. The mortality rate in World War I was 8.5%, and it took several hours for injured soldiers to arrive at a site where they could receive definitive care. In World War II, the mortality rate decreased to 5.8%, and the length of time from injury to definitive care also decreased. The mortality rate in Korea was 2.4%, and the rate in Vietnam was less than 1.7%.[5, 12] Combat experience in Vietnam did show increased survival associated with a reduction in transport time from the battlefield to medical units.[13, 14] A threefold increase in the mortality rate also has been reported for every 30 minutes that elapses without care.[15]

Several factors have contributed to this decrease in the mortality rate: modern surgical techniques, effective anesthesia, a better understanding of the importance of nutrition, and the advent of antibiotics. The most important advance, however, was the recognition that trauma is a time-related disease. The more quickly hemorrhage is controlled and definitive management initiated, the better is the outcome.

The goal of prehospital care is to transport the patient as rapidly as possible to the center that is most appropriately equipped and staffed to handle the specific condition. If distances are great or direct transport is not feasible, the patient should be taken to the nearest facility at which initial resuscitation can be performed. The patient can be transported later, if necessary, to another institution.[16]

Appropriate prehospital assessment and interventions should be performed at the accident site, but any further treatment should be provided during the trip to the hospital. The minimum amount of time possible should be spent in the prehospital setting. There is no indication for prolonged field efforts to stabilize an injured patient who is in hemorrhagic shock. Early, rapid transportation to a trauma care center is essential.

Basic Life Support vs. Advanced Life Support

To discuss the advantages and disadvantages of basic life support (BLS) vs. advanced life support (ALS) for the injured patient in the prehospital setting, the major differences between the two systems must be appreciated (Table 1).

The availability of prehospital paramedic personnel trained to perform invasive resuscitative techniques at accident sites has expanded the setting of early trauma management from the emergency department to the prehospital arena. Controversy exists regarding whether such measures are beneficial or harm the patient by delaying transportation to a trauma facility where definitive operative care is available.

TABLE 1.
Differences Between Basic Life Support and Advanced Life Support Systems*

Basic Life Support	Advanced Life Support
Emergency medical technician	Paramedic
127 hours	400–2,400 hours
National	State
Patient assessment	Basic life support skills plus
Nonendotracheal airway	Endotracheal airway
O_2 administration	Intravenous medication administration
Spine immobilization	
Extremity immobilization	Countershock
Hemorrhage control	Miscellaneous
Cardiopulmonary resuscitation (basic)	
Antishock garment	

*From Rhodes M, Brader AH: Adv Trauma 1989; 4:19–42. Used by permission.

There is a growing belief that it is important to initiate resuscitation as soon as possible and to perform a limited number of definitive interventions to stabilize an injured patient before transporting him or her to a trauma care facility.[17-19] Such ALS procedures may include definitive protection of the airway by endotracheal intubation and initial resuscitation from hypovolemic shock by peripheral venous access line placement, intravenous fluid administration, and pneumatic antishock garment inflation. The rationale is that these components of definitive care are possible in the prehospital environment and that they help to improve patient outcome after severe trauma.

A second school of thought is that ALS has no place in the prehospital management of trauma victims, despite the fact that prehospital ALS has been demonstrated to be more effective than BLS in the management of cardiac emergencies.[20, 21] Those who support this belief claim that it is more appropriate to minimize medical attention and transport trauma victims quickly to a hospital. Their rationale is that the hospital is the definitive place for surgical attention, and that a patient's clinical condition is unlikely to deteriorate during the short time required for rapid transportation. Time to definitive operative treatment is believed to be the single most vital factor in influencing patient outcome after injury.

Prehospital treatment is the first phase of professional trauma care, and definitive care for injured patients cannot be provided in the way it can for those with life-threatening cardiac arrhythmias. ALS interventions require prehospital time for clinical patient assessment, contact with an on-line physician for medical direction, and execution of the pertinent ALS skills. Time also is required for BLS care, however. This includes locating the patient, securing the scene, mobilizing the appropriate resources, extricating the patient in cases of blunt motor vehicle trauma, assessing the patient and determining the vital signs, controlling hemorrhage, immobilizing the spine and suspected fractures, and securing the patient on the stretcher in such a way as to protect against further spinal or long-bone injury. It also includes moving from the scene of the injury to the ambulance and traveling to the trauma center.

Several studies have shown that ALS interventions, carried out in synchrony with BLS care, do not require significant additional time and are associated with more favorable short- and long-term outcomes after major trauma.[17, 18, 22] This requires properly trained and certified personnel, however, in addition to good medical control. The use of advanced skills in the care of injured patients has been shown to require much practice, experience, and dedication on the part of the provider. Procedures requiring such skills should not be attempted by anyone with less training than an emergency medical technician (EMT) paramedic, and then only with on-line medical control and off-line medical review. EMT personnel with only basic training cannot perform endotracheal intubation.[16] Good knowledge of the pathophysiology of trauma as well as education and experience in the treatment of injured patients are essential.

Field resuscitation should be tailored to the circumstances and the needs of the patient; the location of the most appropriately staffed and equipped hospital, the mechanism and severity of the injury, the extrication time, and the training of the emergency medical personnel all should be taken into account.

A patient with a penetrating chest wound who is a few minutes away from a trauma center will benefit most from a "scoop-and-run" approach. An apneic patient with a closed head injury will benefit most from early endotracheal intubation (ALS).

Each task must be carried out as efficiently and quickly as possible, however, based on the knowledge and judgment of the provider. Some tasks can be performed en route to the trauma center. Time is of the essence and it cannot be wasted.

Airway Management

Airway control is a vital component of prehospital care that may affect patient morbidity, mortality, and functional outcome substantially.[17, 23-25] It also is the most challenging prehospital task and carries some risks in injured patients. The preferred method of airway control in critically injured patients is endotracheal intubation.[23, 26, 27] Indications for the intubation of a patient in the prehospital environment include inability to maintain a patent airway, inadequate oxygenation and ventilation, need for hyperventilation, prevention of aspiration of blood or secretions, necessity of a conduit for medications, and potential for airway compromise en route to the destination facility.[28] Problems specific to endotracheal intubation in the injured patient include inability to position the patient optimally because of the need to maintain in-line cervical traction, head injury associated with combativeness and trismus, facial or laryngeal fractures obstructing passage of the tube, blood or vomitus in the oropharynx precluding adequate visualization of the vocal cords, and suboptimal illumination and suction equipment at the scene of the incident.[26, 29] Trauma victims characteristically are young males who are muscular and have full dentition. These factors combine to present a major challenge to intubation. Although there are risks associated with the intubation of trauma patients, definitive control of the airway is essential for optimal care, especially in cases of head injury. As many as 65% of patients with head injuries who are not intubated are hypoxemic on arrival at the emergency department, despite their apparent lack of respiratory distress.[23] Extension of brain injury is thought to occur with prolonged hypoxemia and the presence of persistently high intracranial pressure.[30, 31] Aspiration of blood or vomitus and depressed respiratory function cause hypoxemia in patients with head injury. These factors may be controlled by intubation of the airway. Because head injury is the primary contributor to early mortality in patients with multiple injuries,[32] earlier intubation of the airway may improve outcome.[26]

Success rates for endotracheal intubation in injured patients have been reported to exceed 90%.[26, 33, 34] Because of these high success rates, combined with low complication rates, endotracheal intubation is widely accepted as the best method of obtaining definitive airway control before arrival at the hospital.[28] Although they are in widespread use and require minimal training for insertion, the esophageal obturator airway (EOA) and esophageal gastric tube airway (EGTA) fail to provide optimal airway control and have significant associated complications: inability to intubate the esophagus, unrecognized tracheal intubation, inadequate mask seal, balloon leakage, rupture, esophageal laceration, excessively proximal esophageal balloon location causing tracheal compression, anterior displacement of the larynx, gastric rupture, and emesis or removal of the device.[35] A disadvantage of the EOA is that it may require two people to ventilate the patient adequately: one to secure the mask in place and another to squeeze the bag.[36] A prospective study comparing arterial blood gas levels from patients with the EGTA in the prehospital setting with samples obtained after endotracheal intubation in the emergency department showed significant impairment of both oxygenation and ventilation with the EGTA.[37] Endotracheal intubation is the optimal method of definitive airway control provided adequate training for the procedure has been established.[23, 26, 27]

A relatively new device, the so-called pharyngeal tracheal lumen airway (PTLA), is being tested. The PTLA consists of two parallel polyvinylchloride tubes, each with an internal diameter of 8 mm. The lengths of these tubes were chosen to prevent the 31-cm tube from entering the right main stem bronchus and the 21-cm tube from occluding the epiglottis. Unlike the EOA, the long tube will work in the trachea as an endotracheal tube (ETT). Instead of a mask, a large balloon cuff is inflated in the mouth and pharynx to seal off the upper airway. An obturator stylet clocks off the larger tube. If the long tube is in the esophagus, ventilation occurs through the shorter tube. If no signs of ventilation occur, the large tube is in the trachea; the obturator stylet is removed, and ventilation is accomplished through the longer tube. There are two purported advantages of the PTLA over the EOA. One is that intubation of the trachea is desirable (albeit not mandatory), and the second is that, if the large tube is in the esophagus, a face mask seal is not required.[38]

Frass and colleagues, in Austria, have developed a similar tube known as the esophageal tracheal combitube.[39] This is a twin-lumen tube with two balloons. It is designed to provide adequate ventilation after esophageal or tracheal placement. Double-lumen devices (the PTLA and the combitube) have the advantage of minimizing manipulation of the neck in trauma patients. One of their disadvantages is that the endotracheal route for administration of medication is lost when the device is in the esophageal position. These devices also are more complex than are endotracheal tubes and are difficult to insert, especially in the uncontrolled prehospital environment. Large-scale field trials by prehospital personnel are necessary before any recommendations can be made.

Intravenous Line Placement in the Field

In view of the fact that trauma is a time-related disease and that quick and efficient prehospital care results in improved outcomes, a tremendous amount of controversy has surrounded the topic of intravenous line placement in the field. Many authors have voiced a concern that intravenous line placement in the field delays transportation, and that provides little benefit to the patient because only a minimal amount of fluid can be infused during short prehospital times.[20, 21, 40]

Several studies have addressed this topic. Even though some initial results indicated that the average time required to start an intravenous line in the field was more than 10 minutes, prospective studies since have shown that, with well-trained paramedics and good medical control, this can be accomplished in less than 3 minutes.[18, 41, 42] Data also have shown that success rates for establishing intravenous lines exceed 90%.[18, 41, 42]

Several studies have revealed that en route placement can be accomplished with equally good results, leading to the recommendation that, unless there is a prolonged extrication time, time in the field should not be extended by multiple attempts to place an intravenous line.[41, 43–45] Patients benefit most from rapid transportation and intravenous line placement en route to the trauma center.

To study the amount of fluid that can be infused in the prehospital setting, Lewis designed a computer-based model for which a maximal bleeding rate of 100 mL/min was set and a maximum infusion rate of 100 mL/min was allowed. This study did not show any benefit from prehospital administration of intravenous fluids unless the time in the field exceeded 30 to 45 minutes.[40] Studies have revealed, however, that 400 mL/min to more than 1,000 mL/min can be delivered to the patient using large-bore intravenous lines and pressure infusion.[46–50]

Certain factors in the prehospital setting restrict the amount of fluid that can be infused, including the internal diameter of the catheter used, the use or avoidance of pressure cuffs, and other priorities that may take precedence over intravenous fluids during transportation. Still, time is saved in the emergency department if the catheter is already in place on arrival; blood has been drawn for typing, crossmatching, and other studies; and the patient has received a fluid challenge.

The use of hypertonic/hyperoncotic solutions in the hypotensive injured patient is under investigation. Data seem to indicate that these fluids in lesser amounts than isotonic saline can raise the blood pressure quickly, at least transiently.[51–55] Whether this will improve patient outcome remains to be determined. Concern that increasing the blood pressure with fluids before hemorrhage is controlled by surgical means has led to studies evaluating the efficacy of delaying fluid resuscitation until the time of operation. Results are pending and this practice remains investigational.[57]

Pneumatic Antishock Garment

The pneumatic antishock garment is a simple, trouserlike device that can be easily applied by emergency medical personnel. The suit is designed with three compartments, one for each leg and one for the abdomen, which can be individually inflated with a pump. The suit is placed on the stretcher and the patient is positioned on the suit. The leg sections are inflated first, then the abdominal section.[58]

It was initially thought that the device functioned as an exsanguinating tourniquet that transfused the patient's own blood from the legs and lower abdomen into the intravascular space and preferentially perfused the heart, head, and upper torso. Subsequent data revealed that the autotransfusion effect was small and that the major component of systolic blood pressure elevation was the result of vasoconstriction.[59–61]

The reported complication rate of the device is low, estimated at less than 1 in 10,000.[62] Complications that have been reported include hypotension on rapid deflation without adequate volume replacement, associated compartment syndrome, pulmonary edema, diaphragmatic herniation, air embolism, and worsening of lumbar fractures.[62, 63] The latter was reported with the earlier devices.

Controversy still surrounds the use of the pneumatic antishock garment. In a review of more than 200 studies involving the use of this device, McSwain cited improved survival.[62] He recommended its use to increase blood pressure and thereby improve brain and heart perfusion; control intra-abdominal, pelvic, and thigh hemorrhage; and stabilize pelvic and femoral fractures in the presence of concomitant hypotension. Other studies also have shown a benefit of the pneumatic antishock garment for immobilizing and controlling hemorrhage resulting from unstable pelvic or long-bone fractures.[64, 65]

In a prospective, randomized study involving mostly penetrating injuries in 911 patients, Mattox concluded that application of the pneumatic antishock garment did not improve survival.[66] Patients with thoracic injuries, including cardiac and major thoracic vascular trauma, actually had a worse outcome when the device was used.

More prospective, randomized studies are needed, especially in patients with blunt trauma, before definitive recommendations can be made. Use of the pneumatic antishock garment currently is limited to patients with unstable pelvic or proximal long-bone fractures in combination with hypotension and a lengthy transport time (>30 minutes).[67]

Immobilization

The basic principle of spinal immobilization is to secure the bony vertebral column sufficiently to prevent any movement that may injure the spinal cord or its nerve pathways.

Because injury to the vertebral column can be diagnosed definitively only by a roentgenogram in the hospital, it is accepted practice to immobilize any patient with a suspected injury to the vertebral column. Unnecessary or inappropriate movement of the patient in the field may permanently damage the spinal cord, with subsequent loss of neurologic function and permanent paralysis of the extremities or the diaphragm.

Soft collars are ineffective and have no place in the prehospital setting for spinal immobilization during extrication or transportation of the patient. They do not provide the necessary restriction of flexion, extension, and rotation.

Rigid collars are frequently used for cervical immobilization. The rigid Philadelphia collar is easy to apply because it comes in two premolded pieces. The anterior and posterior parts are easily fastened with a Velcro strap. A particular advantage of this collar is that the anterior portion can be removed to allow inspection of the neck while the posterior portion maintains immobility.

The Stiffneck collar (California Medical Products Inc., Long Beach, Calif.) also is a rigid collar made of polyethylene. It has an enlarged opening in its anterior portion that permits examination of the pulse and prevents constriction of the jugular veins.

Several studies have shown that even the Philadelphia (De Royal Industries, Powell Tenn.), Stiffneck, and other rigid collars allow about 60% of normal rotary and lateral head motion and 40% of normal cervical spine movement in the anteroposterior direction.[68-71]

The Cervical Immobilizer Device (Medical Products, Irvine, Calif.) is a combination of foam blocks and straps that can be used with a long or short board as well as with the scoop-type stretcher. This device is lightweight and radiolucent, but can be used only for adults.

The long spinal board with sandbags and a 3-in. adhesive tape was found to provide better immobilization than any collar tested in a series by Podolsky and colleagues.[70] The backboard used in combination with a Philadelphia collar allowed the least amount of motion in all planes, however.

Rigid collars should not be used alone, but in combination with a short or long backboard if maximum immobilization is to be obtained.[68, 72] The short backboard is used as an extrication device and the long backboard is used for transportation.

The backboard should adequately immobilize the entire spine and should follow the basic orthopaedic principle that any fracture must be immobilized from the joint above to the joint below the fracture site. Thus, to immobilize the complete spine adequately and safely, the head, thorax, abdomen, and pelvis must be immobilized.[68]

Several other devices are available for spinal immobilization. An alternative to the short spine board is the Ferno-Kendrick Extrication Device (KED) (Medical Products, Irvine, Calif.) Made of a ribbed fabric, the KED is designed to wrap around the patient. Chin and forehead restraints, chest and leg straps, and a neck roll restrict patient movement. The KED is designed for quick application and for use in confined spaces. The Reeves

Sleeve is a spinal immobilization device that has an opening to allow the insertion of a rigid board. Once the board has been inserted, the patient is placed on the sleeve and the chest and lower extremity vests are wrapped around the patient and fastened with Velcro closures. The Build-A-Board is a three-section metal device that consists of a seat section, a back support, and a headboard. It is designed for use with a seated patient. A scoop stretcher can be attached to a Build-A-Board. Long boards are available in aluminum, plywood, and plastic.

A vacuum immobilizer, the Coquille, is used almost exclusively for spinal immobilization in France and other European countries. The Coquille is an airtight, radiolucent envelope full of tiny plastic balls. After the device is slid around the patient, a small, manually operated vacuum pump is used to withdraw all the air from the envelope. As air is withdrawn, the balls create a rigid mold around the patient's body, locking the patient into the envelope. The weight of the patient's body is distributed evenly over the envelope, reducing the risk of tissue damage from pressure. The plastic balls also act as thermal insulators to prevent heat loss. This device can be used for a seated or supine patient.

Any fracture or suspected fracture/dislocation must be immobilized to decrease pain, reduce blood loss, and prevent further neurovascular damage. The splints should extend one joint above and below the site of injury.

Extremity trauma is rarely life-threatening; thus, splinting of extremity injuries must be deferred until life-threatening conditions have been addressed. This can be done during transportation to the trauma center without causing a delay.

Conclusions

Data indicate that well-organized trauma systems that provide quick response and transportation, and are staffed with experienced paramedics who can perform ALS without delaying transportation favorably affect the outcome of seriously injured patients.

Airway management is the most important component of prehospital care. Endotracheal intubation is the airway control method of choice; no other device has proved superior.

Intravenous lines should be placed during transportation to the trauma center. This ensures the availability of ready intravenous access on arrival in the emergency department as well as blood for typing and crossmatching. The patient also may benefit from a fluid challenge, especially when transport times are lengthy. Lactated Ringer's solution remains the fluid of choice. Hypertonic/hyperoncotic solutions and fluid restriction until surgical control of the hemorrhage is achieved are under investigation.

More prospective, randomized studies of the pneumatic antishock garment are necessary, especially in patients with blunt trauma, before definitive recommendations can be made. The usefulness of this device presently is limited to patients with unstable pelvic or proximal long-bone fractures in combination with hypotension and a lengthy transport time (>30 minutes).

Spinal immobilization is a basic procedure in the field, but one that is essential to prevent spinal cord injury. Patients should receive immediate manual control of the cervical spine, followed by the application of a rigid cervical collar long backboard, and Cervical Immobilizer Device to prevent disability.

Extremity fractures should be splinted during transportation to the trauma center if time permits.

The emergency medical system has improved substantially over the last 2 decades. Careful scientific scrutiny of new devices and practices will assure continued advances in the quality of prehospital care.

Acknowledgment

Special thanks to Mark Libby, RN, BSN, CCRN, CEN, CFRN, EMT-P, Florence Leishman, Eva Smith, and Irene Sywenkyj, without whose help this manuscript would not have been possible.

References

1. *Advanced Trauma Life Support Instructor Manual*. American College of Surgeons, Chicago, 1989.
2. Schwartz RJ, Jacobs LM, Yaezel D: Impact of pretrauma center care on length of stay and hospital charges. *J Trauma* 1989;29:1611–1615.
3. National Committee for Injury Prevention and Control-Injury Prevention: Meeting the challenge. *Am J Prev Med* 1989;3(suppl):1.
4. *Injury in America: A Continuing Public Health Problem*. Washington, DC, National Academy Press, 1985.
5. Trunkey DD: Trauma. *Sci Am* 1983;249:28–35.
6. Rhodes M, Brader AH: Organization of a trauma resuscitation system. *Adv Trauma* 1989;4:18–42.
7. West JG, Cales RH, Gazzaniga AB: Impact of regionalization: The Orange County experience. *Arch Surg* 1983;118:740–744.
8. Cales RH: Trauma mortality in Orange County: The effects of the implementation of a regional trauma system. *Arch Emerg Med* 1984;13:1–10.
9. Shackford SR, Hollingworth-Fridlung P, Cooper GF, et al: The effects of regionalization upon the quality of trauma care as assessed by concurrent audit before and after institution of a trauma system. *J Trauma* 1986;26:812–820.
10. Clemmer TP, Orme Jr JF, Thomas PO, et al: Outcome of critically injured patients treated at level I trauma centers versus full-service community hospitals. *Crit Care Med* 1985;13:861–863.
11. West JG, Trunkey DD, Lim RC: Systems of trauma care—a study of two counties. *Arch Surg* 1979;114:455–460.
12. Jacobs LM: Initial management and evaluation of the multisystem injured patient, part I. *J Natl Med Assoc* 1987;79:361–370.
13. Eiseman B: Combat casualty management in Vietnam. *J Trauma* 1967;7:53–63.

14. McNabney WK: Vietnam in context. *Ann Emerg Med* 1981;10:659-661.
15. Cowley RA, Hudson F, Scanlan E, et al: An economical and proved helicopter program for transporting the emergency critically ill and injured patient in Maryland. *J Trauma* 1973;13:1029-1038.
16. *Resources for Optimal Care of the Injured Patient.* American College of Surgeons, Committee on Trauma, Chicago, 1990.
17. Jacobs LM, Sinclair A, Beiser A, et al: Prehospital advanced life support: Benefits in trauma. *J Trauma* 1984;24:8-13.
18. Cwinn AA, Pons PT, Moore EE, et al: Prehospital advanced trauma life support for critical blunt trauma victims. *Ann Emerg Med* 1987;16:399-403.
19. Ornato JP, Craren EJ, Nelson NM, et al: Impact of improved emergency medical services and emergency trauma care on the reduction in mortality from trauma. *J Trauma* 1985;25:575-579.
20. Smith JP, Bodai BI, Hill AS, et al: Prehospital stabilization of critically injured patients: A failed concept. *J Trauma* 1985;25:65-70.
21. Border JR, Lewis FR, Aprahamian C, et al: Panel: Prehospital trauma care—stabilize or scoop and run. *J Trauma* 1983;23:708-711.
22. Pons PT, Honigman B, Moore EE, et al: Prehospital advanced trauma life support for critical penetrating wounds to the thorax and abdomen. *J Trauma* 1985;25:828-832.
23. Pepe PE, Copass MK, Joyce TH: Prehospital endotracheal intubation: Rationale for training emergency medical personnel. *Ann Emerg Med* 1985;14:1085-1092.
24. Copass MK, Oreskovich MR, Bladergroen MR, et al: Prehospital cardiopulmonary resuscitation of the critically injured patient. *Am J Surg* 1984;48:20-26.
25. Trunkey DD: Is ALS necessary for pre-hospital trauma care (editorial)? *J Trauma* 1984;24:86-87.
26. Gabram SGA, Jacobs LM, Schwartz RJ, et al: Airway intubation in injured patients at the scene of an accident. *Conn Med* 1989;53:633-637.
27. Tortella BJ: Airway management. *Emerg Care Q* 1991;7:1-12.
28. Gabram SGA, Grant HI, Jacobs LM: The current practice of prehospital endotracheal intubation. *Emerg Care Q* 1991;7:23-37.
29. Furgurson JE, Meislin HW: Airway problems in the trauma victim. *Top Emerg Med* 1979;1:9-27.
30. Clifton GL, McCormick WF, Grossman RG: Neuropathology of early and late deaths after head injury. *Neurosurgery* 1981;8:309-314.
31. Lutz HA, Becker DP, Miller JD, et al: Monitoring, management, and the analysis of outcome, in Grossman RG, Gildenbert PL (eds): *Head Injury: Basic and Clinical Aspects.* New York, Raven Press, 221-228, 1982.
32. Baxt WG, Moody P: The differential survival of trauma patients. *J Trauma* 1987;27:602-606.
33. Jacobs LM, Berrizbeitia LD, Bennett B, et al: Endotracheal intubation in the prehospital phase of emergency medical care. *JAMA* 1983;250:2175-2177.
34. Stewart RD, Paris PM, Winter PM, et al: Field endotracheal intubation by paramedical personnel—success rates and complications. *Chest* 1984;85:341-345.
35. Hawkins ML: The esophageal obturator airway and related airway devices. *Emerg Care Q* 1991;7:13-22.
36. White RD: Controversies in out-of-hospital emergency airway control: Esophageal obturator or endotracheal intubation? *Ann Emerg Med* 1984;13:778-781.
37. Auerbach PS, Geehr EC: Inadequate oxygenation and ventilation using the

esophageal gastric tube airway in the prehospital setting. *JAMA* 1983;250:2067–2071.
38. Jacobs LM: The importance of airway management in trauma. *J Natl Med Assoc* 1988;80:873–879.
39. Frass M, Frazer R, Zdrahal F, et al: The esophageal tracheal combitube: Preliminary results with a new airway for CPR. *Ann Emerg Med* 1987;16:7.
40. Lewis FR: Prehospital intravenous fluid therapy: Physiologic computer modeling. *J Trauma* 1986;26:804–811.
41. Jones SE, Nesper TP, Alcouloumre E: Prehospital intravenous line placement: A prospective study. *Ann Emerg Med* 1989;18:244–246.
42. Pons PT, Moore EE, Cusick JM, et al: Prehospital venous access in an urban paramedic system—A prospective on scene analysis. *J Trauma* 1988;28: 1460–1463.
43. O'Gorman M, Trabulsy P, Pilcher DB: Zero-time prehospital IV. *J Trauma* 1989;29:84–86.
44. McSwain NE: Controversies in prehospital care. *Emerg Med Clin North Am* 1990;8:145–154.
45. MacLeod BAS, Leaberg DC, Paris PM: Prehospital therapy past, present, and future. *Emerg Med Clin North Am* 1990;8:57–74.
46. Mateer JR, Thompson BM, Tucker J, et al: Effects of high pressure and large-bore tubing on IV flow rates. *Ann Emerg Med* 1984;13:405–406.
47. Mateer JR, Thompson BM, Aprahamian C, et al: Rapid fluid resuscitation with central venous catheters. *Ann Emerg Med* 1983;12:149–152.
48. Mateer JR, Perry BWQ, Thompson BM, et al: Effects of rapid infusion with high pressure and large-bore IV tubing on red blood cell lysis and warming. *Ann Emerg Med* 1985;14:966–969.
49. Hausbrough JF, Cain TF, Millikan JS: Placement of 10 gauge catheter by cutdown for rapid fluid replacement. *J Trauma* 1983;23:231–234.
50. Fried SJ, Satiari B, Zeeb P: Normothermic rapid volume replacement for hypovolemic shock: An in vivo and in vitro study utilizing a new technique. *J Trauma* 1986;26:183–188.
51. Rocha e Silva M, Negraes GA, Soares AM, et al: Hypertonic resuscitation from severe hemorrhagic shock: Patterns of regional blood flow. *Circ Shock* 1986;19:165–175.
52. Vasser MJ, Fischer RP, the Multicenter Group for the Study of Hypertonic Saline in Trauma Patients: A multicenter trial for resuscitation of injured patients with 7.5% sodium chloride—the effect of added dextran 70. *Arch Surg* 1993;128:1003–1013.
53. Mattox KL, Maningas PA, Moore EE, et al: Prehospital hypertonic saline/dextrose infusion for post-traumatic hypotension—the U.S.A. multicenter trial. *Ann Surg* 1991;213:482–491.
54. Holcroft JW: The physiolgoic basis for the use of hypertonic solutions in the resuscitation of patients in hemorrhagic shock, in Najarian JS, Delaney JP (eds): *Progress in Trauma and Critical Care Surgery.* St Louis, Mosby, 1992, pp 19–24.
55. Tominaga GT, Waxman K: Resuscitation solutions, in Gamelli RL, Dries DJ (eds): *Medical Intelligence Unit—Trauma 2000 strategies for the New Millenium.* RG Landes, Austin, 1992, p 920–929.
56. Halvorsen L, Kramer GC, Holcroft JW: Prehospital fluid resuscitation with hypertonic saline solutions; in Trunkey DD, Lewis Jr FR (eds): *Current Therapy of Trauma,* 3rd ed. BC Decker, St. Louis, 1991, pp 125–130.
57. Martin RR, Bickell WH, Pepe PE, et al: Prospective evaluation of preoperative

fluid resuscitation in hypotensive patients with penetrating truncal injury: A preliminary report. *J Trauma* 1992;33:354–362.
58. Jacobs LM, Lydon P, Sinclair A: The pneumatic antishock garment. *Med Instrum* 1982;16:194.
59. Bivins HG, Knopp R, Tiernan C, et al: Blood volume displacement with inflation of antishock trousers. *Ann Emerg Med* 1982;11:409–412.
60. Gaffney FA, Thal ER, Taylor WF: Hemodynamic effects of medical antishock trousers. *J Trauma* 1981;21:931–937.
61. Niemann JT, Stapczynski JS, Rosborough JP, et al: Hemodynamic effects of pneumatic external counterpressure in canine hemorrhagic shock. *Ann Emerg Med* 1983;12:661–667.
62. McSwain NE: Pneumatic antishock garment: State of the art, 1988. *Ann Emerg Med* 1988;17:506–525.
63. Aprahamian C, Gessert G, Bandyk DF, et al: MAST-associated compartment syndrome (MACS): A review. *J Trauma* 1989;29:549–555.
64. Batalden DJ, Wickstrom PH, Ruiz E, et al: Value of the G suit in patients with severe pelvic fractures. *Arch Surg* 1974;109:326–328.
65. Mucha Jr P: Pelvic fractures, in Moore EE, Mattox KL, Feliciano DV (eds): *Trauma*, 2nd ed. Appleton & Lange, Norwalk, Conn, 1991, 558–559.
66. Mattox KL, Bickell W, Pepe PE, *J Trauma* 1989;29:1104–1112.
67. Fantini GA, Shires III GT, Shires GT: Management of shock, in Moore EE, Mattox KL, Feliciano DV (eds): *Trauma*, 2nd ed. Appleton & Lange, Norwalk, Conn, 1991, 153.
68. McSwain JR NE: Prehospital emergency medical systems and cardiopulmonary resuscitation, in Moore EE, Mattox KL, Feliciano DV (eds): *Trauma*, 2nd ed. Appleton & Lange, Norwalk, Conn, 1991, 104-105.
69. McSwain NE: Cervical collars—do they work? *Emerg Med Tech J* 1981;5:243–244.
70. Podolsky S, Baraff LJ, Simon RR: Efficacy of cervical spine immobilization methods. *J Trauma* 1983;23:461–465.
71. Cline JR, Scheidel E, Bigsby EF: A comparison of methods of cervical spine immobilization in patient extrication and transport. *J Trauma* 1985;25:649–653.
72. McSwain NE: Acute management in cervical spine trauma, in McSwain NE, Martinez JA, Timberlake GA (eds): *Cervical Spine Trauma: Evaluation and Acute Management*. New York, Thieme Medical Publishers, 1989, pp 105–118.

Diagnosis, Temporary Stabilization, and Definitive Treatment of Injuries to the Cervical Spine

John B. Catalano, M.D.

Fellow in Orthopaedic Traumatology, Department of Surgery, University of Medicine and Dentistry of New Jersey/Robert Wood Johnson Medical School-Camden, Cooper Hospital/University Medical Center, Camden, New Jersey

Christopher T. Born, M.D.

Associate Professor of Clinical Surgery, Department of Surgery, University of Medicine and Dentistry of New Jersey/Robert Wood Johnson Medical School-Camden, Cooper Hospital/University Medical Center, Camden, New Jersey

Steven E. Ross, M.D.

Associate Professor of Surgery, Department of Surgery, University of Medicine and Dentistry of New Jersey/Robert Wood Johnson Medical School-Camden, Cooper Hospital/University Medical Center, Camden, New Jersey

Injuries to the cervical spine and spinal cord were recognized by the ancients, with written records appearing as early as 3,000 B.C. in the Edwin Smith Papyrus. Egyptian, Greek, and Roman records indicate recognition of such injuries, as well as their poor prognosis.[1] Historically, cervical fractures have been detected primarily by the presence of pain and neurologic deficit, and they were considered by Hippocrates to be uniformly fatal. Ambrose Pare, the father of modern surgery, proposed surgical treatment of cervical fractures in the 16th century.[2] Modern treatment of such injuries began in the late 19th century with attempts at surgical stabilization.[3]

Although cervical spine injury occurs as a result of sporting accidents, falls, and other "accidental" causes, most of these injuries result from vehicular trauma. Spinal injury has been estimated to occur in about 54,000 patients yearly in the United States alone, with neurologic injury occurring in 14% of all trauma patients who require hospitalization.[4] Neurologic injury is seen in 40% of patients with injury to the cervical spine.[5] The incidence of cervical spine injury has been estimated to be as high as 20% in patients with major head injury,[6] and the *Advanced Trauma Life Support Manual*[7] reports a 10% incidence of such injury in patients who have lost consciousness. Although the incidence of cervical injury has been reported to be as high as 16% to 24% in patients dying after motor vehicle accidents, Huelke[4] demonstrated that severe neck injuries were sustained by 1 of every 300 individuals involved in crashes in which a vehicle had to be towed from the scene.[8-10] When ejection from the vehicle was included, the rate rose to 1 in 14 individuals.

Clinical Risk Factors

Because the incidence of spinal cord trauma is so high among individuals involved in motor vehicle accidents, those who sustain blunt injury (particularly to more than one system) should be evaluated routinely for cervical spine involvement.[7] Although the likelihood of such injury is well recognized, reports of "occult" and overlooked injury continue to appear in the medical literature.[11, 12] As many as 10% of patients with spinal cord injury are neurologically intact initially, with a deficit developing during the hospital course.[13] In addition, 3% of all spinal cord injuries result from errors in treatment after the institution of initial emergency medical care.[14]

Even at well-established trauma centers, fractures of the cervical spine often are overlooked. This occurs because of failure of the patient to seek medical care, failure of the physician to obtain radiographs, inadequate standard cervical spine radiographs, and misread radiographs.

Adequate standard radiographs usually reveal cervical spine injury.[15, 16] Therefore, significant effort has been directed toward developing criteria for the use of cervical spine radiography in victims of blunt trauma. The clinician's need for highly sensitive criteria for the clinical suspicion of cervical spine injury must be balanced against the goals of reducing unnecessary radiation exposure to both the patient and the clinical team and keeping medical costs low.[17] These diverse objectives have stimulated a search for a highly sensitive and specific set of criteria with which to identify patients who need radiographic evaluation for possible injury to the cervical spine.

The Advanced Trauma Life Support Course recommends that a lateral cervical spine radiograph be obtained in all patients with blunt trauma who have evidence of injury above the clavicle.[7] Many authors consider this recommendation to be too broad, however.[18-24] Most have attempted to address several types of risk factors in refining the indications for spinal radiography in this patient population. The mechanism of injury, level of consciousness, and individual signs and symptoms of injury to the neck are often considered in appraising the risk of injury. In 1987, Cadoux and associates described a series of 749 patients who underwent neck radiography after blunt trauma.[21] They found motor vehicle accidents to be associated with a high risk for cervical spine injury. These authors also noted that no cervical injuries occurred among restrained passengers in their study group. Unfortunately, not all patients with a blunt, high-energy injury who were seen at their institution during the course of the study had radiographs of the cervical spine. Jacobs and Schwartz prospectively evaluated 233 patients with head or neck injury.[20] Injury to the cervical spine was noted in 24 cases. The only mechanism of injury found to be significant as a predictor of cervical spine trauma was a fall of less than 10 ft. This appears to have been an artifact based on triage criteria of the trauma center, however, because patients sustaining such falls are not referred routinely to trauma centers based on mechanism of injury alone unless a severe injury is identified by emergency medical personnel. In 1991, Cohn and colleagues evaluated the Advanced Trauma Life Support guidelines for the use of cervical spine radiography.[19] They concluded that all patients with evidence of head or neck trauma should be immobilized and evaluated radiographically, as recommended by the American College of Surgeons. We have noted 13 unstable injuries in 410 patients evaluated prospectively for injury to the cervical spine, and have found no association between a specific mechanism of injury and absence of risk for such trauma.[18] Based on the extant literature, the mechanism of injury is not sensitive enough to identify patients who do not require temporary immobilization or radiographic evaluation.

Clinical indicators appear to be more useful in identifying patients who are at high risk for cervical spine injury. Fischer evaluated 226 awake, alert patients who were able to follow simple commands and respond to simple questions regarding symptoms of tenderness, pain, and neurologic deficit.[22] The 5 patients who had cervical spine injury were identified by the presence of some clinical sign or symptom of injury. He concluded that, in the absence of pain, cervical neurologic deficit, or spinal tenderness, there was no risk of injury and radiography was not indicated. This conclusion has generated a significant amount of controversy. Reports of occult stable and unstable injuries to the cervical spine continue to appear in the literature.[25] A recent publication described three patients with occult fractures documented at autopsy after normal results were obtained on extensive radiographic evaluation of the cervical spine.[26]

Because most "occult" cervical spine fractures appear to be related to an inadequate index of suspicion, many authors believe that a history of loss of consciousness (including amnesia for events or evidence of cerebral concussion) is an indication for radiography. In 1986, Jacobs and colleagues recommended that patients with any cervical neurologic deficit, neck pain, or tenderness be evaluated radiographically.[20] Roberge[24] indicated that pain, tenderness, and neurologic deficit identified only 93% of unstable cervical spine injuries, and similar results have been obtained in other series.[18, 23, 27] An association of cervical spine injury with facial fracture or laceration, however, has not been identified.[18, 27, 28]

Specific reference to major head injury as a high risk factor for spine injury has been made by both the Advanced Trauma Life Support Course and other sources.[7] Nevertheless, a distinction between major head injury and lesser brain injury (e.g., cerebral concussion) in association with the risk of cervical spine injury has not been drawn conclusively. O'Malley and associates concluded that patients with major head injury were at no greater risk than were those with minor or no head injury.[29] Hills and Deane, however, identified a 67% higher incidence of cervical spine injury in patients with Glasgow Coma Scale scores of 8 or greater compared with those with less severe head injuries.[27] The absence of *major* head injury cannot be used to rule out cervical spine trauma without radiography. Patients with minor head injury also are at significant risk for neck injury. Vandemark attempted to develop a list criteria indicating a high risk of cervical spine injury.[30] He included high-velocity blunt trauma, multiple severe fractures of long bones, direct neck injury, altered mental status, fall from greater than 10 ft, severe head or facial injury, neck pain or tenderness, abnormal neurologic examination, thoracic or lumbar vertebral injury, and history of preexisting vertebral disease as factors that mandated radiography. Other authors have confirmed the necessity of total spine radiography in the presence of an identified vertebral injury at any level.[31] The presence of underlying vertebral disease, especially congenital or surgical fusion or ankylosing spondylitis, has been associated with an increased risk of injury to the cervical spine.[32]

Factors such as specific mechanism of injury or normal cerebral function at the time of arrival at the hospital (in association with signs of minor head injury such as amnesia or documented loss of consciousness at the time of injury) cannot be used to exclude neck injury. We maintain initial immobilization of the neck and perform cervical radiography on all patients with any evidence of head injury, cervical tenderness or pain, or neurologic deficits referable to the cervical cord or a nerve root. Although patients with facial lacerations and facial fractures may not require urgent cervical spine radiography, they typically have "distracting" injuries. Therefore, facial injury must be considered a possible indication for spine radiography, even in the absence of evidence of head or neck trauma.

Initial Radiographic Evaluation

As advocated by the Advanced Trauma Life Support Course, the cross-table lateral view of the cervical spine generally is believed to be the definitive initial study for ruling out an unstable injury to this area.[7, 33] Although the cross-table lateral view has a demonstrated sensitivity of only about 83%, many physicians continue to use this view exclusively for evaluating the cervical spine in all patients.[34–36] It is critical that this film be technically adequate and include the cervicothoracic junction, because injuries at this level have been reported to comprise 3% to 9% of all cervical spine injuries.[37–39] In as many as one fourth of patients with multiple injuries, obtaining a technically adequate lateral cervical radiograph is impossible. The swimmer's view, computed tomography (CT), or thin-section tomography may be used in these cases.[34, 40–42] The swimmer's view may be contraindicated, however, in patients in whom the suspicion of injury is high because of an incomplete neurologic deficit, or in those with unstable fractures of the thoracic or lumbar spine. Bilateral supine oblique films may be used to visualize the lower cervical spine in these individuals.[43] Freemyer and associates found bilateral supine oblique views to add little to the initial evaluation.[44] They detected no injuries using a five-view cervical spine series that were not identified on the initial three-view series.

Because of the low sensitivity of the lateral cervical view when it is used alone, additional views of the cervical spine are necessary. Many authors recommend a three-view cervical spine series including anteroposterior, open-mouth odontoid, and lateral cervical films. The anteroposterior radiograph evaluates the overall alignment of the spine, including the posterior spinous processes and the lateral masses. The lateral radiograph, which is the most useful view in the acute setting, also evaluates the occipitoatloid alignment, the C1 and C2 articulation (including the atlanto-dens interval), the odontoid, and the alignment of the lower cervical spine. Subtle findings such as swelling of the prevertebral soft tissue and displacement of the spinous processes also can be useful. The open-mouth view better evaluates the ring of C1, as well as the odontoid. Each of these views is discussed later as it applies to specific injury patterns.

If these radiographs are technically adequate and the results are normal, the sensitivity can approach 100%.[34] Some centers, however, have reported significant limitations of plain radiographs of the neck. Woodring and Lee found that 61% of cervical spine fractures and 36% of subluxations and dislocations were not detected by the three-view cervical spine series.[45] They recommended the routine use of thin-section polytomography and CT scanning in any patient meeting high-risk clinical criteria for spine radiography. Patients who continue to complain of neck pain after bony injury has been ruled out should undergo flexion-extension radiography under direct physician control to evaluate for unstable ligamentous injury. Physician-assisted flexion-extension radiographs are performed with the patient voluntarily moving the neck and have a limited role in the acute setting. They can demonstrate injury to the transverse ligament at C1–C2, however, or posterior spinous ligamentous disruption in the lower cervical spine.[46]

The routine use of additional radiographic studies for the urgent evaluation of patients at risk for cervical spine injury is controversial. CT scanning has largely replaced polytomography in the identification of cervical spine injuries, with the exception of fractures of the dens. In this instance, the fracture often is in the same plane as the CT scan, making it more difficult to identify.[41] Before CT became widely available, thin-section tomography was the standard of care for evaluating both suspected and identified fractures and was advocated for the routine evaluation of patients with high risk or suspicion of injury.[41, 47] Tomographs can elucidate subtle bony injuries and remain the gold standard for occipital-atlantal dislocations, subluxation of the vertebral bodies, and fractures of the lateral masses, facet joints, and odontoid.[45] Based on a series of 20 patients, Mace recommended that CT be used in certain high-risk cases, even if plain radiographs are normal.[48] Although CT is useful logistically, especially in patients who require urgent head evaluation, using it indiscriminately for all patients at risk is expensive, time-consuming, and probably not indicated.

CT of the neck is invaluable in defining the anatomy of identified or radiographically suggested injury.[42] In a prospective study of 104 patients who underwent CT scanning for the evaluation of suspected cervical spine trauma at our center (including 56 who had inadequate plain radiographs and 31 who had radiographs suspicious for injury), we found an overall sensitivity of 0.78 and a specificity of 0.95.[40] Limited, directed CT of the neck was a valuable adjunct when plain radiographs were technically inadequate or limited by intubation. It also was useful in the evaluation of patients with an established diagnosis. CT of C1 and C2 with 15-degree rotational views may be helpful in assessing patients for atlantoaxial rotatory subluxation.[49] Other authors have confirmed the value of using CT in this manner during the initial evaluation of cervical trauma.[45]

Magnetic resonance imaging (MRI) is useful in cervical spine trauma as a tertiary study to identify cord injury. If neurologic injury is present and bony pathology is ruled out, the MRI scan can be used to define injury to the disk or soft tissues. Acute herniation alone can occur with trauma and may be associated with unilateral or bilateral joint facet injury. Edema and contusion of the spinal cord can be visualized with MRI and aid in determining the patient's prognosis. MRI also may help to identify the locked facet joints.[50] MRI scanning has largely replaced cervical myelography in the evaluation of injured patients in the acute setting. For patients in whom MRI is not technically possible because of monitoring, ongoing therapy, or considerations such as pacemakers or metallic implants, CT myelography is a suitable alternative.

If clinical suspicion of a specific injury is raised, CT, polytomography, MRI, and myelography all are useful for detecting spinal cord injury and bony or ligamentous instability.

Temporary Spinal Immobilization

Spinal immobilization must be maintained during all initial treatment and radiographic evaluation. Until the presence of unstable injury has been excluded definitively, spine boards, semirigid cervical collars, or cervical skeletal immobilization or traction devices must be used. Most patients who are transported to emergency departments after motor vehicle accidents or other types of major blunt trauma are placed in a variety of different devices for spinal immobilization by emergency care providers. These devices also are used for initial temporary immobilization of the cervical spine after arrival at the hospital. None of the cervical immobilization collars provides total control of the injured cervical spine. Prospective studies have been done in the field to evaluate the "short board technique," various "extrication devices," and semirigid, plastic cervical collars. Short board spinal immobilization devices and extrication devices were found to be superior to the use of a collar alone.[51] Various modifications of collars also have individually been tested and found to vary significantly in their ability to restrain motion of the cervical spine. Soft foam collars provide no restraint whatsoever. The semirigid Philadelphia collar (Technol, Fort Worth, Tex) provides better control of motion in all planes compared to the soft foam collar; however, other polyethylene collars (sold commercially under several trade names) provide even greater control. For patients who are at high risk but have apparently normal neck radiographs, immobilization with a semirigid cervical collar may be appropriate until full clearance of the cervical spine is achieved. Patients with identified unstable injuries require a more aggressive approach to initial stabilization, such as initial halo fixation. The halo allows the patient to be moved safely for operative intervention and diagnostic studies, without risk to the spinal cord from unstable bony injury.[52]

After a diagnosis of fracture of the cervical spine has been established, treatment must be tailored to address the specific nature of the injury. Protecting the spinal cord and neural elements from further injury is the first priority. The degree of instability caused by the injury governs the type of immobilization used and the need for surgical stabilization or decompression. We discuss later the various techniques of external immobilization and examine each injury pattern in terms of its mechanism, classification, and treatment.

Specialty Beds for Immobilization of the Spine

The selection of a bed for a patient with a cervical spine injury is based on the patient's general condition, including concomitant injuries, and on the method of reduction needed. A standard hospital bed with a foam pad is generally acceptable for patients with stable fracture patterns. For those with multiple system involvement, a Flexicare or Rotorest bed (Kinetic Concepts, San Antonio, Tex) may be more appropriate. Log rolling may be done as other injuries allow, but the alignment of the cervical spine must be maintained by manual positioning. Decubiti can be prevented by frequent position changes and the use of an air pressure or sand mattress; these modifications, however, do not permit the use of traction.

The Stryker frame (Stryker, Kalamazoo, Mich) allows traction to be maintained while the patient is turned along the longitudinal axis. It also can be used in the operating room to "place" a patient in the prone position. In the presence of unstable fractures, it must be used with caution because of the potential for displacement of the cervical spine with change from the supine to the prone position.

The Rotorest bed allows multidirectional traction. Decubiti are avoided by turning the patient along the longitudinal axis. In addition, the hatches allow access to the back and sacrum. This bed is favored for trauma patients with multiple injuries, especially those who are at risk for or already have pulmonary complications.

Traction, Collars, or the Halo for Cervical Immobilization in the Hospital

Head halter traction may be helpful in treating soft-tissue injuries, but it has a limited role in cervical spine fractures or dislocations. The standard of care with unstable fracture patterns is skeletal traction, most commonly with Gardner-Wells type tongs. This device uses calibrated, spring-loaded pins to fix the outer table of the skull.[53] The goal of traction is to restore alignment of the bony elements and relieve pressure on the neural elements. The application of these tongs is dependent on the patient's general condition but should be done as soon as possible to restore bony alignment. The specific application of cervical traction in the various injury patterns is discussed later in this chapter.

Several devices can be used in the hospital to immobilize the cervical region, including the foam collar, the hard or Philadelphia collar, two- or four-point sternal occipital mandibular immobilization (SOMI) braces, and the halo vest. Johnson and coworkers have compared the effectiveness of these restraints.[54, 55] They found that the halo vest performed best, although it provided less stability with lower cervical injuries.

The Philadelphia collar provides adequate cervical spine immobilization in the acute setting; it is inadequate for unstable fracture patterns, however, because it loses its effectiveness over time.[53] SOMI braces are relatively effective in controlling flexion but fail to control the spine adequately in extension and rotation.

The most useful appliance for acute immobilization of the injured cervical spine is the halo vest. Several types are available, but all rely on skeletal fixation of the skull by halo pins to a plastic, molded body vest. Several investigators have evaluated the effectiveness of this system and have concluded that the standard vest provides effective stabilization for lesions at C4 or above, whereas a vest extension to below the twelfth rib is required for levels of injury between C5 and C7.[55, 56] Known complications of halo vests include minor pin tract infections, pin loosening, or the rare occurrence of pin penetration of the inner table of the skull and intracranial injuries.[57] These complications can be avoided with proper pin site care and initial positioning.

Specific Injury Patterns and Treatment

Fracture of the Occipital Condyles

The occipital condyles can be injured either in isolation or in combination with fractures of the C1–C2 complex.[58] This fracture pattern occurs when a severe deceleration force causes axial compression and anterior or lateral shear forces. Clinically, patients with such an injury are unconscious, with trauma to the lower cranial nerves and quadriparesis, respiratory compromise, or death.[59] Goldstein and associates reported a mortality rate of 44%

with this injury.[60] Lower cranial nerve deficits were noted in 22% of surviving patients. Radiographic diagnosis with plain films is difficult because of the overlying facial bones; therefore, CT scanning or tomography must be used.[59, 60]

Anderson and Montesano described these injuries using a three-part classification system.[61] Type I fractures are nondisplaced, axial compression fractures that maintain their ligamentous stability and can be treated with a halo. Type II injuries represent an extension of a basilar skull fracture into the condyles. These also are relatively stable lesions and should be treated with a halo vest. Type III injuries represent a more unstable pattern, resulting from a lateral bending or shear force that avulses the alar ligaments from the condyles.[59] These patients should be treated with a halo and observed closely for displacement. Operative indications are not defined clearly, but relative indications include compression of the brain stem or instability after adequate immobilization.[62]

Occipital-atlantal Injuries

Occipital-atlantal injuries are extremely rare, with only 21 reported cases since 1989.[63] This figure probably is an underestimate, however, because most of these injuries are fatal. Alker and coworkers performed autopsies on 312 victims of multiple trauma and found 19 (6%) occipital-atlantal dislocations.[64] Similarly, Bucholz and Burkhead reported the results of postmortem examinations of 112 patients and noted 9 (8%) cranial atlantal dislocations.[65] The mechanism of injury is controversial, but some studies have implicated distraction hyperextension. A higher percentage of these injuries were found in children (15%) than in adults (6%) in one study.[63]

The clinical presentation may vary from no neurologic deficit to severe involvement of the brain stem, upper cervical spinal cord, and cranial nerves.[59, 66, 67] In those patients who are neurologically intact, the diagnosis may be difficult to make. The presence of a suboccipital hematoma and severe posterior neck pain are suggestive of this injury.

Radiographic signs can be subtle and include prevertebral soft-tissue swelling (increased from the normal 1 to 7 mm) at the C2 level.[68] The most commonly used method of evaluating this injury is Power's ratio (Fig 1).[69] This is determined by comparing the distance from the basion to the anterior border of the posterior arch of C1 divided by the distance from the opisthion to the posterior border of the anterior arch of the atlas. The normal ratio is .77, with 1 as the upper limit of normal. If this ratio is greater than 1, anterior occipital-atlantal dislocation is present.

The treatment of this injury pattern is guided by the amount of displacement that is present. Traynelis and associates classified these injuries into three types.[70] Type I involves pure distraction of the occipital-atlantal articulation without subluxation and can be treated with a halo vest. Type II is the most common type of injury and involves anterior subluxation or dislocation of the occipital-atlantal articulations. After gentle reduction with Gardner-Wells tongs or a halo ring, immediate conversion to a halo vest is

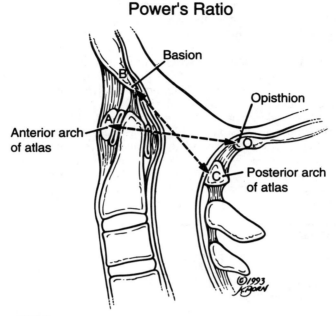

FIG 1.
Power's ratio for identifying craniocervical injury.

required. Type III injuries involve posterior subluxation or dislocation and are reduced in a similar fashion. Some authors suggest that immediate occipital cervical fusion is required because of the instability of this fracture pattern. Wertheim and Bohlman recommend using a 16- to 18-gauge wire passed through bur holes in the external occipital protuberance and sublaminar C1 wires augmented with a corticocancellous autologous bone graft.[71] Halo immobilization then is provided for 3 months.

Fractures of C1

Fractures of the C1 ring, or atlas, are relatively uncommon, representing only 3% to 13% of injuries of the cervical spine[72] and 25% of injuries of the C1–C2 complex.[73] In 53% of patients, this injury occurs with other fractures of the cervical spine, primarily fractures of C2 and its odontoid process.[73] Fracture of the posterior arch is the most common injury and results from hyperextension and axial compression.[74]

Because of the size of the neural canal at this level, the incidence of neurologic injury is low.[58, 72, 75] If a deficit is present, it usually involves injury to cranial nerve VI, IX, X, XI, or XII.

The stability of these fractures is determined by the presence or absence of injury to the transverse ligament. Displacement of the lateral masses of greater than 6.9 mm on the open-mouth view is indicative of disruption of the transverse ligament and represents a more unstable pattern of injury.[76]

Radiographic evaluation of a C1 fracture is primarily done with plain films and CT scanning. Tomography also can be helpful if further clarification of the injured anatomy is required.

The most useful classification scheme is a modification of Gehweiler's original proposal[68] by Segal and coworkers.[77] In this description, type I and type II fractures involve only the anterior or posterior arch, respectively, whereas type III fractures involve the lateral masses. The classic Jefferson type injury is a burst fracture with both anterior and posterior breaks in the ring and represents a type IV fracture. Type V fractures involve the transverse processes of C1. The type VI fracture was added by Segal's group and is a comminuted fracture with a double-ring break and an associated fracture of the lateral mass. The type VI fracture carries the worst prognosis, with a rate of nonunion exceeding 50% and a marked decrease in range of motion.[78]

Treatment of type I or II fractures is generally conservative, involving halo or collar immobilization. Type III or IV fractures are generally treated with halo immobilization, after a period of axial tong traction if significant displacement is present. After 2 months in a halo vest, dynamic flexion-extension films are required for patients with transverse ligament disruption. If significant instability is present, C1–C2 fusion or occiput-to-C2 fusion is undertaken.[78]

Atlantoaxial Rotation Injuries

Atlantoaxial rotatory subluxation is reported most often in the pediatric population but can be seen in adults as well. Patients with this abnormality have suboccipital pain and restricted C1–C2 rotation. The "cock robin" deformity with the skull rotated 20 degrees in one direction and tilted 20 degrees in the opposite direction is a classic presentation. The diagnosis is made by the open-mouth radiographic view on the basis of displacement of the lateral masses of C1 in relationship to the odontoid process. Asymmetry of the C1–C2 articulation or a "wink" sign also is suggestive of this lesion. Dynamic rotational CT scanning or CT scanning with sagittal or three-dimensional reconstruction also may be helpful.[49]

A classification system for this entity was proposed by Fielding and Hawkins in 1977.[79] Type I injuries, usually seen in children, are most common. Rotation is fixed within the physiologic range of motion. Type II lesions, also seen in children, represent an anterior displacement of one C1 lateral mass by 305 mm on the intact contralateral C1–C2 articulation. Type III injuries are more severe and involve anterior displacement by more than 5 mm of both C1 articular processes and a marked increase in the atlanto-dens interval on the lateral radiographic view. A type IV injury is a rare lesion that includes an odontoid fracture and posterior C1 ring displacement on C2. A type V lesion was added to Fielding's scheme by Levin and Edwards and consists of bilateral rotatory dislocations.[80]

Treatment usually consists of gentle head halter or skeletal traction with mild sedation until reduction is complete. This usually requires 5 lb in children and as much as 25 lb in adults.[79, 81] Pain and spasm are relieved immediately by reduction, and the patient usually hears a popping sound.[81] Immobilization with a hard collar, Minerva cast, or halo then is indicated. Reduction of a fixed deformity is controversial and beyond the scope of this review.

Odontoid Fractures

Odontoid fractures are relatively common, occurring in 5% to 15% of all cervical spine injuries.[82] The incidence has recently increased, the male-to-female ratio is 3:1,[83] and patients are usually in their fifth decade.[84, 85] The mechanism of injury has extensively been studied and appears to be an axial compression load coupled with flexion and either an anterior or posterior translation vector.[64, 86, 87]

The most popular classification system for defining odontoid fractures was proposed by Anderson and D'Alonzo in 1972.[83] A type I fracture involves avulsion of the alar ligament from the tip of the dens. Although it is extremely rare, this injury can be associated with a more ominous ligamentous injury to the occipital-atlantal junction.[66, 83] Type II fractures, the most commonly reported, are located at the junction of the dens with the body of C2. Because of a limited fracture surface and precarious blood supply, these fractures progress to nonunion more often than do type I or type III fractures. Type III fractures occur within the body of C2 and can extend into the superior articulating surfaces of the axis.

Clinically, affected patients are usually neurologically intact, although symptoms ranging from greater occipital nerve irritation to quadriplegia and respiratory compromise have been reported.[86]

Radiographic evaluation involves standard anteroposterior, lateral, and open-mouth views, as well as lateral and anteroposterior tomography. CT scanning must include sagittal reconstruction because the transaxial cuts may miss the type II fracture.[85, 88]

Odontoid fractures are treated according to their particular type. Isolated type I fractures are stable injuries that can be treated in a rigid cervical orthosis. The treatment of type II fractures is more controversial because of the significant rate of nonunion (as high as 32%).[89] Risk factors include initial displacement of the odontoid by more than 5 mm or angulation of greater than 10 degrees. These patients were initially treated with a halo and union was reported in 68% of cases. Because of this poor nonunion rate, Anderson and D'Alonzo recommend primary surgical fusion for all type II fractures.[83] In a review of 70 consecutive patients treated between 1980 and 1990, Cotler noted that 30 progressed to nonunion (43%).[90] Of the type II fractures treated in halo immobilization, 75% went on to nonunion compared to the 100% union rate seen after primary arthrodesis. The direction of displacement affected the rate of nonunion: a 70% nonunion rate was reported in those fractures that initially were displaced posteriorly compared with a 33% nonunion rate in fractures with initial anterior displacement. Patients were initially treated with Gardner-Wells tongs traction to reduce displacement, then were converted to halo vests. The author suggested that risk factors for nonunion included displacement of greater than 5 mm posteriorly or anteriorly, patient age greater than 60 years, and loss of previous reduction. Patients exhibiting these factors should be considered for primary surgical fusion and placement of a halo. The treatment of a type II fracture should include a period of traction with 10 to 15 lb of weight for reduction, frequent radiographic evaluation, and conversion to halo immobilization for 3 months. Healing then is documented by tomography. Nondisplaced type III fractures should be treated with a halo for 3 months.

Displaced type III fractures are treated with Gardner-Wells tong reduction for as long as 6 weeks, followed by conversion to a halo vest for 3 months. The rate of union for this fracture pattern is higher than for type II fractures because of the rich blood supply to the C2 body and the larger fracture surfaces.

Hangman's Fracture

Originally described by Garber in 1964, the term "traumatic spondylolisthesis of the axis" refers to a fracture bilaterally through the pars interarticularis of the axis.[91] Classically described as a "hangman's fracture," the lesion that results from a motor vehicle accident differs significantly from the injury inflicted by a hangman's noose. In judicial hanging, violent extension and axial distraction occurs, with transection of the cord. Extension and axial compression is more common in a motor vehicle accident.

Axis fractures occur in 12% to 18% of all cervical spine injuries and are rarely associated with neurologic deficits because of the large diameter of the spinal canal in this area.[92–94] Axis fracture is associated with other injuries of the cervical spine in 14% to 33% of cases.[95–97] Injuries to the face, trachea, and thorax also are common.[94] Clinically, these patients have associated head and neck trauma, neck pain, and, occasionally, pain from compression of the greater occipital nerve. The diagnosis is made by lateral plain films CT, or tomography.

A classification system developed by Levin and Edwards has been used widely in the orthopaedic literature.[97] A type I fracture is one that occurs through the pars bilaterally, with less than 3 mm of fracture displacement, no angulation, and no gross instability. This fracture is usually associated with a fracture of the C1 ring, odontoid, or C1 lateral mass.[97] The type II fracture has greater than 3 mm of displacement, with angulation and wedging anteriorly of the C3 body. Although subtypes exist, the presence of angulation and instability on flexion/extension radiographic views indicates a more unstable pattern of injury. Type III injuries involve bilateral pars fractures with associated facet dislocation of C2 on C3 either unilaterally or bilaterally. This injury represents significant disruption of both the anterior and posterior longitudinal ligaments and makes reduction by closed methods extremely difficult. Frequently, operative reduction and internal fixation are required.

A type I fracture can be treated for 3 months in a rigid cervical orthosis or halo.[89] Physician-assisted flexion/extension radiographic views with the patient moving voluntarily can aid in making the diagnosis as well as document osseous union. Type II fractures involve more significant soft-tissue injury and usually require a period of skeletal tong traction, with postural manipulation occasionally needed to achieve final reduction. The optimal duration of traction before halo application is controversial, as is the appropriate amount of translation or angulation. Recently, Fielding and colleagues reported a 94% healing rate in type II fractures with no significant difference between patients treated with immediate halo immobilization, 2 weeks of traction before halo application, or 6 weeks of traction before halo immobilization.[96] He did report nonunion in six of seven patients with greater than 11 degrees of angulation.

Treatment of the type III fracture includes open reduction of the facet dislocation and internal fixation through a posterior approach. This fixation must occasionally be supplemented with an oblique wire from the inferior facet of C2 to the spinous process of C3, depending on the location of the pars fracture.[97]

Injuries to the Lower Cervical Spine

In the lower cervical spine, injuries are classified not by anatomic level, but by mechanism of injury. The five major categories include flexion, flexion rotation, axial load, extension, and penetrating trauma (Fig 2). The goal of both initial and long-term therapy is to protect the neural elements from further injury and to establish a stable osseous structure. Injuries at this level often cause neurologic deficits; therefore, stability is of paramount importance to prevent new or further neurologic impairment.

Pure flexion injuries usually result in a less than 25% compression fracture of the vertebral body. Because this fracture does not compromise the posterior height of the vertebral body, there is no retropulsion of bone. In the absence of shear or rotation forces, the posterior ligamentous structures remain intact. Subluxation or translation of the body on the adjacent vertebra does not occur because of the intact posterior ligaments and facets. These injuries can be treated successfully in a cervical orthosis for 4 to 8 weeks if posterior ligamentous injury is not present.[98]

In pure flexion injuries with loss of more than 25% of the anterior vertebral height, dynamic instability from injury to the posterior ligaments must be ruled out. Late progression of deformity, kyphosis, and cervical myelopathy and radiculopathy can occur if this injury is not diagnosed. To define these criteria further radiographically, White and coworkers developed a checklist for use in determining stability (Table 1).[99] Major criteria, worth two points each, include the presence of sagittal plane translation of greater than 3.5 mm, rotation of greater than 11 degrees, spinal cord damage, and destroyed anterior or posterior elements. Minor criteria, worth

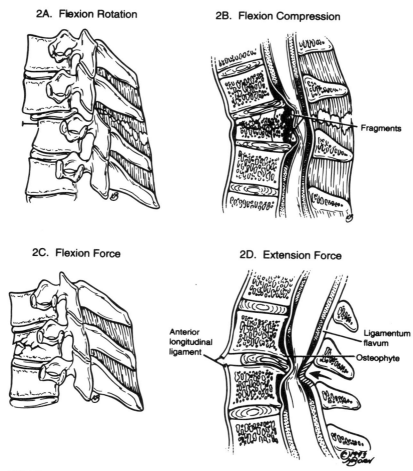

FIG 2.
Biomechanical etiology of injuries to the lower cervical spine.

one point each, include nerve root damage, abnormal disk narrowing, and expectation of dangerous loading. If a total of five points is accumulated, the spine is unstable. Using these radiographic criteria in conjunction with flexion/extension radiographic views when indicated and a good clinical examination, spinal stability can be determined.

Treatment of patients with demonstrated instability resulting from posterior ligamentous disruption should include posterior cervical fusion with a bone graft from the iliac crest.[100] The use of a cervical orthosis or halo alone may lead to late displacement and instability, especially in the presence of an anterior compression fracture.[101, 102] Techniques for posterior cervical fusion range from the classic triple-wire method to posterior cervi-

TABLE 1.
Radiographic and Clinical Criteria for Instability of the Cervical Spine*†

Major (2 points)	Minor (1 point)
1. Anterior elements destroyed	1. Nerve root damage
2. Posterior elements destroyed	2. Abnormal disc narrowing

3. Relative sagittal plane
   Translation >3.5 mm
   Rotation >11 degrees
	3. Dangerous loading expected

4. Positive stretch test	
5. Spinal cord damage	

*From White AA, Southwick WO, Panjabi MM: Clinical instablity in the lower cervical spine: A review of past and current concepts. Spine 1976; 1:15. Used by permission.
†Five or more points (total) = unstable spine injury.

---

cal plates. Regardless of the technique chosen, a cervical orthosis is used for 8 to 12 weeks postoperatively. Once serial radiographs show incorporation of the bone graft, the external support can be discontinued. Flexion/extension radiographs then are obtained to check for residual instability.

Injury by flexion rotation may cause unilateral or bilateral facet dislocation or facet fracture. In the absence of facet fracture, unilateral dislocation results in anterior translation of the superior vertebral body on the inferior body by about 25%, whereas bilateral dislocation causes 50% or greater subluxation. With facet fracture, any degree of subluxation can be present.

The head of a patient with unilateral facet dislocation is locked in a position looking away from the "jumped" side. On the lateral radiograph, 25% subluxation of the cephalad vertebra can be seen. On the anteroposterior radiograph, the spinous processes are rotated at the level of the dislocation. Tomographs or reconstruction CT scans demonstrate facet fracture and dislocation most reliably. Neurologic injury is common in this injury pattern, particularly with bilaterally dislocated facets.

In general, reduction is accomplished with tongs and is initiated with 10 to 15 lb of weight. Lateral radiographs should be obtained at intervals of 15 to 30 minutes to avoid excessive distraction and to check for reduction. The amount of weight used has been a controversial topic in the orthopaedic literature. Initially, Cotler recommended 5 lb per cervical level after 10 lb were added for the head[103] (i.e., 15 lb for a C1–C2 fracture or 40 lb for a C6–C7 injury). These weight limits have been increased in recent reports and now range from 70 lb to 100 lb.

Manipulation also may be used to facilitate reduction. Evans[104] advocates manual reduction under general anesthesia, whereas Miller and associates[105] believe that judicious use of manipulation is beneficial in certain cases. In the latter series, manipulation was performed without anesthesia. More recently, closed reduction under general anesthesia has been replaced by open reduction of irreducible fractures.

Treatment of unilateral facet dislocation is begun with the application of skeletal traction in the form of Gardner-Wells tongs or a halo ring. The tongs are positioned 1 cm above the pinna and 1 cm posterior to the external auditory meatus. This posterior position allows a flexion movement to be placed on the neck, thus helping to reduce the facets. This reduction is accomplished best on a Stryker frame or Rotorest bed and begins with about 10 lb of traction. At this point, a lateral radiograph is obtained to evaluate the ligamentous integrity of the occiput C1–C2 level. This film, at a relatively small weight, helps prevent excessive distraction of the cervical spine.[106] Weights are added in 10-lb increments and radiographs are obtained at 15- to 20-minute intervals between weight additions. Serial neurologic examinations are performed to monitor the patient's neurologic status. Small doses of muscle relaxants can be used cautiously, but care must be exercised to avoid excessive sedation because this may interfere with the neurologic examination. Bilateral "jumped" facets require less weight to reduce than do unilateral lesions because of secondary soft-tissue disruption.[97] Facet fractures require a variable amount of weight, and postural reduction or manual manipulation may be necessary to obtain anatomic alignment.

The role of manipulation in unreduced dislocations of the cervical spine is controversial. Although it is widely accepted in Europe, its use in this country is more limited. Manipulation can be attempted using intravenous sedation and serial neurologic examinations.[107, 108] If compromise occurs, further attempts are abandoned. Reduction under general anesthesia also has been described.[107, 108] This technique precludes neurologic monitoring, however.

The presence of an irreducible unilateral facet dislocation is an indication for operative reduction. A posterior approach with controlled open reduction and posterior cervical fusion is the procedure of choice.

Treatment of a reduced unilateral facet dislocation may vary from halo immobilization alone to posterior cervical fusion. If a facet fracture is present, however, immobilization alone carries a higher rate of recurrent displacement.[102, 109] Therefore, posterior cervical fusion should be considered for facet fractures of the cervical spine. Bilateral facet dislocation involves much more soft-tissue disruption, including the disc space. The patient should be studied by MRI or CT scanning enhanced with myelography to determine whether disk material has been extruded into the spinal canal. If no impingement is present, a halo should be applied and posterior fusion performed, especially in cases involving an anterior compression fracture.[101] If disc material is present in the spinal canal after reduction, a combination anterior and posterior decompression and fusion is performed.[110, 111] Another approach is an anterior decompression and strut grafting supplemented by anterior cervical plate fixation.[112, 113] If rigid fixation by plating of the anterior column can be achieved, the need for posterior fusion may be eliminated. The role of this technique is still being investigated in the literature.

When an axial compressive load is placed on the cervical spine, a burst fracture pattern frequently occurs. The most common fracture is at C5, and an associated neurologic injury often is present. The anteroinferior portion of the vertebral body may be split coronally, resulting in a characteristic "teardrop" fragment. The posterior portion of the body may be driven back into the canal, compromising the neural elements. If a severe flexion movement also was present, the posterior elements may be disrupted. The prognosis for neurologic recovery in these patients is poor, even with thorough surgical decompression.

Treatment begins with cervical traction. In flexion injuries, a rolled towel is placed beneath the shoulders and as much as 40 to 50 lb is applied in 10-lb increments, with serial radiographs obtained between each addition of more weight. The height of the vertebra is usually restored; however, the fragment that underwent retropulsion may remain in the canal. In the absence of neurologic deficit, the patient is treated with traction for 2 weeks before being converted to a halo for 2 to 3 months. In more than 50% of cases, spontaneous fusion will occur. When a neurologic deficit is present, skeletal traction is applied and the spinal canal is assessed by MRI or CT scanning. If neurologic recovery is obtained with traction and realignment, conservative treatment with traction and a halo is considered. If the neurologic deficit remains unchanged and posterior stability is present, early anterior decompression and fusion can be performed. Early realignment, decompression, and fusion are required in patients in whom reduction cannot be achieved. If posterior stability is not present, early posterior fusion with either staged or simultaneous anterior decompression and fusion is necessary. Operative stabilization always should be augmented by external halo vest immobilization.

Although major extension-type injuries of the cervical spine are uncommon, elderly patients with preexisting cervical spondylosis or congenitally small canals are predisposed to injury by this mechanism. In these patients, the cord is "pinched" between the degenerative disk or osteophyte anteriorly and the buckled ligamentum flavum posteriorly. The neurologic deficit is usually a central cord syndrome, with the upper extremities (especially the hands) affected more than the lower extremities. There is a 50% chance of recovery to the point of independent ambulation; however, significant spasticity in the lower extremities can occur. Upper extremity involvement remains more profound, with permanent lower motor neuron paralysis of the hands. The typical patient retains bowel and bladder control, with spastic gait and poor return of fine motor control of the upper extremities.

Treatment of these patients is controversial. Some authors suggest nonsurgical therapy,[114] whereas others recommend decompressive surgery for patients with a permanently deformed spinal cord.[115] The timing of surgery also is a matter of debate.

Penetrating Trauma to the Cervical Spine

In many urban centers, penetrating injuries to the cervical spine by low-velocity gunshot or knife wounds are common. Only rarely is the stability of the bony elements compromised, but damage to the cervical cord and contamination of the spinal column by tracheoesophageal contents may occur. With penetrating wounds near the spinal canal, a CT scan is used to determine the pathway of the projectile. If the cord has been traversed, no decompression is required; however, some controversy exists regarding the indications for removal of metallic objects from the spinal canal. Some authors believe that, because the stability of the column is not compromised and the likelihood of return of neural function is minimal, removal of the projectile is unwarranted.[116] Others believe that retained metallic fragments within the spinal canal can cause a delayed myelopathy.[58] In addition, a recent study has raised concerns abut an abscess-like reaction to copper metallic fragments in an animal model.[117] Finally, osteomyelitis is a rare, but real, concern in the treatment of gunshot wounds to the cervical spine. To prevent its occurrence, a protocol has been developed for the treatment of these injuries.[118] This regimen mandates exploration of any missile wound of the spine that has a documented transoral or transpharyngeal path. Debridement of soft tissue and bone fragments is performed after closure of the pharyngeal or esophageal wound. Removal of easily accessible metallic objects is indicated. Appropriate antibiotics, including an aminoglycoside, should be administered. Immobilization is governed by the bony stability of the spinal column and may be accomplished with a Philadelphia collar or a halo. Using this approach, cervical vertebral osteomyelitis has largely been eliminated.[119]

References

1. Garfin SR, Katz MM: The vertebral column: Experimental aspects, in Nahum AM, Melvin J (eds): *The Biomechanics of Trauma.* Norwalk, Connecticut, Appleton-Century-Crofts, 1985, pp 301–340.
2. Pare A: *The Apologie and Treatise.* London, Falcon Educational Books, 1951.
3. Hadra B: Wiring of the vertebra as a means of immobilization in fracture and Pott's disease. *Medical Times and Register* 1891.
4. Huelke DF, O'Day J, Mendelsohn R: Cervical injuries suffered in automobile crashes. *J Neurosurg* 1981; 54:316–322.
5. Riggins RS, Kraus JF: The risk of neurologic damage with fractures of the vertebrae. *J Trauma* 1977; 17:126–133.
6. Toberts JR: Trauma of the cervical spine. *Top Emerg Med* 1979; 1:63–77.
7. American College of Surgeons, Committee on Trauma: *Advanced Trauma Life Support Manual.* Chicago, American College of Surgeons, 1993.
8. Bucholz RW, Burkhead WZ, Graham W, et al: Occult cervical spine injuries in fatal traffic accidents. *J Trauma* 1979; 19:768–771.
9. Bivins HG, Ford S, Beznalinovic Z, et al: The effect of axial traction during

orotracheal intubation of the trauma victim with an unstable cervical spine. *Ann Emerg Med* 1988; 17:25–29.
10. Alker GJ, Oh Ys, Leslie EV, et al: Postmortem radiology of head and neck injuries in fatal traffic accidents. *Radiology* 1975; 114:611–617.
11. Born CT, Ross SE, Iannacone WM, et al: Delayed identification of skeletal injury in multisystem trauma. The "missed" fracture. *J Trauma* 1989; 29:1643.
12. Enderson BL, Reath DB, Meadors J, et al: The tertiary trauma survey: A prospective study of missed injury. *J Trauma* 1990; 30:666.
13. Rogers WA: Fractures and dislocations of the cervical spine: An end result study. *J Bone Joint Surg [Am]* 1957; 39:341–376.
14. Geisler WC, Wynne-Jones MM, Jousse AT: Early management of the patient with trauma to the spinal cord. *Med Serv J Canada* 1966; 23:512–522.
15. Reid DC, Henderson R, Saboe L, et al: Etiology and clinical course of missed spine fractures. *J Trauma* 1987; 27:980–986.
16. Davis JW, Phreaner DL, Hoyt DB: The etiology of missed cervical spine injuries. *J Trauma* 1993; 34:342–346.
17. Singer CM, Baraff LJ, Benedict SH, et al: Exposure of emergency medicine personnel to ionizing radiation during cervical spine radiography. *Ann Emerg Med* 1989; 18:822–825.
18. Ross SE, O'Malley KF, DeLong WG: Clinical predictors of unstable cervical spinal injury in multiply injured patients. *Injury* 1992; 23:317–319.
19. Cohn SM, Lyle WG, Linden CH, et al: Exclusion of cervical spine injury: A prospective study. *J Trauma* 1991; 31:570–574.
20. Jacobs LM, Schwartz R: Prospective analysis of acute cervical spine injury: A methodology to predict injury. *Ann Emerg Med* 1986; 15:44–49.
21. Cadoux CG, White JD, Hedberg MC: High-yield roentgenographic criteria for cervical spine injuries. *Ann Emerg Med* 1987; 16:738–742.
22. Fischer RP: Cervical radiographic evaluation of alert patients following blunt trauma. *Ann Emerg Med* 1984; 13:905.
23. Hoffman JR, Schriger DL, Mower W, et al: Low-risk criteria for cervical-spine radiography in blunt trauma: A prospective study. *Ann Emerg Med* 1992; 21:1454–1460.
24. Roberge RJ, Wears RC: Evaluation of neck discomfort, neck tenderness, and neurologic deficits as indicators for radiography in blunt trauma victims. *J Emerg Med* 1992; 10:539–544.
25. Mace SE: Unstable occult cervical-spine fracture. *Ann Emerg Med* 1991; 20:1373–1375.
26. Sweeney JF, Rosemurgy AS, Gill S, et al: Is the cervical spine clear? Undetected cervical fractures diagnosed only at autopsy. *Ann Emerg Med* 1992; 21:1288–1290.
27. Hills MW, Deane SA: Head injury and facial injury: Is there an increased risk of cervical injury? *J Trauma* 1993; 34:549–554.
28. Luce EA, Tubb TD, Moore AM: Review of 1,000 major facial fractures and associated injuries. *Plast Reconstr Surg* 1979; 60:26–30.
29. O'Malley KF, Ross SE: The incidence of injury to the cervical spine in patients with craniocerebral injury. *J Trauma* 1988; 28:1476–1478.
30. Vandemark RM: Radiology of the cervical spine in trauma patients: Practice pitfalls and recommendations for improving efficiency and communication. *AJR Am J Roentgenol* 1990; 155:465–472.
31. Scher AT: Double fractures of the spine—an indication for routine radio-

graphic examination of the entire spine after injury. *S Afr Med J* 1978; 52:411–413.
32. MacMillan M, Stauffer ES: Traumatic instability in the previously fused cervical spine. *J Spinal Disord* 1991; 4:449–454.
33. Bucholz RW: Fracture-dislocations of the cervical spine, in Meyers MH (ed): *The Multiply Injured Patient With Complex Fracture.* Philadelphia, Lea & Febiger, 1984, pp 179–195.
34. Ross SE, Schwab CW, David ET, et al: Clearing the cervical spine: Initial radiologic evaluation. *J Trauma* 1987; 27:1055–1060.
35. Shaffer MA, Doris PE: Limitation of the cross table lateral view in detecting cervical spine injuries: A retrospective analysis. *Ann Emerg Med* 1981; 10:508–513.
36. Streitweiser DR, Knopp R, Wales LR, et al: Accuracy of standard radiographic views in detecting cervical spine fractures. *Ann Emerg Med* 1983; 12:538–542.
37. Miller MD, Gehweiler JA, Martinez S, et al: Significant new observations on cervical spine trauma. *AJR Am J Roentgenol* 1978; 130:659–663.
38. Evans DK: Dislocations at the cervicothoracic junction. *J Bone Joint Surg Br* 1983; 65 124–127.
39. Nichols CG, Young DH, Schiller WR: Evaluation of cervicothoracic junction injury. *Ann Emerg Med* 1987;16:640–642.
40. Schleehauf K, Ross SE, Civil I, et al: Computed tomography in the initial evaluation of the cervical spine. *Ann Emerg Med* 1989; 18:815–817.
41. Maravilla KA, Cooper PR, Sklar FH: The influence of thin-section tomography on the treatment of cervical spine injuries. *Radiology* 1978; 127: 131–139.
42. Post MJ, Green BA, Quencer RM, et al: The value of computed tomography in spinal trauma. *Spine* 1982; 7:417–431.
43. Teretsky DB, Vines FS, Clayman DA, et al: Technique and use of supine oblique views in acute cervical spine trauma. *Ann Emerg Med* 1993; 22:685–689.
44. Freemyer B, Knopp R, Piche J, et al: Comparison of five-view and three-view cervical spine series in the evaluation of patients with cervical trauma. *Ann Emerg Med* 1989; 18:818–821.
45. Woodring JH, Lee C: The role and limitations of computed tomographic scanning in the evaluation of cervical trauma. *J Trauma* 1992; 33:698.
46. Lewis LM, Docherty M, Ruoff BE, et al: Flexion-extension views in the evaluation of cervical-spine injuries. *Ann Emerg Med* 1991; 20:117–121.
47. Anderson LD, Smith BL, DeTorre J, et al: The role of polytomography in the diagnosis and treatment of cervical spine injuries. *Clin Orthop* 1982; 165:64–68.
48. Mace SE: Emergency evaluation of cervical spine injuries: CT versus plain radiographs. *Ann Emerg Med* 1985; 14:973–975.
49. Iannacone WM, Delong WG Jr, Born CT, et al: Dynamic computerized tomography of the occiput atlas-axis complex in trauma patients with odontoid lateral mass asymmetry. *J Trauma* 1990; 30:1501–1505.
50. Hall AJ, Wagle VG, Raycroft J, et al: Magnetic resonance imaging in cervical spine trauma. *J Trauma* 1993; 34:21.
51. Graziano AF, Scheidel EA, Cline JR, et al: A radiographic comparison of prehospital cervical immobilization methods. *Ann Emerg Med* 1987; 16:1127–1131.

52. Heary RF, Hunt CD, Krieger AJ, et al: Acute stabilization of the cervical spine by halo/vest application facilities evaluation and treatment of multiple trauma patients. *J Trauma* 1992; 33:445–450.
53. Botte MJ, Byrne TP, Garfin SR: Application of the halo device for immobilization of the cervical spine utilizing an increased torque pressure. *J Bone Joint Surg [Am]* 1987; 69:750–752.
54. Johnson RM, Hart DL, Simmons EF, et al: Cervical orthosis. *J Bone Joint Surg [Am]* 1977; 59:332–339.
55. Johnson RM, Owen JR, Hart DL, et al: Cervical orthosis. *Clin Orthop* 1981; 154:34–45.
56. Krag MH, Beynnon BD: A new halo-vest: Rationale, design and biomechanical comparison to standard halo-vest designs. *Spine* 1988; 12:228–235.
57. Garfin SR, Botte MJ, Waters RL, et al: Complications in the use of the halo fixation device. *J Bone Joint Surg [Am]* 1986; 68:320–326.
58. Levine AM, Edwards CC: Traumatic lesions of the occipito-atlanto-axial complex. *Clin Orthop* 1989; 239:53–68.
59. Desai SS, Coumas JM, Danylevich A, et al: Fracture of the occipital condyle: Case report and review of the literature. *J Trauma* 1990; 30:240–241.
60. Goldstein SJ, Woodring JA, Young AB: Occipital condyle fracture associated with cervical spine injury. *Surg Neurol* 1982; 17:350–352.
61. Anderson PA, Montesano PX: Morphology and treatment of occipital condyle fractures. *Spine* 1988; 13:731–736.
62. Harding-Smith J, MacIntosh PK, Sherbon KJ: Fracture of the occipital condyle. *J Bone Joint Surg [Am]* 1981; 63:1170–1171.
63. Bohlman HH: Acute fractures and dislocations of the cervical spine. An analysis of three hundred hospitalized patients and review of the literature. *J Bone Joint Surg [Am]* 1979; 61:1119–1142.
64. Alker GJ Jr, Oh YS, Leslie EV: High cervical spine and craniocervical junction injuries in fatal traffic accidents. *Orthop Clin North Am* 1978; 9:1003–1010.
65. Bucholz RW, Burkhead WZ: The pathologic anatomy of fatal atlanto-occipital dislocations. *J Bone Joint Surg [Am]* 1979; 61:248–250.
66. Eismont FJ, Bohlman HH: Posterior atlanto-occipitial dislocation with fractures of the atlas and odontoid process. Report of a case with survival. *J Bone Joint Surg [Am]* 1978; 60:1397–1399.
67. Montane I, Eismont FJ, Green BA: Traumatic occipitoatlantal dislocation. *Spine* 1991; 16:112–116.
68. Gehweiler JA, Osborne RL Jr, Becker RF: *The Radiology of Vertebral Trauma.* Philadelphia, WB Saunders, 1980.
69. Powers B: Traumatic anterior-occipital dislocations. *Neurosurgery* 1979; 4:12–17.
70. Traynelis VC, Marano GD, Dunker RO, et al: Traumatic atlanto-occipital dislocation. Case report. *J Neurosurg* 1986; 65:863–870.
71. Wertheim SB, Bohlman HH: Occipitocervical fusion. Indications, techniques and long-term results in thirteen patients. *J Bone Joint Surg [Am]* 1987; 69:833–836.
72. Levine AM, Edwards CC: Fractures of the atlas. *J Bone Joint Surg [Am]* 1991; 73:680–691.
73. Libson SJ: Fractures of the atlas associated with fractures of the odontoid process and transverse ligament ruptures. *J Bone Joint Surg* 1977; 59A:940–943.

74. Jefferson E: Fracture of the atlas vertebra. Report of four cases and a review of those previously recorded. Br J Surg 1920; 7:407–422.
75. Keterson L, Benzel E, Orrison W, et al: Evaluation and treatment of atlas burst fractures (Jefferson fractures). J Neurosurg 1991; 75:213–220.
76. Pierce DS, Barr JS: Fractures and dislocations at the base of the skull and upper cervical spine, in Cervical Spine Research Editors Committee (eds): The Cervical Spine. Philadelphia, JB Lippincott, 1989, pp 312–324.
77. Segal LS, Grimm JO, Stauffer SE: Nonunion of fractures of the atlas. J Bone Joint Surg [Am] 1987; 69:1423–1433.
78. Wilber RG, Peters JG, Likaver MJ: Surgical techniques in cervical spine surgery, in Errico TJ, Bauer RD, Waugh T (eds): Philadelphia, JB Lippincott, 1991, pp 145–158.
79. Fielding JW, Hawkins RJ: Atlanto-axial rotatory fixation. J Bone Joint Surg [Am] 1977; 59:37–44.
80. Levin AM, Edwards CC: Treatment of injuries to the C1-C2 complex. Orthop Clin North Am 1986; 17:31–44.
81. Fielding JW, Francis WR, Hawkings RJ, et al: Atlantoaxial rotary deformity. Semin Spine Surg 1991; 3:33–83.
82. Ackerson TT, Patzakis MJ, Moore TM, et al: Fractures of the odontoid: A ten year retrospective study. Contemp Orthop 1982; 4:54–67.
83. Anderson LD, D'Alonzo RT: Fractures of the odontoid process of the axis. J Bone Joint Surg [Am] 1974; 56:1663–1674.
84. Paradis GR, Jones JM: Post traumatic atlantoaxial instability: The fate of the odontoid process fracture in 46 cases. J Trauma 1973; 13:359–363.
85. Schatzker J, Rorabeck CH, Waddel JP: Fractures of the dens (odontoid process). An analysis of thirty-seven cases. J Bone Joint Surg [Br] 1971; 53:392–405.
86. Anderson LD, Clark CR: Fractures of the odontoid process of the axis, in Cervical Spine Research Society Editors Committee (eds): The Cervical Spine, 2nd ed. Philadelphia, JB Lippincott, 1989, pp 325–343.
87. Southwick WO: Current concept review: Management of fractures of the dens (odontoid process). J Bone Joint Surg [Am] 1980; 62:482–486.
88. El-Khoury GY, Kathol MH: Radiographic evaluation of cervical spine trauma. Semin Spine Surg 1991; 3:3–23.
89. Clark CR, White AA: Fractures of the dens: A multicenter study. J Bone Joint Surg [Am] 1985; 67:1340–1348.
90. Craft DV, Cotler JM, Bauerle W: A rational approach to the management of type II and type III odontoid fractures. Presented at the AAOS Annual Meeting, San Francisco, 1993.
91. Garber JN: Abnormalities of the atlas and axis vertebrae: Congenital and traumatic. J Bone Joint Surg [Am] 1964; 46:1782–1791.
92. Hadley MN, Dickman CA, Browner CM, et al: Acute axis fractures: A review of 229 cases. J Neurosurg 1989; 71:642–647.
93. Bucholz RW: Unstable Hangman's fractures. Clin Orthop 1981; 154:119–124.
94. Francis WR, Fielding JW, Hawkins RJ, et al: Traumatic spondylolisthesis of the axis. J Bone Joint Surg [Br] 1981; 673:313–318.
95. Effendi B, Roy D, Cornish B, et al: Fracture of the ring and axis. A classification based on the analysis of 131 cases. J Bone Joint Surg [Br] 1981; 63:319–327.

96. Fielding JW, Francis WR, Hawkins RJ, et al: Traumatic spondylolisthesis of the axis. *Clin Orthop* 1989; 239:47–52.
97. Levin AM, Edwards CC: The management of traumatic spondylolisthesis of the axis. *J Bone Joint Surg [Am]* 1985; 67:217–226.
98. White AA, Panjabi M: *Clinical Biomechanics of the Spine.* Philadelphia/Toronto, JB Lippincott, 1978.
99. White A, Southwick W, Panjabi M: Clinical instability in the lower cervical spine. A review of past and current concepts. *Spine* 1976; 1:15.
100. Stauffer S: Wiring techniques of the posterior cervical spine for the treatment of trauma. *Orthopedics* 1988; 11:1543.
101. Stauffer S: Management of spine fractures C3–C7. *Orthop Clin North Am* 1986; 17:45.
102. Cooper P, Cohen A, Rosiello A: Halo immobilization of cervical spine fractures. Indications and results. *J Neurosurg* 1979; 51:603.
103. Cotler HB, Miller LS, DeLucia FA, et al: Closed reduction of cervical spine dislocations. *Clin Orthop* 1987; 214:185–199.
104. Evans DL: Reduction of cervical dislocation. *J Bone Joint Surg [Br]* 1961; 43:552–555.
105. Miller LS, Cotler HB, DeLucia FA, et al: Biomechanical analysis of cervical distraction. *Spine* 1987; 12:831–837.
106. Cotler H, Miller L, DeLucia F: Closed reduction of cervical spine dislocations. *Clin Orthop* 1987; 214:185.
107. Burke D, Berryman D: The place of closed manipulation in the management of flexion-rotation dislocation of the cervical spine. *J Bone Joint Surg [Br]* 1971; 53:165.
108. Evans D: Reduction of cervical dislocations. *J Bone Joint Surg [Br]* 1961; 43:552.
109. Whitehill R, Richman J, Glaser J: Failure of immobilization of the cervical spine by the halo vest. *J Bone Joint Surg [Am]* 1986; 68:326.
110. Cloward R: Treatment of acute fractures and fracture dislocations of the cervical spine by vertebral-body fusion. *J Neurosurg* 1961; 18:201.
111. Stauffer S, Kelly E: Fracture-dislocations of the cervical spine-instability and recurrent deformity following treatment by anterior interbody fusion. *J Bone Joint Surg [Am]* 1977; 59:45.
112. Oliveira J: Anterior plate fixation of traumatic lesions of the lower cervical spine. *Spine* 1987; 121:324.
113. Bohler J, Gaudernak T: Anterior plate stabilization for fracture-dislocations of the lower cervical spine. *J Trauma* 1980; 20:2031.
114. Schneider RC: Surgical indications and contraindications in spine and spinal cord trauma. *Clin Neurosurg* 1960; 8:157–183.
115. Bose B, Northrup BE, Osterholm JL, Cotler JM, DiTunno JF: Reanalysis of central cervical cord injury management. *Neurosurgery* 1984; 15:367–372.
116. Yashon D, Jane JA, White RJ: Prognosis and management of spinal cord and cauda equina bullet injuries in sixty-five civilians. *J Neurosurg* 1970; 32:163–170.
117. Schaefer S, Bucholz R, Jones R, et al: Management of transpharyngeal gunshot wounds to the cervical spine. *Surg Gynecol Obstet* 1981; 152:17–29.
118. Wigle RL: The reaction of copper and other projectile metals in body tissues. *J Trauma* 1992; 33:14.
119. Jones R, Bucholz R, Schaeffer S: Cervical osteomyelitises complicating transpharyngeal gunshot wounds to the neck. *J Trauma* 1979; 19:630.

Practical Approaches to Hypothermia

Larry M. Gentilello, M.D.

Assistant Professor of Surgery, Harborview Medical Center, University of Washington School of Medicine, Seattle, Washington

Definitions

Hypothermia is defined as a core body temperature that is below normal in a homeothermic organism. To allow for the normal diurnal temperature variation of 1° C to 2° C, hypothermia is considered to be present in humans when the core temperature drops below 35° C.[1] Hypothermia is classified into zones of severity according to the criteria outlined in Table 1.[2, 3] These zones are based on the physiologic changes that usually occur within each range of temperatures (Fig 1). During mild hypothermia, the body begins to lose its ability to maintain normal function, but the danger is minimal because heat production and conservation mechanisms remain intact.[4] As the core temperature reaches 32° C, cardiac conduction disturbances become apparent, and at 28° C, the risk of dysrhythmias rises rapidly.[5] Below 28° C, heat production and conservation mechanisms are extremely impaired. Shivering is abolished, metabolism decreases, heat loss is passively accepted, and the body behaves in an ectothermic (cold-blooded) fashion. At 20° C, virtually all patients are asystolic. Deep hypothermia is an artificial classification that is incompatible with life except when it is therapeutically induced for medical reasons.

It is important to note that the physiologic effects of hypothermia cannot

TABLE 1.
Classification of Hypothermia

Classification	Celsius Temperature	Fahrenheit Temperature
Mild hypothermia	<35°–32°	<95.0°–89.6°
Moderate hypothermia	<32°–28°	<89.6°–82.4°
Severe hypothermia	<28°–20°	<82.4°–68.0°
Profound hypothermia	<20°–14°	<68.0°–57.2°
Deep hypothermia	Below 14°	Below 57.2°

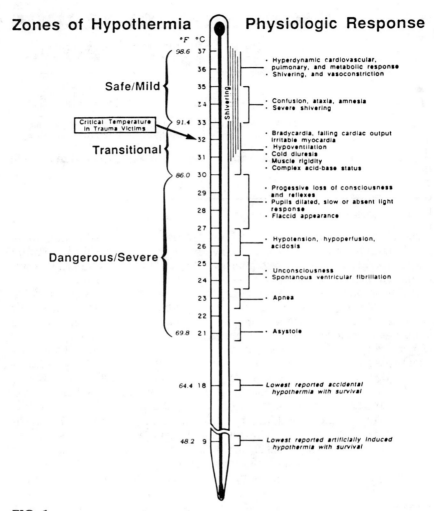

FIG. 1.
Physiologic responses to hypothermia. (From Jurkovich GJ: Hypothermia in the trauma victim, in *Advances in Trauma and Critical Care*, vol 4. St Louis, Mosby, 1989, pp 111–140. Used by permission.)

be strictly assigned to zones, because they vary not only according to its depth, but in relation to its duration and rapidity of onset, the underlying medical condition of the patient, and a variety of other factors. Hypothermia is generically classified as follows: Primary accidental hypothermia occurs when thermoregulation and heat production are normal, but the patient becomes cold as a result of overwhelming environmental cold stress (e.g., cold water immersion). Secondary accidental hypothermia occurs despite mild cold stress and results from illness- or injury-induced alterations in thermoregulation and heat production (e.g., hypothyroidism, drug intoxication, trauma). Induced hypothermia is used for therapeutic reasons usually to allow a period of circulatory arrest.

Hypothermia in the Trauma Victim

In a study performed at Harborview Medical Center in Seattle, the average initial temperature of intubated trauma victims on arrival at the emergency department was 35° C, with no seasonal variation, and 23% of patients had an initial core temperature of 34° C or less.[6] Even in the temperate climate of San Diego, hypothermia was reported to occur in 21% of seriously injured patients, and as many as 46% of trauma victims who require laparotomy leave the operating room with some degree of hypothermia.[7,8]

A multicenter review of 401 cases of hypothermia resulting from exposure reported only 21% mortality among patients admitted with a core temperature between 27.8° C and 32.2° C, with virtually all deaths attributable to underlying diseases rather than to the hypothermia.[9] In contrast, studies on outcome from hypothermia after trauma indicate that a core body temperature of 32° C or less carries a high mortality rate, and that any hypothermia is a poor prognostic sign (Fig 2).[10-12]

It appears that the alterations in homeostasis produced by even mild degrees of hypothermia are poorly tolerated when they are superimposed on patients with shock, hemorrhage, or major tissue injury. Compared to other patient populations, the mortality rate associated with hypothermia in

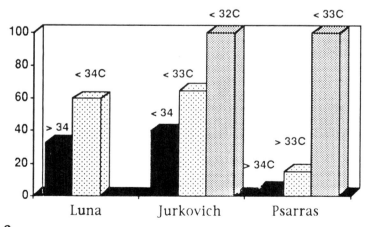

FIG. 2.
Correlation between core body temperature and mortality rate in trauma victims. (From Gentilello LM, Jurkovich GJ, Moujaes S: *Perspectives in General Surgery* 1991; 2:25–55. Used by permission.)

trauma victims is so high that classifying it as a distinct form of hypothermia is probably justified. The following zones of severity have been proposed[13]: (1) mild hypothermia, < 36° C to 34° C (<96.8° F to 93.2° F); (2) moderate hypothermia, <34° C to 32° C (<93.2° F to 89.6° F); and (3) severe hypothermia, below 32° C (below 89.6° F).

Because hypothermia is more common and more profound in more seriously injured patients, controversy exists regarding whether the high mortality rate is primarily attributable to the hypothermia itself or to the underlying injuries. Some have proposed that hypothermia is protective in injured patients, and that mortality rates would not be higher in cold patients if all other factors were equal.[7,14] For example, in the report from San Diego, 21% of injured patients with an Injury Severity Score (ISS) of 9 or greater were hypothermic (<35° C) on arrival at the emergency department.[15] Although hypothermic patients had a mortality rate of 63% and none of the euthermic patients died, the higher death rate in the hypothermic group was attributed to the presence of more severe injuries. When severity of injury was controlled by stratifying injury severity using a combination of anatomic and physiologic data (TRISS methodology), patients who became hypothermic had the same mortality rate as did patients who remained warm.

It may be inappropriate, however, to use physiologic data to stratify injury severity in hypothermic patients, because hypothermia itself has a deleterious effect on physiology. This would result in an overestimation of the severity of injury in cold patients, and mildly injured hypothermic patients would be compared with more severely injured euthermic ones. In this same study, when patients were stratified using the ISS (a strictly anatomic index of injury severity), hypothermic patients had significantly higher mortality rates than did patients with the same ISS who remained warm.

A deleterious effect of hypothermia on survival also was noted in a study that stratified not only by ISS, but by blood and fluid requirements, and by the presence or absence of shock (Table 2).[10] Patients who became hypothermic had significantly higher mortality rates than did similar patients who remained warm. Mortality was 100% if core body temperature dropped to 32° C, even in mildly injured patients. In another study confined to victims of penetrating trauma, all patients who had a core temperature of 33° C or less died.[11]

Even mildly hypothermic injured patients have a higher mortality rate than do normothermic patients sustaining the same degree of trauma. Nevertheless, it is impossible to prove cause and effect using retrospective studies. A reduction in body temperature occurs naturally during the process of dying, and progressive hypothermia may simply identify patients who are succumbing to their injuries. Only prospective studies using treatment of hypothermia as an independent variable can answer this question. In one recent prospective study, aggressive rewarming of trauma victims did lower mortality rates, and also decreased blood loss, fluid requirements, episodes of organ failure, and length of intensive care unit stay

TABLE 2.
Percent Mortality in Hypothermic Patients Stratified by Injury Severity Score (ISS), Fluid Requirements, and Shock*†

	34° C		33° C		32° C	
	Colder	Warmer	Colder	Warmer	Colder	Warmer
All patients	40	7*	69	7*	100	10*
ISS						
25–39	33	0*	50	4*	100	3*
40–49	33	67	67	33	100	38
>50	66	100	100	25*	100	40*
Fluids						
> 5 L crystalloid	46	12*	79	10*	100	15*
> 5 U packed red blood cells	48	9*	79	9*	100	15*
Shock	52	21*	79	17*	100	21*

*From Jurkovich GJ, Greiser WB, Luterman A, et al: *J Trauma* 1987; 27:1019–1024. Used by permission.
†The asterisk indicates a statistically significant figure.

compared to a control group of patients who were rewarmed much less aggressively.[16] Two additional prospective studies have demonstrated improvements in outcome when protocols designed to minimize heat loss were used.[17,18]

Thermoregulation

Humans have a remarkable capacity to dissipate heat by evaporating body water, as was demonstrated more than 200 years ago when a human volunteer was placed inside a 150° F chamber for 2 hours, along with a raw cut of meat.[19] The volunteer emerged dehydrated but otherwise well, but the meat was cooked. Our tropical evolutionary heritage, however, has provided us with a relatively poor capacity for heat production. The thermoneutral temperature (28° C or 82.4° F) is defined as the ambient temperature at which the basal rate of thermogenesis is sufficient to offset ongoing heat losses. Maintaining euthermia when the temperature around the body drops below the thermoneutral zone requires an increase in heat production. Because humans produce heat by combustion, additional oxygen is needed as substrate.

When tissue oxygen consumption is limited by shock, any heat that is lost as a result of cold emergency and operating room environments, resuscitation with cold fluid, alcohol-induced vasodilation, and open thoracic and abdominal cavities cannot be offset by increasing heat production, and body temperature decreases. A reduced supply of oxygen is further aggravated by anesthetic and paralyzing agents that, in effect, produce an ectothermic state in which heat loss is passively accepted.

Body temperature is controlled by the preoptic region of the hypothalamus, which balances the equilibrium between heat production and heat loss, and determines the temperature "set point" for shivering.[20] Although complex neural mechanisms are involved, hypothalamic nuclei respond directly to changes in blood temperature, and to peripheral thermosensitive receptors located in the skin that provide feedback control of body temperature.[6, 21] The central nervous system also is responsible for generating the sympathetic response that results in peripheral vasoconstriction, which effectively increases the depth of the body's insulating layers.

There is some evidence that injury actually elicits hypothermia as a compensatory response.[15, 22-24] Shivering is inhibited during episodes of hypotension or hypoxemia.[25, 26] This inhibition in shivering is apparently the result of decrease in the temperature that the body accepts as being thermoneutral. Downward extension of the thermoneutral zone to accommodate a decrease in core temperature without increasing oxygen demand for thermogenesis may spare oxygen-sensitive organs during shock. This has been proposed as a teleologic mechanism designed to gain the protective effect of hypothermia during periods of limited oxygen supply. In one study, shivering was noted to occur in only 1 of 82 severely injured hypothermic trauma victims.[15] Central inhibition of temperature control may explain the strong relationship between injury severity and degree of hypothermia.[27, 28]

An alternative proposed mechanism for the frequent finding of hypothermia in injured patients is that inadequate oxygen delivery results in metabolic failure. The metabolic response to injury was originally described in terms of an "ebb phase" during which a reduction in oxygen consumption and a fall in body temperature occurred.[29, 30] After restoration of perfusion, a "flow phase" ensued that was characterized by hypermetabolism and increased heat production. It is now clear that the response to injury can best be explained in terms of the adequacy of tissue oxygenation, rather than by ebb and flow phenomena.[31]

When tissue oxygen delivery falls below a critical level, the capacity of maximal tissue oxygen extraction is exceeded, and oxygen consumption and heat production decrease in a linear fashion.[32-34] In fully resuscitated injured patients, measurements of oxygen consumption are usually elevated, even when they are obtained shortly after injury.[31, 35] The ebb phase, and the fall in body temperature that occurs after injury, may simply represent inadequate resuscitation and a nonphysiologic shock-inducing uncoupling of oxidative phosphorylation, which results in diminished heat production. The frequent presence of lactic acid accumulation in cold, seriously injured patients supports this hypothesis.

Hypothermia and Oxygen Consumption

Body temperature has a significant effect on oxygen uptake. Oxygen consumption ($\dot{V}O_2$) is highest when humans are placed in a cold environment, and increases dramatically with any fall in body temperature. When involuntary muscle contractions in the form of shivering occur, oxygen consumption increases by as much as threefold to fivefold.[36-38]

Understanding the relationship between body temperature and oxygen consumption requires familiarity with the concept of specific heat. Specific heat is defined as the number of kilocalories required to raise the temperature of 1 kg of a substance by 1° C. For example, the specific heat of water is 1.0 kcal/kg/° C. To raise the temperature of 1 L (kg) of water from 30° C to 37° C requires 7 kcal:

$$Q = 1 \text{ kg} \times 1.0 \text{ kcal/kg/° C} \times (37° \text{ C} - 30° \text{ C}) = 7.0 \text{ kcal}$$

Because the specific heat of the human body is known, the amount of heat lost by a hypothermic patient can be similarly calculated:

$$Q = mc(t_2 - t_1)$$

in which Q equals heat loss (kcal), m equals mass of the patient (kg), c equals specific heat of the patient (0.83 kcal/kg/° C), and $t_2 - t_1$ equals change in temperature (° C).

A 70-kg patient with an average body temperature of 32° C has a heat deficit of 290.5 kcal:

$$Q = 70 \text{ kg} \times 0.83 \text{ kcal/kg/° C} \times (37° \text{ C} - 32° \text{ C}) = 290.5 \text{ kcal}$$

Because combustion is the only means of increasing heat production, the heat deficit can be thought of as the amount of oxygen that will have to be consumed to restore body temperature to 37° C if the patient does not receive exogenous heat. On a mixed-fuel diet, heat is generated at a rate of 1 kcal for every 198 mL of O_2 consumed.[39, 40]

Because the resting $\dot{V}O_2$ for a 70-kg patient is roughly 225 mL/min, 69.75 kcal, or about 1 kcal/kg, is produced each hour. A heat deficit of 290.5 kcal, therefore, is equivalent to the total amount of heat a resting patient produces in 4.16 hours. The resting rate of heat production is just sufficient to offset ongoing heat losses, and body temperature remains constant. The heat deficit represents *additional* heat production above the basal level that must be generated for the temperature of the body mass to increase. Stated another way, if the rate of heat loss is unchanged, heat production would have to increase by twofold for 4.16 hours for spontaneous rewarming to 37° C to occur. This also would require a twofold increase in oxygen consumption, with the transport and utilization of an additional 57,408 mL of oxygen during that period.

The actual amount of heat required for rewarming may differ because the body's heat-conserving mechanisms will retain heat more effectively.

On the other hand, the only means humans have of increasing heat production significantly is by muscular activity such as shivering. This is inefficient because such heat is produced near the surface of the body, causing most of it to be lost to the environment, with less than 45% being retained by the patient.[20]

The thermoregulatory drive is such a powerful one that it takes precedence over many other homeostatic functions and may deprive vital organs of needed oxygen, resulting in anaerobic metabolism, acidosis, and significant cardiopulmonary stress.[41, 42] This effect was demonstrated experimentally when injured rats placed in a 10° C ambient environment were noted to consume significantly more oxygen and to have higher mortality rates than injured rats treated in a 20° C or 30° C environment.[25]

Clinical reports also have described the oxygen costs of hypothermia. One study noted a 35% increase in oxygen consumption and a 65% increase in CO_2 production in postoperative patients after resolution of anesthesia, when the thermostatic drive reappeared.[43] In another study, a core temperature decrease of as little as 0.3° C in postoperative patients was associated with a 7% increase in V_{O_2}, and temperature reductions between 0.3° C and 1.2° C were associated with a 92% increase, with proportional increases in minute ventilation.[44]

Temperature and Metabolism

The hypermetabolic response that occurs after injury is primarily a result of an increase in the oxidative breakdown of protein. In a study on the effect of environmental temperature on the metabolic response to injury (femur fracture), animals kept in a thermoneutral (30° C) environment failed to show the characteristic increase in urinary nitrogen excretion that normally follows such an injury in animals kept at room temperature (20° C to 22° C).[45] The warmed animals also demonstrated significantly faster wound healing than did the cold animals. The authors suggest that the catabolic response to injury, with its attendant increase in heat production, is increased by the imposition of cold stress.[46, 47]

A similar effect was noted in rats subjected to burn injury. Those kept in an ambient temperature of 30° C did not have a hypermetabolic response, whereas animals with similar injuries maintained at 20° C had a high mortality and negative nitrogen balance.[48] Caldwell demonstrated a similar finding in humans when the hypermetabolic response to burn injury was greatly attenuated by using insulating dressings and ambient temperatures of 28° C. He postulated that cold stress imposed by an increase in evaporative and radiational heat loss is the major drive for hypermetabolism after burn injury.[49–51]

Carli noted that maintaining patients in a thermoneutral environment during and immediately after hip surgery also reduces postoperative nitrogen excretion.[52] In another study, patients undergoing abdominal surgery were placed randomly into one of two groups.[53] One group received warm intravenous fluids, warm inspired gases, heating blankets, and other measures to prevent hypothermia, and remained warm throughout surgery. The second group did not receive these measures, and had an average core temperature decrease of 2.2° C. Throughout the first 4 postoperative days, the warmed group had significantly less muscle protein degradation and nitrogen loss than did the cold group. It appears that demands on body reserves for extra energy, and the accelerated rate of nitrogen loss and consequent increase in oxygen utilization, can be attenuated by controlling environmental factors that lead to heat loss.[54]

Induced Hypothermia

In contrast to accidental hypothermia, oxygen consumption is decreased when anesthetics and neuromuscular blocking agents are used to block the thermoregulatory response. This phenomenon is known as the Q_{10} effect, which describes the change in oxygen consumption (V_{O_2}) per 10° C change in body temperature. In humans, hypothermia reduces oxygen consumption by 7% per degree. Therefore, a 32° C patient would have a V_{O_2} that is only 69% of normal.[55] Although a decrease in cardiac output accompanies the reduction in temperature, oxygen extraction and arteriovenous oxygen content difference remain relatively unchanged during cooling, which suggests that the reduction in cardiac output is proportional to the change in V_{O_2}.

Although it has been demonstrated that the balance between oxygen supply and demand is initially preserved during hypothermia, only a few studies have assessed oxygen balance during the rewarming phase and after return to normal body temperature. Steen cooled dogs to 29° C for 24 hours and found that V_{O_2} increased during rewarming, but cardiac output did not, which resulted in severe tissue hypoxia, acidosis, and death in some animals.[56]

Morray studied the cardiovascular effects of dogs subjected to acute (4 hours) and prolonged (24 hours) hypothermia.[38] In both groups, the increase in cardiac index and oxygen delivery that occurred during rewarming failed to keep pace with the more rapid rise in V_{O_2}, resulting in an increase in oxygen extraction. In addition, after rewarming, V_{O_2} in the prolonged hypothermia group rose significantly above the pre-hypothermia induction value, despite shivering blockade. The authors postulated that an oxygen debt was present, and that lactate reentered normal oxidative pathways after restoration of perfusion, consuming oxygen in the process.

Other studies show that, with continued cooling for 72 hours, a severe coagulopathy occurs and animals die of hemorrhage and multiple organ failure.[57,58] Although brief episodes of induced hypothermia generally are well-tolerated by humans, similar phenomena have been noted after prolonged hypothermia.[59-61] Most studies also demonstrate a metabolic acidosis after rewarming, which suggests a "washout" phenomenon involving lactate as circulation improves.[38,62]

It appears that, despite the use of anesthetics and neuromuscular blocking agents, the safe use of hypothermia for protective purposes is limited to a relatively brief period. When adenosine triphosphate (ATP) synthesis is reduced by anaerobic conditions, loss of transport function in the cell membrane occurs, causing Na+ influx and K+ efflux, and the loss of ionic gradients across the cell membrane. This opens voltage-dependent calcium channels, and excessive cytosolic calcium activates phospholipases that destroy membranes and lead to cell death.[63, 64] During prolonged cold exposure, progressive Na+ and K+ equilibration occurs across the cell membrane, which ultimately leads to cellular disruption by the same mechanisms that lead to cell death during hypoxia, namely, failure of ATP-dependent pumping mechanisms.[65, 66] In other words, although hypothermia decreases the rate of ATP utilization, it reduces the rate of ATP synthesis to an even greater extent and, therefore, is ultimately lethal.

In spite of the risks, brief periods of induced hypothermia using drugs to mitigate the endothermic response to heat loss may some day play a role in trauma surgery, as it has in other disciplines.[67, 68] Previously irreparable injuries may be treated using hypothermic circulatory arrest to provide a bloodless field.[69-74] One of the limitations, however, will be the bleeding diathesis that occurs as a result of impairment of platelet function, activation of the fibrinolytic cascade, and inhibition of the kinetics of clotting enzymes associated with cooling of the blood.[75-79] These issues are less of a concern during cardiac surgery, in which controlled hemorrhage into a single body cavity is amenable to blood salvaging and autologous transfusion. Noncavitary hemorrhage resulting from such conditions as multiple fractures may be exacerbated by hypothermia, and may limit its application to a select number of patients.

Perhaps the most promising area for the use of hypothermia in injured patients lies in the realm of traumatic brain injury. Poor reproducibility of pathologic findings in brain ischemia models led to the discovery that small variations in brain temperature critically affect the extent of histopathologic injury. Ischemic cell injury has been noted to be absent in rats in areas of the brain exposed for electroencephalographic recordings, presumably as a result of brain exposure to environmental cooling.[80-82] In fact, the need to monitor brain temperature during ischemia in models is critical to decreasing experimental variability. It appears that drastic reductions in brain temperature are not necessary to reduce the degree of ischemic central nervous system tissue damage.[83]

Numerous studies confirm the improved ability of moderately hypothermic animals to withstand better a variety of ischemic insults to the central nervous system[84-88]; however, most studies used preischemic cooling. The therapeutic window for hypothermia induction appears to be narrow. One study showed a benefit to postischemic cooling if it was instituted within 10 minutes, but no benefit when it was begun after 30 minutes.[81] In another study, hypothermia induced immediately with reperfusion after cardiac arrest improved functional and morphologic outcome in dogs, but a delay of 15 minutes in initiating cooling eliminated any protective effect.[89] Hypothermia also appears to be more protective after transient rather than prolonged focal ischemia, because extended ischemia seems to initiate events that are not amenable to hypothermic protection.[80]

Widespread therapeutic application of moderate brain cooling may require methods to cool the brain selectively in short periods in patients with multiple injuries. Local cooling with ice packs or cooling of the cerebrospinal fluid is unlikely to cool rapidly a brain with intact warm blood circulation, and may induce harmful temperature gradients.[90, 91] Isolation of the cerebral circulation for selective cooling would require heparin, contraindicating its use for traumatic brain injury.

As with hypothermic circulatory arrest, the use of deep hypothermia as a means of cerebral protection during neurosurgical procedures has proven challenging, with one of the major problems being intracranial hemorrhage caused by an induced bleeding diathesis.[92-95] The major benefit may be obtained with only slight cooling, because this may prevent the rise in intracranial temperature that often occurs after injury. Intracranial temperature may be as much as 2° C warmer than body temperature, and the resulting accelerated cerebral metabolic rate may predispose to secondary injury.[96]

Except for isolated case reports, schemes for reaping any potential benefit of hypothermia in trauma patients have not been identified. Hypothermia has only one accepted application in the trauma victim. After traumatic limb amputation, the ischemic limb is maintained in a hypothermic state until surgical reimplantation, because this has been shown both clinically and experimentally to prolong the viability of ischemic muscle. Nevertheless, the concept of using hypothermia for tissue protection in injured patients is a tantalizing one.

Detrimental Effects of Hypothermia

The body's general response to hypothermia mimics intense sympathetic stimulation, with tremulousness, profound vasoconstriction, tremendous increases in oxygen consumption, and acceleration of the heart rate and minute ventilation.[97-100] Although hypothermia in trauma victims usually is too mild to elicit most of the symptoms described below, the following major organ system effects may occur.

Cardiovascular

The initial cardiovascular response is one of tachycardia, followed by progressive bradycardia that starts at about 34° C and results in a 50% heart rate decrease at 28° C. Stroke volume is relatively well preserved, and the decline in cardiac output that occurs results primarily from the effect of hypothermia on heart rate. Blood pressure is maintained initially by intense vasoconstriction, but then begins to fall when the reduction in cardiac output becomes severe.

The conduction system is particularly sensitive to hypothermia, and the PR, then the QRS, and finally the QT interval become progressively prolonged.[101] The effect of hypothermia on the ST segment is highly variable. An Osborne wave, or J wave (hypothermic hump), is occasionally present at the junction of the QRS and ST segment in leads II and V6. It occurs in patients with a temperature of less than 32° C, and increases in size with falling temperature. J waves are not pathognomonic of hypothermia and carry no prognostic significance, but may aid in its diagnosis.[102-104]

Because the normal conductive pathways are slowed to a greater extent than is transmyocardial conduction, a rerouting of stimuli through the muscle occurs that predisposes to reentrant dysrhythmias.[105] At temperatures less than 32.5° C, a variety of atrial and then predominantly ventricular dysrhythmias occur. Asystole usually occurs at less than 25° C. Although "freezing to death" generally is thought to imply ventricular fibrillation, some have proposed that asystole is the primary fatal rhythm, and that when ventricular fibrillation is present, it often is iatrogenic and the result of therapeutic manipulations such as chest compression.[106] This is supported by the fact that myocardial cooling during cardiac surgery usually causes asystole, rather than fibrillation.

The role of cardiopulmonary resuscitation (CPR) in hypothermic cardiac arrest has not been well defined. Because of reduced chest wall and myocardial compliance, cardiac output during CPR for hypothermic cardiac arrest is only 50% of that achieved during normothermic CPR. The American Heart Association, in conjunction with the Wilderness Medical Society, has developed the following recommendations: CPR should be initiated unless (1) "do not resuscitate" status is previously documented; (2) obvious lethal injuries are present; (3) chest wall compression is impossible; (4) rescuers would be endangered by the delay in the evacuation; and (5) signs of life are present.[107]

Because of the difficulty in palpating weak, bradycardic pulses in cold, stiff, hypothermic patients, the presence of an organized rhythm should be taken as a sign of life that contraindicates CPR, despite the absence of a palpable pulse. Such a rhythm may provide diminished, but sufficient, circulation in patients with severely reduced metabolism, and the risk of converting it to fibrillation through vigorous chest compression is not justified. If a patient lacks an organized rhythm and CPR cannot be instituted because of field conditions, rewarming, with its attendant increase in metabolic rate, should probably not be undertaken until effective chest compression is possible. It also is important to remember that, almost every winter, there are reports of patients with hypothermic cardiac arrest who have successfully been resuscitated after many hours of CPR.

Endotracheal intubation is *not* a known risk factor for ventricular fibrillation, and should be undertaken according to standard indications.[9] Trismus often requires nasal intubation or cricothyrotomy. There is a theoretic risk of precipitating fibrillation with pulmonary artery catheterization, but little evidence to back this assertion.[108]

Hypothermia affects the reactivity of inotropic and antiarrhythmic drugs given for cardiac support. Increased protein binding of such agents reduces their effectiveness, and higher doses may be required. Because renal and hepatic clearance rates are reduced, toxicity may occur during rewarming. In most cases, bradycardia and mild hypotension are physiologically appropriate for the reduced metabolic rate and, other than rewarming, no specific treatment is necessary. Vasoconstrictors may be arrhythmogenic, may deleteriously affect frostbitten tissues, may decrease the effectiveness of external rewarming techniques, and should be used only for refractory hypotension that does not respond to fluids and rewarming.

Antiarrhythmics are generally ineffective at temperatures less than 30° C to 32° C. As a result of slowed conduction, atrial arrhythmias do not produce a rapid ventricular rate, are generally inconsequential, and resolve with rewarming. Procainamide has been reported to increase the risk of fibrillation in patients with ventricular dysrhythmias, and lidocaine is reported as being ineffective.[109-111] Bretylium is the only agent known to be effective in controlling ventricular fibrillation caused by hypothermia, although data are sparse and the optimal dosage is unknown.[112-114]

Respiratory System

Respiratory drive is increased during the early stages of hypothermia, but progressive respiratory depression occurs at temperatures lower than 33° C, resulting in a decline in minute ventilation. This is usually not a significant problem until temperatures less than 29° C are reached. Transalveolar exchange of oxygen and carbon dioxide is not affected seriously by hypothermia; however, hypothermia may intensify abnormalities in gas exchange that already are present as it attenuates hypoxic pulmonary vasoconstriction.[115] Occasionally, hypothermia results in the production of a large amount of mucus (cold bronchorrhea).[116] Because ciliary action and the cough reflex also are depressed, this predisposes to atelectasis and aspiration.

Noncardiogenic pulmonary edema also is frequently reported, especially in elderly patients and after prolonged periods of hypothermia.[117] Two mechanisms have been proposed. Intense vasoconstriction shunts blood to central vessels, resulting in an increase in circulating volume relative to the available vascular bed. In addition, hypothermia results in intracellular fluid shifts that are proportional to the depth and duration of cooling. These fluid shifts reverse during rewarming, and a rapid rate of fluid return to the circulation may cause pulmonary edema.

Perhaps the greatest controversy regarding the pulmonary effects of hypothermia revolves around the need to correct blood gases to the patient's hypothermic body temperature. Arterial blood gas samples always are warmed to 37° C before measurement. A nomogram then is used to estimate the blood gas values at the patient's actual body temperature. With each 1° C temperature reduction, the following changes occur: the pH increases by 0.015 pH units, the $P{CO_2}$ decreases by 4.4%, and the $P{O_2}$ decreases by 7.2%.

A blood gas measured at 37° C with a PCO_2 of 40 and a PO_2 of 70 in a 32° C patient will be reported as having a PCO_2 of 32 and a PO_2 of 48 after temperature correction. These changes occur with cooling, even if the blood is kept in an airtight syringe. The decrease in partial pressure is related to the increased solubility of gases in cold fluids and does not result from a change in the content or level of carbon dioxide, oxygen, or serum bicarbonate. Because the partial pressure of oxygen in the tissues is affected to the same extent, the capillary-to-tissue PO_2 gradient that is necessary to maintain oxygen uptake is unchanged.

Clinicians often assume that the normal PCO_2 and PO_2 at 37° C are the values that should be attained at all temperatures. If normothermic end points for PCO_2 are attained in a hypothermic patient using temperature-corrected blood gases, however, the patient would have a respiratory acidosis and increased total body CO_2 stores, which would be manifest by an elevated $PaCO_2$ and a low pH after rewarming. Likewise, attempts to increase a PO_2 that reflects normal oxygen content at a lower temperature also are inappropriate.

If blood gases are to be temperature-corrected, the physician not only must know what the "normal" blood gas values are at each temperature, but also must be aware of the normal value at each temperature change that occurs during rewarming. A far simpler strategy is to assess the blood gases at 37° C without temperature correction. Values that are normal and acceptable when reported at 37° C correspond to normal values and contents when "corrected" for hypothermic temperatures.

Temperature correction of blood gases for pH management also is unnecessary. A pH of 7.40 at 37° C would be temperature-corrected to 7.47 in a 32° C patient, which may prompt the physician to reduce the intensity of ventilator support. A pH of 7.40 is not normal at all temperatures, however. At 37° C, the acid–base balance of water is neutral (pH = pOH) when the pH is 6.8. The body functions optimally when its pH is offset 0.6 pH units above the neutral point of water, or it has a relatively alkaline pH of 7.40. The pH of water rises with cooling, causing the pH of blood to rise by 0.015 pH units per degree Celsius, without a change in bicarbonate content.[118–120] Treating a 30° C patient with a pH of 7.40 fails to maintain the normal pH offset above the neutral point of water (relative alkalinity) and results in an acidotic cellular and chemical environment. Because blood with a pH of 7.40 assessed at 37° C will be reported as having a pH of 7.47 when it is temperature-corrected to 32° C, the simplest strategy when confronted with a 32° C patient is to assess the blood gas at 37° C only, and to use the normal 37° C uncorrected pH value for treatment.[121, 122]

Central Nervous System

As core temperature falls, confusion, slurred speech, and incoordination progressively occur. Patients are often amnestic at temperatures less than 32° C and frequently lose consciousness at temperatures between 31° C and 27° C. Pupillary dilatation and loss of cerebral autoregulation occur at temperatures less than 26° C. Shivering increases cerebral oxygen uptake by roughly twofold, but shivering and deep tendon reflexes are usually abolished at temperatures less than 31° C.[123] Although hypothermia may reduce intracranial pressure by decreasing cerebral blood flow, it occasionally causes cerebral edema.

The electroencephalogram becomes abnormal at temperatures less than 33.5° C and is silent at 19° C to 20° C.[124] These findings, combined with an undetectable pulse and apparent rigor mortis, may cause the patient to appear dead. It is important to remember that patients have been revived from core temperatures as low as 17° C; therefore, the saying that, "no one is dead until warm and dead" remains true, except after prolonged underwater submersion.[125] It also is important to note that cold has been used to alleviate pain since antiquity. As a result of the anesthetic effects of cold, hypothermic patients may be unaware of injuries that would be sensed if they were euthermic.

Renal

Reductions in blood pressure and cardiac output decrease the glomerular filtration rate, but urinary output is maintained because of an impairment in renal tubular Na+ reabsorption (cold diuresis).[126, 127] Vasoconstriction also results in an initial increase in central blood volume that prompts a diuresis. Normal cellular volume is dependent on the continued pumping of Na+ out of the cell. Cold-induced suppression of Na+/K+ adenosine triphosphatase leads to Na+ leakage into the cell and to intracellular hypertonicity.[128] This causes "third spacing" of fluids, which compounds hypovolemia.[129, 130] Cellular swelling is a major limiting factor in the use of hypothermia for organ preservation for transplantation.[131]

Renal blood flow and filtration may take as long as 24 hours to return to normal after rewarming.[126] The kidneys comprise only a few kilograms of body weight, but they receive 25% of the total cardiac output and consume a proportionally large amount of oxygen. They appear to be particularly sensitive to hypothermia, because they undergo a far greater reduction in oxygen uptake during cooling than does any other organ. This suggests that the body views the kidneys as more dispensable than other organ systems during hypothermia, just as it does during hemorrhagic shock.

Gastrointestinal

Hypothermia causes depression of smooth-muscle motility throughout the gut, and gastric dilatation, ileus, and colonic distention are frequently seen. Splanchnic blood flow decreases and hepatic dysfunction occurs, with its attendant effects on the metabolism of anesthetics and other drugs.[132] Gastric mucosal erosions are common, but seldom cause significant bleeding. Acute pancreatitis also has been reported after hypothermia, and some degree of pancreatic necrosis is found at autopsy in as many as 82% of patients who die of hypothermia.[133-137]

Endocrine

Hypothermia inhibits insulin release and insulin uptake at receptor sites, making hyperglycemia a relatively common finding, especially at temperatures less than 30° C.[138] Exogenous insulin administration is unwarranted and may result in "rebound hypoglycemia" during rewarming. Glucose-containing solutions also should be used judiciously. On the other hand, hypoglycemia is an occasional cause of mild hypothermia, particularly when it is related to alcohol use, and as many as 50% of patients admitted with hypoglycemia are cold.

Serum electrolyte changes are unpredictable, but serum potassium often is increased in hypothermic patients as a result of renal tubular dysfunction, acidosis, and the breakdown of liver glycogen.[139] Calcium levels may be elevated in some patients or decreased to the point of tetany in shivering patients with hyperventilation. In either case, cardiac dysrhythmias may result.

Serum corticosteroids are invariably increased in hypothermic patients.[140, 141] There is no evidence to support the routine administration of exogenous steroids, although one study noted unexpectedly low corticosteroid levels in two patients who were exhausted from prolonged outdoor exposure.[142]

Blood

The viscosity of blood is increased by hypothermia. In uncomplicated cases, a reduction in plasma volume occurs that increases the hematocrit by 2% for each 1° C temperature reduction.[143] The leukocyte count can be low, normal, or high, and cannot be reliably used to predict infection. Although splenic leukocyte sequestration and impaired phagocytosis occur, the effect of hypothermia on immunity is unknown.

Thrombotic complications are seen in severe cases of hypothermia. Many studies, including several recent ones, have claimed erroneously that coagulation is not impaired until the temperature drops to less than 26° C.[144-150] The extent to which hypothermia intensifies bleeding from coagulopathy has been elucidated only recently. Tests such as the partial thromboplastin time, prothrombin time, and thrombin time are temperature-standardized to 37° C. Devices that measure coagulation parameters contain a thermal block that heats the plasma and reagents to 37° C before initiating the assay. Thus, tests of coagulation provide quantitative information about the depletion of clotting factors, but are corrected for any potential effect of hypothermia.

Using a fibrometer that was modified to permit coagulation assays at temperatures other than 37° C, Reed showed that temperatures less than 35° C significantly prolong clotting times.[151] For example, during and after major surgical procedures, patients with factor IX deficiency (hemophilia B) are treated with sufficient plasma to raise factor IX levels to between 50% and 100% of normal. When the partial thromboplastin time is assayed at

35° C, 33° C, and 32° C, it is prolonged to the same extent as occurs when factor IX levels are reduced to 39%, 16%, and 2.5%, respectively, of normal.[152]

Platelets sequester in the portal circulation during hypothermia and are nearly absent from the peripheral circulation at temperatures less than 20° C.[153] Cold-mediated platelet dysfunction also may result in bleeding from coagulopathy, despite a normal platelet count. In patients with coagulopathy, the amount of nonsurgical blood loss correlates most closely with the bleeding time (Duke or Ivy method), which is primarily a measure of platelet function.[154] Valeri induced systemic hypothermia to 32° C in baboons, but kept one forearm warm using heating lamps and a warming blanket.[77] Simultaneous bleeding time measurements in the warm and cold arm were 2.4 and 5.8 minutes, respectively.

A dilutional coagulopathy often coexists with hypothermia in the trauma patient. Low concentrations of platelets and coagulation factors, combined with hypothermia-induced alterations in their activity, may make all attempts at achieving hemostasis futile. Recognition that the clinical appearance of nonsurgical bleeding may not correlate with laboratory coagulation tests and platelet counts in cold patients can prevent futile attempts at staunching hemorrhage. It also should prompt consideration of an abbreviated laparotomy and transfer to the intensive care unit for rewarming.

Mechanisms of Heat Loss and Heat Transfer

The physical principles that govern heat loss or gain are important in preventing hypothermia and developing effective rewarming strategies. There are four primary means of heat loss or transmission.

Conduction

Conduction is the transfer of heat between two masses in contact with one another. The rate of heat transfer is dependent on the temperature gradient at the interface, the size of the contact area, and the "thermal conductivity" (insulating properties) of the material. Conductive heat transfer also is inversely proportional to the distance the heat must travel and, in patients, relates to the thickness of the skin and subcutaneous tissue. If there are two parallel surfaces across which heat is flowing, and the process can be considered at steady state (fixed in time), then:

$$Q_{cond} = k A (t_1 - t_2)/l$$

in which k equals thermal conductivity (kcal/m/hr/°C); A equals area of contact (m^2); t_1 and t_2 equal temperature at surfaces 1 and 2, respectively; and l equals length (m).

Because metals and liquids have high thermal conductivity, lying on a metallic surface can increase dramatically the rate of heat loss from the body, and lying on a wet surface is one of the fastest ways to lose body heat.

Convection

Convection is the transfer of heat through the flow of liquids or gases over a surface. When warm air overlying a patient is continuously swept away, convective heat loss to the environment occurs. Convective heat loss is analogous to the wind chill factor, and is proportional to the body surface area, the temperature difference between the body and the fluid flowing over it, and the air velocity. By introducing a constant to describe variables such as turbulence and air velocity, convection can be described as:

$$Q_{conv} = hA\,(t_2 - t_1)$$

in which h equals coefficient of heat transfer (kcal/m^2/hr/°C), A equals surface area (m^2), and $t_2 - t_1$ equals temperature difference from surface to air.

The greatest risk of convective heat loss occurs during patient transport.[155] Helicopter transport of trauma victims can cause convective heat loss if the landing site is close to the patient, because the wind chill effect caused by propeller downdraft can decrease the body temperature of a wet patient by 2°–3° C in several minutes. Transport of the patient in the hospital for diagnostic tests also causes convective heat loss if the patient is not well covered. Operating rooms are cold and, to remove anesthetic gases and minimize contamination, they have an air turnover rate of about 25 times per hour, with 100% exhaust. This produces a wind chill effect that accounts for as much as 30% to 35% of intraoperative heat losses. Keeping operating room doors closed during surgery limits air movement and may reduce convective losses.

Radiation

Transfer of radiant heat is the result of electromagnetic transmission and does not require any intervening mass or fluid. It is proportional to the fourth power of the temperature difference between the body and its surroundings, the surface area of the radiating bodies, and their emissivity (black-body characteristics). It can be expressed as follows:

$$Q_{rad} = EJ\,A\,(t_1^4 - t_2^4)$$

in which E equals emissivity of the skin, J equals Botzmann's constant (kcal/m^2/°K^4), A equals surface area (m^2), and $t_1^4 - t_2^4$ equals temperature difference between the body and the surrounding walls (°K^4).

The fourth power relationship explains the fact that most of the heat loss (55% to 60%) that occurs in fully exposed patients in a cold room is by this route. Cutaneous vasodilatation during anesthesia increases the temperature of the skin, which dramatically increases radiant heat loss. If skin temperature is 33° C and the temperature of nearby solid objects is 21° C, an uncovered patient with a surface area of 1.8 m^2 can lose as much as 114 kcal/hr through radiation.[156]

Evaporation

The rate of heat loss by evaporation of water from the surface of the body is proportional to the change in vapor pressure from the skin surface to ambient air, and to the velocity of air movement.

$$Q_{evap} = 0.577(4.66\ V_{air})\ (pH_2O_{air} - pH_2O_{skin})$$

in which 0.577 equals latent heat of vaporization (kcal/mL H_2O), V_{air} equals air velocity (m/hr), pH_2O_{air} equals partial pressure of water vapor in air (mm Hg), and, pH_2O_{skin} equals partial pressure of water vapor next to skin (mm Hg).

At usual room temperature and humidity, about one third of evaporative heat loss occurs in the lung during the process of saturating inspired air and the rest is from the skin surface. Evaporation usually accounts for less than 10% of total body heat loss, but increases with high minute ventilation, particularly when breathing cold, dry air. Evaporation, however, can become the source of the greatest amount of heat loss from the open abdominal cavity, and the common practice of covering the exposed bowel with moist towels increases evaporative heat loss by nearly 250%.[157] Covering exposed bowel with dry towels or enclosing the intestines in a plastic "bowel bag" is a better strategy for preventing heat loss. Because the heat of vaporization of water is 0.577 kcal/mL, leaving as little as 30 mL of H_2O to vaporize on the skin can result in a heat loss of 18 kcal.

Treatment

The relatively high specific heat of the body makes hypothermia difficult to treat. Early attention to the mechanisms of heat loss as outlined previously remains the best form of therapy. Several reports have described the efficacy of rewarming techniques. These should be examined critically, because most do not take into account the patient's initial body temperature and mass, the rate of endogenous heat production, and the presence or absence of anesthetics, vasodilating agents, shock, or shivering, all of which are important determinants of the rewarming rate. Thermodynamic analyses can be used to measure more accurately the efficacy of heat transfer.[39, 158]

The treatment of hypothermia is classified into three broad categories:

1. Passive external rewarming
2. Active external rewarming
3. Active core rewarming

Passive External Rewarming

Passive external rewarming consists of allowing the patient's own endogenous heat production to restore normothermia. As outlined previously, this requires tremendous energy expenditure and should be reserved for relatively healthy, mildly hypothermic patients. Because the specific heat of the body is 0.83 kcal/kg/° C, a 70-kg patient would have to gain 58.1 kcal to increase average body temperature by 1° C. Because basal heat production is about 1 kcal/kg/hr, endogenous heat production produces a rewarming rate of roughly 1.2° C/hr if the patient is sufficiently insulated to prevent all heat loss. Shivering can increase heat production by threefold, so that a spontaneous rewarming rate of 3.6° C/hr is theoretically possible.

It is important to consider the mechanism of hypothermia when considering passive rewarming. Patients with acute forms of hypothermia such as cold water immersion usually rewarm rapidly. In contrast, patients who are cold and exhausted after being lost in the wilderness for several days will have depleted their energy stores and will be unable to generate a significant amount of heat. Elderly or malnourished patients also demonstrate slower spontaneous rewarming rates.

Anesthetics and neuromuscular blocking agents prevent shivering and decrease heat production by roughly one third. Although this spares oxygen, it prolongs hypothermia, which may be detrimental in patients in whom rapid restoration of clotting and cardiac function are important objectives.

Active External Rewarming

Active external rewarming techniques include fluid-circulating heating blankets, convective warm air blankets, radiant warmers, warm bath immersion, and diathermy. The dissipation of heat from the skin to the core is related to the blood supply through the skin. Because of the poor cutaneous circulation in hypothermic patients, burns can be caused by external rewarming techniques using levels of heat that would not be uncomfortable for a normothermic patient.

Heat always flows from an area of higher temperature to one of lower temperature as a function of the laws of thermodynamics. Skin temperature may be 10° C to 15° C cooler than core temperature in hypothermic patients. External rewarming techniques cannot transfer heat to the core until the temperature of the skin is raised to at least the level of the core. During this lag time, core temperature actually may continue to decrease. This phenomenon, whereby core temperature continues to decline after removal from the cold, is known as the afterdrop and occurs most often when external rewarming techniques are used. Because external rewarming has little immediate effectiveness, it should not be the sole method used when rapid rewarming (e.g., for defibrillation or control of bleeding) is required. In addition, external rewarming provides a sensation of warmth to cutaneous thermoreceptors without actually transmitting a significant amount of heat. This may reduce the patient's own heat generation rate and prolong the duration of hypothermia.

Standard fluid-circulating heating blankets are relatively inefficient because they are only in contact with the occiput, shoulders, presacral region, and heels, which constitute only 20% to 30% of the total body surface area. Using heat flux transducers, English measured 55 kcal/hr of heat transfer with the use of fluid-circulating heating blankets.[156] These measurements, however, were made in a warm room in healthy, euthermic volunteers with well-perfused skin. Skin perfusion can decrease from the normal state of roughly 200 mL/min/m^2 to as little as 4 mL/min/m^2 during hypothermia. This reduces the thermal conductivity of the skin to a level that is roughly equivalent to that of cork.[159, 160]

Based on observed rewarming rates in hypothermic patients, a 2.5 to 4.0 kcal/hr per degree Celsius temperature difference between blanket and skin can be estimated to occur.[161] The blanket should be placed above rather than below the patient. Burns are possible when circulating is diminished, particularly in elderly patients with thin skin, and placing the blanket below the patient causes pressure points that increase the risk of burn injury. Placing the blanket above the patient also is more efficient, because more heat is lost by radiation and convection to the overlying air than by conduction to the underlying mattress, which serves as a good insulator.

Convective air rewarmers provide a larger surface area for heat exchange than do fluid-circulating heating blankets. These devices use a disposable plastic and paper blanket with slits on the patient side through which 43° C air exits. To understand the use of these devices, it is important to understand the difference between heat content and temperature. The density of air is so low that it contains very little heat, even at a high temperature. A hand can be placed safely in a 400° F oven to remove a casserole dish, but touching the 400° F casserole dish itself would result in an immediate burn injury. Heat always flows down a temperature gradient, however, regardless of heat content. For example, a cup of water placed in a hot oven will be heated until its temperature equilibrates with the air temperature, even though the cup of water has a much greater quantity of heat. These principles of heat transfer cause some interesting effects. First, if the temperature of the surrounding environment is warmer than skin temperature, heat loss cannot occur, except by sweating, and cold patients do not sweat. The purpose of a convective warmer is to establish a 43° C environment around the patient. Because almost all heat is lost through the skin surface, this effectively prevents most heat loss.[162] Second, the very low heat-carrying capacity of air means that virtually no heat can be transferred actively to a patient by blowing warm air on the skin surface.

Thus, these devices can be used to prevent hypothermia, but are ineffective methods of treatment. Almost all the warming that occurs will be the result of the patient's own heat generation. To create a 43° C environment around the patient requires coverage of a substantial portion of the body surface (ideally, from the neck to the toes), with fastening of the borders of the blanket around the patient and provision of additional coverage in the form of standard cotton hospital blankets. This limits access to the patient. Merely laying the device next to the patient to blow warm air on the skin while resuscitation lines are placed is of no benefit, and will cool the patient if the skin surface is wet. Although these devices reduce the rate of heat loss, in a randomized study designed to test their effectiveness in rewarming hypothermic patients, they did not rewarm any faster than did standard cotton hospital blankets (Fig 3).[163]

Attempting to prevent or to treat hypothermia by increasing the operating room temperature appears to have relatively little effect, except in pediatric and burned patients.[164, 165] When a patient is lying naked in usual operating room ambient temperatures of 18° C to 20° C, heat loss through convection and radiation alone is estimated to be as high as 284 kcal/hr.[157] This rate is so high that the effect of marginal changes in ambient temperatures cannot be detected. To minimize heat loss significantly, the temperature of the operating room would have to be raised to a level that would be uncomfortable for surgeons, who are wearing two sets of clothing.

Because water has a high specific heat, warm water immersion is the only external rewarming technique that transfers a significant amount of heat. Unfortunately, this technique is associated with a high rate of cardiovascular collapse. The most dangerous time is during removal from the tub. A hydrostatic squeeze occurs, and removal from the water bath often results in a precipitous drop in venous return and blood pressure, resulting in cardiac arrest.[166] Because heat is applied externally, circulation to the skin surface also is required for effective heat transfer, and failure of core

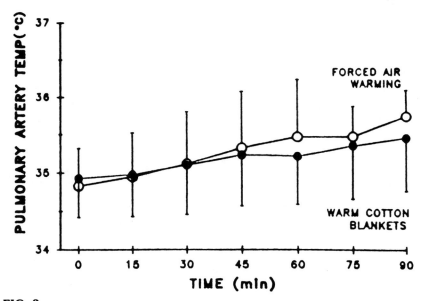

FIG. 3.
Randomized study results comparing convective air rewarming with standard cotton hospital blankets. (From Ereth MH, Lennon RL, Sessler DI: *Aviat Space Environ Med* 1992; 63:1065–1069. Used by permission.)

rewarming may occur in very cold patients or those with absent or diminished circulation.[167] This technique is contraindicated in severely injured patients because it limits access to the patient and is electrically hazardous when patients are intubated and monitored invasively. In the event of ventricular fibrillation, the patient must be removed from the tank and dried thoroughly. Using defibrillation on a wet patient is dangerous, because the charge merely runs over the wet body surface, is ineffective, and may short to the ground and cause burns.[168]

Aluminum space blankets are made of material that often is used as a lining in survival apparel and are designed to reflect emitted photons back to the patient.[169, 170] Their function is to increase the insulating capacity of the blankets covering the patient. The effectiveness of radiant barriers decreases rapidly as the distance between the emitting and reflective surfaces increases. Because the blanket does not conform well to the body surface, a large space often is present between the blanket and the patient. This not only reduces the blanket's effectiveness, but allows air to circulate between the patient and the blanket, resulting in convective and conductive heat losses. Proper use involves wrapping the blanket snugly around the patient and placing an additional standard blanket on top of the space blanket to minimize underlying air movement. It is important to cover the head with some sort of reflective material, particularly in patients with alopecia. Because scalp vessels do not undergo vasoconstriction, even in hypothermic patients, as much as 50% of radiant heat loss occurs above the neck.

Overhead radiant warmers can produce intense local heat in patients with vasoconstriction if the circulation cannot carry the heat away, sometimes causing severe thermal injury. Patients must be exposed fully to receive radiant heat. A blanket is often placed over the patient to diminish the risk of thermal injury, but radiant heat is then supplied only to the blanket and the patient is warmed inefficiently by the air trapped underneath the blanket. Based on observed rewarming rates in hypothermic patients, Henneberg has calculated an approximate heat transfer of 17.7 kcal/hr with the use of an overhead radiant warmer.[171]

Some investigators have used diathermy (ultrasonic, microwave, or short-wave energy transfer) as a means of external rewarming.[172] Ultrasonic diathermy involves the use of acoustic compression waves to cause tissue particle movement or heat, and requires physical contact between the patient and the transducer because the waves cannot propagate through air.[173] Microwave rewarming has poor muscle penetration, even at the lowest frequency range, which results in hot spots at the fat/muscle interface. Clinical experience with this modality is limited. Short-wave diathermy consists of the passage of high-frequency current through the patient, and most researchers advocating diathermy have used this method.[174-176] In one study, dogs were cooled to a core temperature of 25° C, then rewarmed to 30° C. The mean time required was nearly 4 hours using airway rewarming, 3 hours using peritoneal lavage, and 1.5 hours using short-wave diathermy. All dogs survived without adverse sequelae.

Diathermy is unlikely to have widespread clinical application. It cannot be used on patients who may be pregnant or have metallic implants. Determining the proper dosage is difficult because the absorbed power depth varies from patient to patient as a result of differences in subcutaneous fat content. This requires an awake patient who can communicate any sensation of burn injury to the physician. Moisture on the skin can be heated rapidly, particularly with microwave and short-wave rewarming, which can cause scalding. Because of their high water content, moist dressings and areas of edema also must be avoided. With improper dosing, diathermy can cook tissues, and there even have been reports of the heart being burned.[160]

Active Core Rewarming

Active core rewarming includes airway rewarming, heated peritoneal or pleural lavage, warm intravenous fluid infusion, and extracorporeal circulatory rewarming. Heated gastric, bladder, or colonic lavage provides too small a surface area for effective heat transfer.

Airway rewarming is one of the most frequently used core rewarming techniques. The amount of water capable of being held as vapor depends on the temperature of the air. When a hypothermic patient breathes saturated warm air, the humidity condenses on contact with the relatively cold lung surface. Fully saturated 41° C air can hold 0.05 mL of H_2O per liter. At 30° C, air can hold only 0.03 mL of H_2O per liter. Thus, if a 30° C patient inspires 1 L of saturated 41° C air, 0.02 mL of H_2O condenses within the airway. With a minute ventilation of 10 L/min (600 L of air per hour), condensation will equal 12 mL of H_2O per hour. The amount of heat liberated when water condenses (the latent heat of vaporization) is 0.577 kcal/mL of H_2O. Thus, the amount of heat transfer would equal only:

$$0.577 \text{ kcal/mL } H_2O \times 12 \text{ mL } H_2O/hr = 6.92 \text{ kcal/hr}$$

Some additional heat is liberated when the dry air itself and the condensate cool from their original temperature to the temperature of the patient. Little heat is transferred by the condensate because its volume is only 12 mL/hr (1 kcal/kg/° C × 41° C − 30° C × .012 L = 0.132 kcal). At sea level, the density of air is 0.0012 kg/L. If the minute ventilation is 600 L/hr, then 0.72 kg of air per hour enters the respiratory tract. The specific heat of air is 0.24 kcal/kg/° C; thus, the air will transmit only an additional 1.7 kcal/hr (0.24 kcal/kg/° C × 0.72 kg × 41° C − 30° C).

Because 58 kcal is required to raise the temperature of a 70-kg patient by 1° C, airway rewarming has little effect on core temperature. Yet, when air at subzero temperatures, which contains little moisture, is inspired, considerable heat is lost through the airways because patients must warm the air to body temperature and saturate it fully. Thus, breathing warm air can be an effective means of conserving heat during wilderness rescues.

In comparative studies, pleural or peritoneal lavage results in significantly greater heat transfer than does airway rewarming, and should be considered for use in patients who have a deleterious response to hypothermia. The amount of heat transferred depends on the difference between the inlet and outlet water temperatures, and on the water flow rate:

$$Q = mc\,(T_i - T_o)$$

in which m equals mass flow of water per unit time (L/hr), c equals specific heat of water (1 kcal/kg/° C), T_i equals inlet water temperature, and T_o equals outlet water temperature.

If 1 L of 40° C water is infused into a body cavity and exits at 35° C, then 5 kcal of heat will have been left in the body. The rate of rewarming depends on the body cavity used, because the water will exit at a colder temperature if it flows through a well-perfused area, such as the pleural space. Attempting to improve the rewarming rate by increasing the fluid flow rate provides only a small benefit, because a higher outlet temperature results. The outlet temperature also rises as the body rewarms; in common with most rewarming techniques, therefore, body cavity lavage becomes progressively more inefficient as the patient rewarms.

Prolonging the operative time to irrigate the open peritoneal cavity with warm fluids is counterproductive. It takes roughly 15 minutes for 1 L of 44° C fluid to decrease in temperature by 10° C. Most of the 10 kcal of heat transfer that results from this cooling will have been lost to the 21° C operating room environment, rather than to the patient. Because the rate of intraoperative heat loss is so high, rapid abdominal closure and transfer to the intensive care unit is a better rewarming strategy.

The pleural and peritoneal cavities produce roughly equivalent rewarming rates.[177] The pleural cavity may be preferred if an arrhythmia is present because it may warm the heart faster than will peritoneal irrigation. Two ipsilateral chest tubes should be used to enable a continuous flow of water. Peritoneal lavage is more likely to rewarm the liver and may restore its synthetic and metabolic properties more quickly; however, it is not feasible in most patients who have undergone laparotomy. The maximal safe water temperature for lavage has not been determined, but temperatures less than 44° C are considered acceptable in patients with intact circulation.[178, 179] Bowel necrosis has been reported in patients lavaged with fluid temperatures at this level in the setting of cardiac arrest or severely diminished blood flow.

The administration of warm intravenous fluids is a critical step in preventing hypothermia, because the high specific heat of water makes cold intravenous fluid administration the fastest way of inducing hypothermia.[180] A patient must generate 16 kcal to warm 1 L of room-temperature (21° C) crystalloid to 37° C. If the patient cannot generate this additional heat, the loss of 16 kcal will decrease body temperature by 0.28° C, which is enough to cause vigorous shivering. The frequent finding of hypothermia in trauma victims at the time of hospital admission may be a result of the administration of cold fluids in the field.

Warming of blood products is particularly important, because they are stored at 4.0° C. The specific heat of blood is 0.87 kcal/kg/° C; thus, a patient must generate an extra 28.6 kcal to prevent a temperature decrease after receiving 1 L of cold blood. The loss of 28.6 kcal in a 70-kg patient reduces body temperature by 0.49° C.

A bolus of cold fluid placed into the central circulation at high flow rates has the additional effect of increasing cardiac irritability by directly affecting the conducting system.[181–185] The use of warmed intravenous fluids has been associated with a reduction in intraoperative cardiac arrest, coagulopathy, and acidosis, and with better temperature preservation when compared to the administration of fluids at room temperature.[15, 16, 186, 187]

Fluid warmers were first introduced at a time when maximum flow rates of 150 mL/min were considered acceptable. Current trauma protocols often require fluid infusion at rates as high as 1 L/min, and effective methods of warming solutions at these flow rates should be made available.[188, 189] Fluids can be warmed by inserting the intravenous bag into a warm water bath or placing it in an infrared heater or microwave oven. Infrared lamps can be used to warm crystalloid solutions only, because they cause cellular damage, abnormal erythrocyte function, and a fall in the pH level when blood is warmed. These changes may occur with only mild heating (34.8 ° C).[188, 190, 191]

One liter of crystalloid solution at room temperature can be heated to 40° C in 2.5 minutes in an ordinary culinary microwave oven. Considerable variability exists in the heating capacity of these ovens, however, and each institution should experiment with times on its own appliance. Because of the uneven nature of microwave heating, solutions must be shaken vigorously before they are administered. Glucose-containing solutions cannot be heated in a microwave oven because glucose caramelizes at 60° C.[192, 193] Microwave warming can only be performed on solutions that are stored in plastic bags. Glass bottles have metal caps that cannot be used in microwave units. Hansen reported the explosion of such a bottle, which blew the door of the microwave open and sprayed the room with glass.[194]

Standard culinary microwave units should never be used to warm blood products. Numerous complications have resulted from the tendency of microwave ovens to heat unevenly, which causes "hot spots" and results in severe hemolysis and protein degradation. Severe, and even fatal, hemolysis has been reported.[192, 195–198] Recent research has been done on the use of in-line microwave units that warm blood as it passes through intravenous tubing using continuous feedback temperature control monitoring to minimize the risk of overheating.[199, 200]

Blood products can be warmed by admixture with warm saline. Raising the temperature of a unit of 4° C packed erythrocytes to 37° C requires the addition of an equal volume of 70° C saline.[201–203] This reportedly is not deleterious to erythrocytes, but handling a bag of 70° C (170° F) saline during a chaotic trauma resuscitation may be difficult. The 70° C saline would have to be added to the blood immediately because of the rapid cooling that occurs when warm fluids are left at room temperature.

The major problem with prewarming bags of intravenous fluid with ovens and heaters is that the fluid must be administered rapidly. Fluid at 37° C will cool to 34° C within 5 minutes, and to 32° C within 15 minutes if it is kept at room temperature.[204] Warming blood in-line during its passage through a delivery system eliminates this risk of temperature reduction. In-line heaters can be divided into three main categories: those that use dry heat, those that use a still water bath, and those that use a countercurrent water bath. Dry heaters and still water baths require long contact times and long intravenous tubing coils. Little warming of the blood occurs at flow rates greater than 150 to 250 mL/min. In addition, with both dry heat and still water baths, the slow flow rates necessary for adequate contact time result in significant cooling of the blood in the intravenous tubing after it has left the warmer, making normothermic infusion impossible at any flow rate.[205, 206]

Countercurrent fluid warmers pass fluids through a 40° C water bath that flows rapidly in a countercurrent direction to maximize temperature gradients. The fluid passes through the water bath through a length of thin aluminum tubing that has a 1,000 times greater thermal conductivity than does standard plastic intravenous tubing (Fig 4). This enables the infusion of as much as 750 mL of saline or 1 unit of blood per minute at a euthermic temperature.[15, 16, 205, 206]

Warm intravenous fluids not only are important in preventing hypothermia, they also provide the simplest means of transferring significant amounts of heat to patients who require massive fluid resuscitation. Warm intravenous fluids equilibrate with body temperature, liberating heat in the process. One liter of 40° C crystalloid infused into a 32° C patient is equivalent to a transfusion of 8 kcal. Although 8 kcal will increase body temperature by only 0.14° C, when fluid requirements are massive, a significant amount of heat can be transfused into the patient with intravenous fluids. Ten liters of 40° C fluid infused into a 32° C patient provides an intravenous infusion of 80 kcal of heat, which is enough to raise the temperature of a 70-kg patient by 1.4° C.

Cardiopulmonary bypass is the most efficient warming technique, and it relies on the principle of continuous infusion of warmed intravenous fluids.[207, 208] The limitations imposed by the patient's fluid requirements are circumvented by recirculating the patient's own blood. The need for systemic anticoagulation, lack of general availability, and need for large-bore (15- to 20-French) vessel cannulation restricts the use of this technique to all but a few centers.[209]

Continuous arteriovenous rewarming (CAVR) is a newly described means of performing extracorporeal circulatory rewarming that does not require a mechanical pump or heparin.[16, 210, 211] Unlike patients in fibrillation who have hypothermia caused by exposure, trauma victims have an intact circulation and do not require cardiac pump assistance or an oxygenator. The only benefit of cardiopulmonary bypass rewarming relates to the use of the heat exchanger. CAVR is analogous to the use of continuous arteriovenous hemofiltration as an alternative to conventional pump-

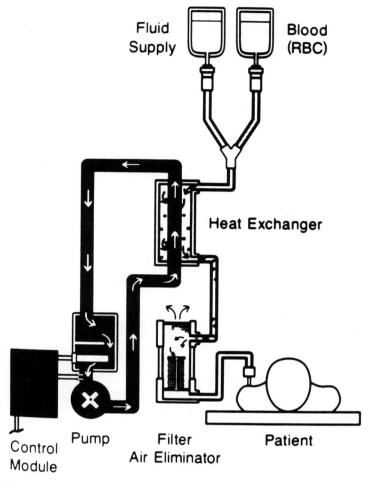

FIG. 4.
Schematic of countercurrent fluid warmer. *RBC* = red blood cell. (From Iserson KV, Huestis DW: *Transfusion* 1991; 31:558–571. Used by permission.)

drive dialysis (CAVH-D) or ultrafiltration in patients with renal failure.[212] It uses 8.5-F femoral arterial and venous catheters placed percutaneously and the patient's own blood pressure to create an arteriovenous fistula through the heating mechanism of a standard countercurrent fluid warmer (Fig 5). The tubing circuit is heparin-bonded and no additional heparinization is necessary.

The effectiveness of CAVR is limited when the arterial pressure is less than 80 mm Hg. Such patients generally require additional fluids that can be "piggybacked" into the heat exchanger to supplement the flow rate of

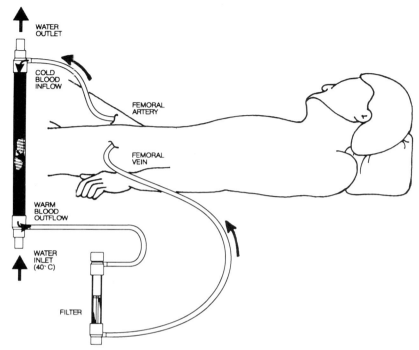

FIG. 5.
Depiction of continuous arteriovenous rewarming (CAVR) technique. (From Gentilello LM, Cotean RA, Offner PJ, et al: *J Trauma* 1992; 32:316–327. Used by permission.)

the fistula (Fig 6). When very rapid administration of a large volume of fluids is necessary, the arterial limb can be clamped and the circuit used as a standard large-bore central venous line. On return of an adequate blood pressure, the arterial limb is unclamped and fistula flow is reestablished.

The typical fistula flow rate is between 250 and 350 mL/min. If the patient's temperature is 32° C and blood is reinfused at a temperature of 39° C, about 6 kcal of heat will be transferred every 3 to 4 minutes. A comparison of heat transfer rates provided by various rewarming methods is shown in Table 3.

In a study involving 34 hypothermic (<35° C) patients admitted to our surgical intensive care unit after trauma (n = 23), major surgery (n = 10), or near-drowning (n = 1), 18 were treated with a combination of airway rewarming, fluid-circulating or convective heating blankets, an aluminized head covering, and warm intravenous fluids, and 16 were treated with CAVR.[16] Time to resolution of hypothermia (≥35° C) was 39 minutes with CAVR and 3.23 hours in the control group. Rapid rewarming resulted in a 57% decrease in blood product requirements and a 67% decrease in crys-

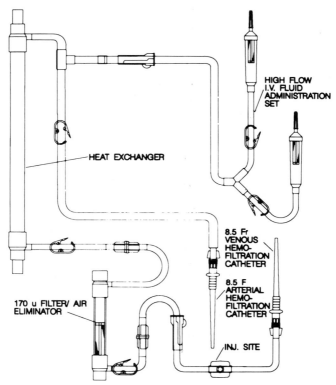

FIG. 6.
Heparinized CAVR set with high-flow intravenous (IV) fluid side port to supplement the fistula flow rate in hypotensive patients. (From Gentilello LM, Cobean RA, Offner PJ, et al: J Trauma 1992; 32:316–327. Used by permission.)

talloid requirements. The rapidly rewarmed group also had better pulmonary function, fewer organ failures, and a shorter intensive care unit stay, and a reduction in mortality was seen in the important subset of trauma patients.

Another method of performing extracorporeal blood rewarming is to use a conventional cardiopulmonary bypass roller pump to drive blood through a countercurrent fluid warmer.[213, 214] The use of a roller pump requires constant attendance by a qualified physician or technician. Loose connections or open stopcocks result in air being drawn into the circuit that then is pumped actively into the patient. Air contained in intravenous bags or tubing also will be pumped into the patient if there is a roller pump, and fatalities may occur during rewarming with this technique.[213] Bubble detectors with an automatic shut-off feature are standard during cardiopulmonary bypass and should be considered a mandatory safety feature.[215, 216]

TABLE 3.
Approximate Rate of Heat Transfer With Available Rewarming Methods

Rewarming Technique	Heat Transfer (kcal/hr)
Airway rewarming	8–12
Overhead radiant warmer	17
Heating blankets	20
Convective warmers	15–26
Body cavity lavage	36
Continuous arteriovenous rewarming	92–139
Cardiopulmonary bypass	710

Kinking or obstruction in the catheter responsible for returning blood to the patient results in a sudden rise in line pressure that may lead to rupture of the circuit. In one small series, rupture secondary to collapse or crimping of the tubing occurred in two of eight patients treated with a veno-venous bypass rewarming system.[214] These systems are similar in concept and operation to conventional dialysis machines and, with adequate safeguards, they may be applicable for use by personnel experienced with extracorporeal perfusion techniques.

Summary

The simplified formulas presented in this chapter for calculating heat gain and loss are considered as instantaneous rates of heat transfer. Because the body temperature increases during rewarming, the difference in temperature between the body and the heat transfer media decreases. Heat transfer, therefore, is a dynamic process. In any case, hypothermia is difficult to treat and early attention to the mechanisms of heat loss remains the best form of therapy. Once hypothermia occurs, every effort should be made to minimize cold stress and rewarm the trauma victim aggressively. Adolph was correct when he stated that "low temperatures have two recognized physiological effects: to prolong life and to kill."[217]

References

1. *Report of Committee on Accidental Hypothermia.* London, Royal College of Physicians, 1966.
2. Moss J: Accidental severe hypothermia. *Surg Gynecol Obstet* 1886; 162:501–513.

3. Wong KC: Physiology and pharmacology of hypothermia. *West J Med* 1983; 138:227–232.
4. Jolly BT, Ghezzi KT: Accidental hypothermia. *Emerg Med Clin North Am* 1992; 10:311–327.
5. Virtue RW: *Hypothermic Anesthesia.* Springfield, Ill, CC Thomas, 1955.
6. Spray DC: Cutaneous temperature receptors. *Annu Rev Physiol* 1986; 48:625–638.
7. Steinemann S, Shackford SR, Davis JW: Implications of admission hypothermia in trauma patients. *J Trauma* 1990; 30:200–202.
8. Gregory JS, Flancbaum L, Townsend C, et al: Incidence and timing of hypothermia in trauma patients undergoing operations. *J Trauma* 1991; 31:795–800.
9. Danzl D, Pozos RS, Auerbach PS, et al: Multicenter hypothermia survey. *Ann Emerg Med* 1987; 16:1042–1055.
10. Jurkovich GJ, Greiser WB, Luterman A, et al: Hypothermia in trauma victims: An ominous predictor of survival. *J Trauma* 1987; 27:1019–1024.
11. Psarras P, Ivatury RR, Rohman M, et al: Presented at the Eastern Association for the Surgery of Trauma, Longboat Key, Fla, 1988.
12. Luna GK, Maier RV, Pavlin EG, et al: Incidence and effect of hypothermia in seriously injured patients. *J Trauma* 1987; 27:1014–1017.
13. Gentilello LM, Jurkovich GJ: Hypothermia in the penetrating trauma victim, in Ivatury R, Cayten G (eds): *Textbook of Penetrating Trauma.* Philadelphia, Lea & Febiger, in press.
14. Britt LD, Dascombe WH, Rodriguez A: New horizons in management of hypothermia and frostbite injury. *Surg Clin North Am* 1991; 71:345–370.
15. Little RA, Stoner HB: Body temperature after accidental injury. *Br J Surg* 1981; 68:221–224.
16. Gentilello LM, Cobean R, Offner PJ, et al: Continuous arteriovenous rewarming: Rapid reversal of hypothermia in critically ill patients. *J Trauma* 1992; 32:316–327.
17. Satiani B, Fried SJ, Zeeb P, et al: Normothermic rapid volume replacement in traumatic hypovolemia: A prospective analysis using a new device. *Arch Surg* 1987; 122:1044–1047.
18. Satiani B, Fried SJ, Zeeb P, et al: Normothermic rapid volume replacement in vascular catastrophes using a new device. *Ann Vasc Surg* 1988; 2:37–42.
19. Blagden: Experiment and observation in a heated room. *Philos Trans R Soc Lond* 1775; 65:111.
20. Lloyd EL: Hypothermia and cold. *Sci Prog* 1989; 73:101–116.
21. Boulant JA, Dean JB: Temperature receptors in the central nervous system. *Annu Rev Physiol* 1986; 48:639–654.
22. Wood SC: Interactions between hypoxia and hypothermia. *Annu Rev Physiol* 1991; 51:71–85.
23. Stoner HB, Marshall HW: Studies on the mechanism of shock: Thermoregulation during limb ischaemia. *Br J Exp Pathol* 1971; 52:650–655.
24. Bastow MD, Rawlings J, Allison SP: Undernutrition, hypothermia, and injury in elderly women with fractured femur: An injury response to altered metabolism? *Lancet* 1983; 1:143–146.
25. Stoner HB: Studies on the mechanism of shock: The impairment of thermoregulation by trauma. *Br J Exp Pathol* 1969; 50:125–138.
26. Stoner HB: Effect of injury on the responses to thermal stimulation of the hypothalamus. *J Appl Physiol* 1972; 33:665–671.

27. Best R, Syverud S, Nowak RM: Trauma and hypothermia. *Am J Emerg Med* 1985; 3:48–55.
28. Little RA: Heat production after injury. *Br Med Bull* 1985; 41:226–231.
29. Cuthbertson DP: Post shock metabolic responses. *Lancet* 1942; 1:433.
30. Stoner HB, Threlfall CJ: *The Biochemical Response to Injury.* Oxford, Blackwell, 1960.
31. Stoner HB: Responses to trauma: Fifty years of ebb and flow. *Circ Shock* 1993; 39:316–319.
32. Shibutani K, Komatsu T, Kubal K, et al: Critical level of oxygen delivery in anesthetized man. *Crit Care Med* 1983; 11:640–643.
33. Weg JG: Oxygen transport in adult respiratory distress syndrome and other acute circulatory problems: Relationship of oxygen delivery and oxygen consumption. *Crit Care Med* 1991; 19:650–657.
34. Vincent JL, Roman A, DeBacker D, et al: Oxygen uptake/supply dependency. *Am Rev Respir Dis* 1990; 142:2–7.
35. Edwards JD, Redmond AD, Nightingale P, et al: Oxygen consumption following trauma: A reappraisal in severely injured patients requiring mechanical ventilation. *Br J Surg* 1988; 75:690–692.
36. Pozos RS, Wittmers LE: *The Nature and Treatment of Hypothermia.* Minneapolis, University of Minnesota Press, 1983.
37. Iampietro PF, Vaughan JA, Goldman RF, et al: Heat production from shivering. *J Appl Physiol* 1960; 15:632–634.
38. Morray JP, Pavlin EG: Oxygen delivery and consumption during hypothermia and rewarming in the dog. *Anesthesiology* 1990; 72:510–516.
39. Gentilello LG, Jurkovich GJ, Moujaes S: Hypothermia and injury: Thermodynamic principles of prevention and treatment, in Levine B, (ed): *Perspectives in Surgery*, vol 2. St Louis, Quality Medical Publishers, 1991, pp 25–55.
40. Weir JB de V: A new method for calculating metabolic rate with special reference to protein metabolism. *J Physiol* (London) 1949; 109:1.
41. Flacke JW: Temperature regulation and anesthesia. *Int Anesthesiol Clin* 1963; 1:43–54.
42. Flacke JW, Flacke WE: Inadvertent hypothermia: Frequent, insidious and often serious. *Seminars in Anesthesia* 1983; 2:183–196.
43. Zwischenberger JB, Kirsh MM, Dechert RE, et al: Suppression of shivering decreases oxygen consumption and improves hemodynamic stability during postoperative rewarming. *Ann Thorac Surg* 1987; 43:428–431.
44. Roe CF, Goldberg MJ, Blair CS, et al: The influence of body temperature on early postoperative oxygen consumption. *Surgery* 1966; 60:85–92.
45. Campbell RM, Cuthbertson DP: Effect of environmental temperature on the metabolic response to injury. *Q J Exp Physiol* 1967; 52:114–129.
46. Campbell RM, Cuthbertson DP: *Nature* 1966; 210:206.
47. Cuthbertson DP: Into the disturbance of protein metabolism following physical injury: *Biochemical response to bacterial injury*, in Stoner HB, Threlfall CJ (eds): Oxford, Blackwell, 1960, p 193–216.
48. Caldwell FT: Metabolic response to thermal trauma: II. Nutritional studies with rats at two environmental temperatures. *Ann Surg* 1962; 155:119.
49. Caldwell FG, Wallace BH, Cone JB, et al: Control of the hypermetabolic response to burn injury using environmental factors. *Ann Surg* 1992;216:485–491.
50. Arturson MC: Metabolic changes following thermal injury. *World J Surg* 1978; 2:203–214.

51. Caldwell FT Jr, Bowser BH, Crabtree JH: The effect of occlusive dressings on the energy metabolism of severely burned children. Ann Surg 1981; 193:579–591.
52. Carli F, Emery PW, Freemantle CA: Effect of preoperative normothermia on postoperative protein metabolism in elderly patients undergoing hip arthroplasty. Br J Anaesth 1989; 63:276–282.
53. Carli F, Itiaba K: Effect of heat conservation during and after major abdominal surgery on muscle protein breakdown in elderly patients. Br J Anaesth 1986; 58:502–507.
54. Carli F: Preoperative normothermia attenuates increase in postoperative metabolic rate in elderly patients. Br J Anaesth 1988; 61:511–512.
55. Blair E, Montgomery AV, Swan H: Posthypothermic circulatory failure. Physiologic observations on the circulation. Circulation 1956; 13:909–915.
56. Steen PA, Milde JH, Michenfelder JD: The detrimental effects of prolonged hypothermia and rewarming in the dog. Anesthesiology 1980; 52:224–230.
57. Fisher B, Russ C, Fedor EJ: Effect of hypothermia of 2 to 24 hours on oxygen consumption and cardiac output in the dog. Am J Physiol 1957; 188:473–476.
58. Clifton GL, Allen S, Berry J, et al: Systemic hypothermia in treatment of brain injury. J Neurotrauma 1992; 9(suppl 2):S487–495.
59. Block M: Cerebral effects of rewarming following prolonged hypothermia: Significance for the management of severe craniocerebral injury and acute pyrexia. Brain 1967; 90:769–784.
60. Physiology of Induced Hypothermia. Proceedings of a Symposium. Washington, DC, National Academy of Sciences, Publication No. 451, 1955.
61. Little DM: Hypothermia. Anesthesiology 1959; 20:842–877.
62. Prakash O, Jonson B, Bos E, et al: Cardiorespiratory and metabolic effects of profound hypothermia. Crit Care Med 1978; 6:165–171.
63. Venkatachalam MA, Patel YJ, Kreisberg JI, et al: Energy thresholds that determine membrane integrity and injury in a renal epithelial cell line. J Clin Invest 1988; 81:743–758.
64. Warnick CT, Lazarus HM: Recovery of nucleotide levels after cell injury. Can J Biochem 1981; 59:116–121.
65. Hochachka PW: Defense strategies against hypoxia and hypothermia. Science 1986; 231:234–241.
66. Michenfelder JD, Theye RA: Hypothermia: Effect on canine brain and whole body metabolism. Anesthesiology 1968; 29:1107–1112.
67. Sori AJ, El-Assuooty A, Rush BF, et al: The effect of temperature on survival in hemorrhagic shock. Am Surg 1987; 53:706–710.
68. Tanaka J, Sato T, Berezsky IK, et al: Effect of hypothermia on survival time and ecg in rats with acute blood loss. Adv Shock Res 1983; 9:219–232.
69. Hartman AR, Yunis J, Frei LW, et al: Profound hypothermic circulatory arrest for the management of penetrating retrohepatic venous injury: Case report. J Trauma 1991; 31:1310–1311.
70. Hickey PR: Deep hypothermic circulatory arrest: Current status and future direction. Mt Sinai J Med 1985; 52:541.
71. Livesay JJ, Cooley DA, Reul GJ, et al: Resection of aortic arch aneurysms: A comparison of hypothermia techniques in 60 patients. Ann Thorac Surg 1983; 36:19.
72. O'Connor JV, Wilding T, Farmer P, et al: The protective effect of profound hypothermia in the canine central nervous system during one hour of circulatory arrest. Ann Thorac Surg 1986; 41:255.

73. Tisherman SA, Safar P, Radovsky A, et al: Profound hypothermia (<10° C) compared with deep hypothermia (15° C) improves neurologic outcome in dogs after two hours of circulatory arrest induced to enable resuscitative surgery. J Trauma 1991; 31:1051–1062.
74. Tisherman SA, Safar P, Radovsky A, et al: Deep hypothermic circulatory arrest during intractable hemorrhagic shock in dogs: A resuscitation modality for "irreparable" injury. J Trauma 1990;30:308–316.
75. Feinberg H, Rosenbaum DS, Levitsky S, et al: Platelet deposition after surgically induced myocardial ischemia: An etiology factor for reperfusion injury. J Thorac Cardiovasc Surg 1982; 84:815–822.
76. Harker LA, Malpass TW, Bronson HE, et al: Mechanism of abnormal bleeding in patients undergoing cardiopulmonary bypass: Acquired transient platelet dysfunction associated with selective alpha-granule release. Blood 1980; 56:824–834.
77. Valeri CR, Feingold H, Cassidy G, et al: Hypothermia-induced reversible platelet dysfunction. Ann Surg 1987; 205:175–181.
78. Yoshihara H, Yamamoto T, Mihara H: Changes in coagulation and fibrinolysis occurring in dogs during hypothermia. Thromb Res 1985; 37:503–512.
79. Reed RL II, Bracey AW Jr, Hudson JD, et al: Hypothermia and blood coagulation: Dissociation between enzyme activity and clotting factor levels. Circ Shock 1990; 32:141–152.
80. Dietrich WD: The importance of brain temperature in cerebral injury. J Neurotrauma 1992; 9:S475–485.
81. Busto R, Dietrich WD, Globus MY-T, et al: Postischemic moderate hypothermia inhibits CA1 hippocampal ischemic neuronal injury. Neurosci Lett 1987; 101:299–304.
82. Vibulsresth S, Dietrich WD, Busto R, et al: Failure of nimodipine to prevent ischemic neuronal damage in rats. Stroke 1987; 18:210–216.
83. Martinez-Arizala A, Green BA: Hypothermia in spinal cord injury. J Neurotrauma 1992; 9(suppl 2):S497–505.
84. Busto R, Dietrich WD, Globus MY-T, et al: Small differences in intra-ischemic brain temperature critically determine the extent of ischemic neuronal injury. J Cereb Blood Flow Metab 1987; 7:;729–738.
85. Clifton GL, Jiang JY, Lyeth BG, et al: Conditions for pharmacologic evaluation in the gerbil model of experimental forebrain ischemia. Stroke 1989; 20:1545–1552.
86. Clifton GL, Jiang JY, Lyeth BG, et al: Marked protection by moderate hypothermia after experimental traumatic brain injury. J Cereb Blood Flow Metab 1991; 11:114–121.
87. Minamisawa H, Smith ML, Siesjo BK: The effect of mild hyperthermia and hypothermia on brain damage following 5, 10, and 15 minutes of forebrain ischemia. Ann Neurol 1990; 28:26–33.
88. Minamisawa H, Nordstrom CH, Smith ML, et al: The influence of mild body and brain hypothermia on ischemia brain damage. J Cereb Blood Flow Metab 1990; 10:365–374.
89. Kuboyama K, Safar P, Radovsky A, et al: Delay in cooling negates the beneficial effect of mild resuscitative cerebral hypothermia after cardiac arrest in dogs: A prospective, randomized study. Crit Care Med 1993; 21:1348–1358.
90. Almond CH, Jones JC, Snyder HM, et al: Cooling gradients and brain damage with deep hypothermia. J Thorac Cardiovasc Surg 1964; 48:890–897.
91. Fisher B, Fedor EJ, Smith VW: Temperature gradients associated with extra-

corporeal perfusion and profound hypothermia. *Surgery* 1957; 188:473–476.
92. Drake C, Joy T: Hypothermia in the treatment of critical head injury. *Can Med Assoc J* 1962; 87:887–891.
93. Drake CG, Barr WK, Coles JC, et al: The use of extracorporeal circulation and profound hyopothermia in the treatment of ruptured intracranial aneurysm. *J Neurosurg* 1964; 21:575–581.
94. Uihlein A, MacCarty CS, Michenfelder JD, et al: Deep hypothermia and surgical treatment of intracranial aneurysms. *JAMA* 1966; 195:127–129.
95. Mullan S, Raimondi AJ, Suwanwela C: Effect of hypothermia upon cerebral injuries in dogs. *Arch Neurol* 1961; 5:545–551.
96. Sternau LL, Thompson C, Dietrich WD, et al: Intracranial temperature observations in the human brain. *J Cereb Blood Flow Metab* 1991; 11(suppl 2): S123.
97. Brantigan CO, Patton B: Clinical hypothermia, accidental hypothermia and frostbite, in Goldsmith HS (ed): *Lewis Practice of Surgery*. New York, Harper & Row Publishers, 1978.
98. Harnett RM, Pruitt JR, Sias FR: A review of the literature concerning resuscitation from hypothermia: Part I—the problem and general approaches. *Aviat Space Environ Med* 1983; 5:425–434.
99. Harnett RM, Pruitt JR, Sias FR: A review of the literature concerning resuscitation from hypothermia: Part II—selected rewarming protocols. *Aviat Space Environ Med* 1983; 5:487–495.
100. Little DM: Hypothermia. *Anesthesiology* 1959; 20:842–877.
101. Trevino A, Razi B, Beller BM: The characteristic electrocardiogram of accidental hypothermia. *Arch Intern Med* 1971; 127:470–473.
102. Rothfield TB: Hypothermic hump. *JAMA* 1970; 213:626.
103. Schwab RH, Lewis DH, Killough JH, et al: Electrocardiographic changes occurring in rapidly induced deep hypothermia. *Am J Med Sci* 1964; 248:290–303.
104. Gould L, Gopalaswamy C, Kim BS, et al: Osborn wave in hypothermia. *Angiology* 1985; 36:125–129.
105. Paton BC: Accidental hypothermia. *Pharmacol Ther* 1983; 22:331–377.
106. Ferguson NV: Urban hypothermia. *Anaesthesia* 1985; 40:651–654.
107. Standards and guidelines for cardiopulmonary resuscitation (CPR) and emergency cardiac care (ECC). *JAMA* 1986; 255:2905–2984.
108. Miller JW, Danzl DF, Thomas DM: Urban accidental hypothermia: 135 cases. *Ann Emerg Med* 1980; 9:456–461.
109. Angelakos ET: Influence of pharmacologic agents on spontaneous and surgically-induced hypothermia ventricular fibrillation. *Ann N Y Acad Sci* 1959; 80:351.
110. Dundee JW, Clarke RSJ: Pharmacology of hypothermia. *J Am Coll Emerg Phys* 1979; 8:48.
111. Nielson KC, Owman C: Control of ventricular fibrillation during induced hypothermia in cats after blocking the adrenergic neurons with bretylium. *Life Sci* 1968; 7:159–168.
112. Danzl DF: Accidental hypothermia, in Rosen P, Baker FJ, Brain GR, et al (eds): *Emergency Medicine: Concepts and Clinical Practice*. St Louis, Mosby-Year Book, 1983, pp 477–497.
113. Kochar G, Kahn SE, Kotler MN: Bretylium tosylate and ventricular fibrillation in hypothermia. *Ann Intern Med* 1986; 105:624.

114. Dronen S, Nowak RM, Tomlanovich MC: Bretylium tosylate and hypothermic ventricular fibrillation. *Ann Emerg Med* 1980; 9:335.
115. Benumof JL, Wahrenbrock EA: Dependency of hypoxic pulmonary vasoconstriction on temperature. *J Appl Physiol* 1977; 42:56–58.
116. Cohen DJ, Cline JR, Lepinski SM, et al: Resuscitation of the hypothermic patient. *Am J Emerg Med* 1988; 6:475–478.
117. Ledingham I McA, Mone JG: Treatment of accidental hypothermia: A prospective clinical study. *BMJ* 1980; 1:1102–1105.
118. Rahn H: Body temperature and acid-base regulation. *Pneumonologie* 1974; 151:87.
119. Rahn H, Reeves RB, Howell BJ: Hydrogen ion regulation, temperature, and evolution. *Am Rev Respir Dis* 1975; 112:165–172.
120. Ream AK, Reitz BA, Silverberg G: Temperature correction of $Paco_2$ and pH in estimating acid-base status: An example of emperor's new clothes? *Anesthesiology* 1982; 56:41.
121. White FN: A comparative physiologic approach to hypothermia. *J Thorac Cardiovasc Surg* 1982; 82:;821–831.
122. Hansen JE, Sue DY: Should blood gas measurements be corrected for the patient's temperature (letter)? *N Engl J Med* 1980; 303:341.
123. Elder PT: Accidental hypothermia, in Shoemaker WC (ed): *Textbook of Critical Care*. Philadelphia, WB Saunders, 1984, pp 85–93.
124. Orlowski JP, Erenberg G, Lueders H, et al: Hypothermia and barbiturate coma for refractory status epilepticus. *Crit Care Med* 1984; 12:367–372.
125. Gregory RT, Patton JF: Treatment after exposure to cold. *Lancet* 1972; 1:377.
126. Moyer JH, Morris GC Jr, DeBakey ME: Hypothermia: Effect of renal hemodynamics and excretion of water and electrolytes in dog and man. *Ann Surg* 1957; 145:26.
127. Anderson M, Nielsen KC: Renal function under experimental hypothermia in rabbits. *Acta Med Scandinav* 1955:151:191.
128. Belzer FO: Kidney preservation. *Surg Clin North Am* 1978; 58:261–272.
129. Fregly M: Water and electrolyte exchange during exposure to cold. *Pharmacol Ther* 1982; 18:199–231.
130. MacKnight AC, Leaf A: Regulation of cellular volume. *Physiol Rev* 1977; 57:510–573.
131. Taylor CA: Surgical hypothermia. *Pharmacol Ther* 1988; 38:169–200.
132. Brauer RW, Holloway RJ, Krebs JS, et al: The liver in hypothermia. *Ann N Y Acad Sci* 1959; 80:395.
133. Duguid H, Simpson RG, Stowers JM: Accidental hypothermia. *Lancet* 1961; 2:1213–1219.
134. Bryant RE, Hood AF, Hood CE, et al: Factors affecting mortality in gram-negative rod bacteremia. *Arch Intern Med* 1971; 127:120–128.
135. Mant AK: Autopsy diagnosis of accidental hypothermia. *J Forensic Med* 1969; 16:126–129.
136. Read AE, Emslie-Smith D, Gough KR, et al: Pancreatitis and accidental hypothermia. *Lancet* 1961; 2:1219–1221.
137. Savides EP, Hoffrand BI: Hypothermia, thrombosis and acute pancreatitis. *BMJ* 1974; 1:245.
138. Curry DL, Curry KP: Hypothermia and insulin secretion. *Endocrinology* 1970; 87:750–755.

139. Axelrod DR, Bass DF: Electrolytes and acid base balance in hypothermia. *Am J Physiol* 1956; 186:31.
140. Stoner HB, Frayn KN, Little RA, et al: Metabolic aspects of hypothermia in the elderly. *Clin Sci* 1980; 59:19–27.
141. MacLean D, Browning MC: Plasma 11-hydroxycorticosteroid concentrations and prognosis in accidental hypothermia. *Resuscitation* 1974; 3:249–256.
142. McInnes C, Rothwell RI, Jacobs HS, et al: Plasma 11-hydroxycorticosteroid and growth hormone levels in climbers. *Lancet* 1971; 1:49–51.
143. Kanter GS: Hypothermic hemoconcentration. *Am J Physiol* 1968; 214:856–859.
144. Sharp KW, LoCicero RJ: Abdominal packing for surgically uncontrollable hemorrhage. *Ann Surg* 1992; 215:467–475.
145. Burch JM, Ortiz VB, Richardson RJ, et al: Abbreviated laparotomy and planned reoperation for critically injured patients. *Ann Surg* 1992; 215:476–484.
146. Blair E: *Clinical Hypothermia* New York, McGraw-Hill, 1964.
147. Bunker JP, Goldstein R: Coagulation during hypothermia in man. *Proc Soc Exp Biol Med* 1958; 97:199.
148. Anstall HB, Huntsman RG: Influence of temperature upon blood coagulation in a cold and a warm-blooded animal. *Nature* 1960; 186:726.
149. Halinen MO, Suhonen RE, Sarajas HS: Characteristics of blood clotting in hypothermia. *Scand J Clin Lab Invest* 1968; 21(suppl 101):65.
150. Kopriva CJ, Sreenivasan N, Stefansson S, et al: Hypothermia can cause errors in activated coagulation time. *Anesthesiology* 1980; 53:585.
151. Reed RL II, Johnston TD, Hudson JD, et al: The disparty between hypothermic coagulopathy and clotting studies. *J Trauma* 1992; 33:465.
152. Johnston TD, Chen Y, Reed RL II: Relative sensitivity of the clotting cascade to hypothermia. *Surgical Forum* 1989; 40:199.
153. Villalobos TJ, Adelson E, Riley PA Jr, et al: A cause of the thrombocytopenia and leucopenia that occurs in dogs during deep hypothermia. *J Clin Invest* 1958; 37:1–7.
154. Czer L, Bateman T, Gray R, et al: Prospective trial of DDAVP in treatment of severe platelet dysfunction and hemorrhage after cardipulmonary bypass. *Circulation* 1985; 72:III-130.
155. Fox JB, Thomas F, Clemmer TP, et al: A retrospective analysis of air-evacuated hypothermia patients. *Aviat Space Environ Med* 1988; 59:1070–1075.
156. English MJM, Farmer C, Scott WAC: Heat loss in exposed volunteers. *J Trauma* 1990; 30:422–424.
157. English MJM, Papenberg R, Forias E, et al: Heat loss in an animal experimental model. *J Trauma* 1991; 31:36–38.
158. Burton A: The application of the theory of heat flow to the study of energy metabolism. *J Nutr* 1934; 7:497.
159. Maclean D, Emslie-Smith D: *Accidental Hypothermia*. Edinburgh, Blackwell, 1977.
160. Lloyd EL: *Hypothermia and Cold Stress*. Rockville, MD, Aspen, 1986.
161. Morrison RC: Hypothermia in the elderly. *Int Anesthesiol Clin* 1988; 26:124–133.
162. Sessler DI, Moayeri A: Skin-surface rewarming: Heat flux and central temperature. *Anesthesiology* 1990; 73:218–224.
163. Ereth MH, Lennon RL, Sessler DI: Limited heat transfer between thermal compartments during rewarming in vasoconstricted patients. *Aviat Space Environ Med* 1992; 63:1065–1069.

164. Joachimsson PO, Hedstrand U, Tabow F, et al: Prevention of intraoperative hypothermia during abdominal surgery. *Acta Anesthesiol Scand* 1987; 31:330–337.
165. Roizen MF, Sohn YJ, L'Hommedieu CS, et al: Operating room temperature prior to surgical draping: Effect on patient temperature in recovery room. *Anesth Analg* 1980; 59:852.
166. Golden F StC: Problems of immersion. *Br J Hosp Med* 1980; 24:371–374.
167. Jessen K, Hagelson JO: Peritoneal dialysis in the treatment of profound accidental hypothermia. *Avia Space Environ Med* 1978; 49:426–429.
168. Marcus P: The treatment of acute accidental hypothermia: Proceedings of a symposium held at the RAF Institute of Aviation Medicine. *Aviat Space Environ Med* 1979; 50:834–843.
169. Radford P, Thurlow AC: Metallized plastic sheeting in prevention of hypothermia during surgery. *Br J Anaesth* 1979; 51:237–239.
170. Bourke DL, Wurm H, Rosenberg M, et al: Intraoperative heat conservation using a reflective blanket. *Anesthesiology* 1984; 60:151–154.
171. Henneberg S, Eklund A, Joachimsson PO, et al: Effects of a thermal ceiling on postoperative hypothermia. *Acta Anaesthesiol Scand* 1985; 29:602–606.
172. Harnett RM, Pruitt JR, Sias FR: A review of the literature concerning resuscitation from hypothermia: Part II—selected rewarming protocols. *Aviat Space Environ Med* 1983; 54:487–495.
173. Lehman JF, Johnson EW: Some factors influencing the temperature distribution in thighs exposed to ultrasound. *Arch Phys Med* 1958; 39:347–356.
174. Lehman JF: Diathermia, in *Handbook of Physical Medicine and Rehabilitation*, 2nd ed. Philadelphia, WB Saunders, 1971.
175. White JD, Butterfield AB, Greer KA, et al: Controlled comparison of radio wave regional hyperthermia and peritoneal lavage rewarming after immersion hypothermia. *J Trauma* 1985; 25:989–992.
176. White JD, Butterfield AB, Greer KA, et al: Comparison of rewarming by radio wave regional hyperthermia and warm humidified inhalation. *Aviat Space Environ Med* 1984; 55:1103–1106.
177. Otto RJ, Metzler MH: Rewarming from experimental hypothermia: Comparison of heated aerosol inhalation, peritoneal lavage, and pleural lavage. *Crit Care Med* 1988; 16:;869–875.
178. Patton J, Doolittle W: Core rewarming by peritoneal dialysis following induced hypothermia in the dog. *J Appl Physiol* 1972; 33:800–804.
179. Jessen K, Hagelsten J: Peritoneal dialysis in the treatment of profound accidental hypothermia. *Aviat Space Environ Med* 1978; 49:426.
180. Slotman GJ, Jed EH, Burchard KW: Adverse effects of hypothermia in postoperative patients. *Am J Surg* 1985; 149:495–500.
181. Ozinsky J: Hypothermic ventricular fibrillation and halothane. *S Afr Med J* 1963; 37:110–112.
182. Hoffman EF: Hypothermia and vulnerability. *Ann N Y Acad Sci* 1959; 80:348–350.
183. Boyan CP, Howland WS: Cardiac arrest and temperature of bank blood. *JAMA* 1963; 183:58–60.
184. Boyan CP: Cold or warmed blood for massive transfusions. *Ann Surg* 1964; 160:282–236.
185. Dinnick OP: Deaths associated with anaesthesia: Observations on 600 cases. *Anaesthesia* 1964; 19:536–556.
186. Dybkjaer E, Elkjaer P: The use of heated blood in massive blood replacement. *Acta Anaesthesiol Scand* 1964; 8:271–278.

187. Dumham CM, Belzberg H, Lyles R, et al: The rapid infusion system: A superior method for the resuscitation of hypovolemic trauma patients. *J Trauma* 1989; 29:1724.
188. Iserson KV, Huestes DW: Blood warming: Current applications and techniques. *Transfusion* 1991; 31:558–570.
189. Mateer JR, Thompson BM, Tucker J, et al: Effects of high infusion pressure and large-bore blood tubing on intravenous flow rates. *Am J Emerg Med* 1985; 3:187–189.
190. Strauss RG, Bell EF, Snyder EL, et al: Effects of environmental warming on blood components dispensed in syringes for neonatal transfusions. *J Pediatr* 1986; 109:109–113.
191. Opitz JC, Baldauf MC, Kessler DL, et al: Hemolysis of blood in intravenous tubing caused by heat. *J Pediatr* 1988; 112:111–113.
192. Staples PJ, Griner PF: Extracorporeal hemolysis of blood in a microwave blood warmer. *N Engl J Med* 1971; 285:317–319.
193. Werwath DL, Schwab CW, Scholten JR, et al: Microwave ovens: A safe new method of warming crystalloids. *Am Surg* 1984; 50:656–659.
194. Hansen G: Microwave oven explosion. *Hosp Pharm* 1979; 14:12.
195. Linko K, Hynynen K: Erythrocyte damage caused by the Haemotherm microwave blood warmer. *Acta Anaesthesiol Scand* 1979; 23:320–328.
196. Inoue K, Reichelt W, Kleesiek K: Transfusion reaction following blood-warming with a microwave blood warmer. *Anaesthesist* 1987; 36:180–181.
197. McCullough J, Polesky HF, Nelson C, et al: Iatrogenic hemolysis: A complication of blood warmed by a microwave device. *Anesth Analg* 1972; 51:102–106.
198. Leonard PF, Restall CJ, Taswell HF, et al: Microwave warming of banked blood. *Anesth Analg* 1971; 50:302–305.
199. Paddock H, Connolly RJ, Medina M, et al: Continuous microwave warming in an ex-vivo extracorporeal circuit. *Crit Care Med* 1993; 4(suppl):S181.
200. Schwaitzberg SD, Allen MJ, Connolly RJ, et al: Rapid in-line blood warming using microwave energy. *J Surg Res* 1991; 51:505.
201. Wilson EB, Knauf MA, Iserson KV: Red cell tolerance of admixture with heated saline. *Transfusion* 1988; 28:170–172.
202. Wilson EB, Knauf MA, Donohoe K, et al: Red cell survival following admixture with heated saline: Evaluation of a new blood warming method for rapid transfusion. *J Trauma* 1988; 28:1274–1277.
203. Iserson KV, Knauf MA, Anhalt D: Rapid admixture blood warming: Technical advances. *Crit Care Med* 1990; 18:1138–1141.
204. Linkow K, Palosaari S: Warming of blood units in water bath and cooling of blood at room temperature. *Acta Anaesthesiol Scand* 1979; 23:97–102.
205. Fried SJ, Satiani B, Zeeb P: Normothermic rapid volume replacement for hypovolemic shock: An in vivo and in vitro study utilizing a new technique. *J Trauma* 1986; 26:183–188.
206. Flancbaum L, Trooskin SZ, Pedersen H: Evaluation of blood-warming devices with the apparent thermal clearance. *Ann Emerg Med* 1989; 18:355–359.
207. Fruehan A: Accidental hypothermia. *Arch Intern Med* 1960; 105:218.
208. Kugelberg J, Schuller H, Berg B: Treatment of accidental hypothermia. *Scand J Thorac Cardiovasc Surg* 1967; 1:142.
209. Del Rossi A, Cernainu AC, Vertrees RA, et al: Heparinless extracorporeal bypass for treatment of hypothermia. *J Trauma* 1990; 30:79–82.
210. Gentilello LM, Cortes V, Moujaes S, et al: Continuous arteriovenous rewarm-

ing: Experimental results and thermodynamic model simulation of treatment for hypothermia. *J Trauma* 1990; 30:1435–1449.
211. Gentilello LM, Rifley WJ: Continuous arteriovenous rewarming: Report of a new technique for treating hypothermia. *J Trauma* 1991, 31:1151–1154.
212. Kramer P, Bohler J, Kehr A, et al: Intensive care potential of continuous arteriovenous hemofiltration. *Trans Am Soc Artif Intern Organs* 1982; 28:28–32.
213. Gregory JS, Bergstein JM, Aprahamian C, et al: Comparison of three methods of rewarming from hypothermia: Advantages of extracorporeal blood warming. *J Trauma* 1991; 31:1247–1252.
214. Gregory JS, Flancbaum L, Smead WL, et al: Extracorporeal venovenous recirculation for the treatment of hypothermia during elective aortic surgery: A phase 1 study. *Surgery* 1993; 114:40–45.
215. Zwischenberger JB, Cilley RE, Hirschl RB, et al: Life-threatening intrathoracic complications during treatment with extracorporeal membrane oxygenation. *J Pediatr Surg* 1988; 23:599–604.
216. Chapman RA, Bartlett RH: *Extracorporeal Life Support Manual,* 1st ed. Ann Arbor, University of Michigan, 1991.
217. Adolph EF: *The Physiology of Induced Hypothermia: Proceedings of a Symposium.* Washington, DC, National Academy of Sciences, Publication 451, 1956.

Protective Surgical Wear

Reginald W. Martin, M.D.

Assistant Professor of Surgery, Department of Surgery, University of Mississippi Medical Center, Jackson, Mississippi

Robert S. Rhodes, M.D.

James D. Hardy Professor and Chairman, Department of Surgery, University of Mississippi Medical Center, Jackson, Mississippi

Modern forms of protective surgical attire bear little resemblance to the original types of surgical theater dress. The evolution of surgical attire reflected increasing scientific knowledge and concern about disease transmission in the health care setting. Before the microbial basis of sepsis was understood, operating rooms resembled auditoriums in which the surgeon's street clothes, often soiled and reused, sufficed as acceptable attire. The introduction of surgical attire focused on asepsis rather than antisepsis. In 1865, Lister attempted to attain this state using carbolic spray. In 1886 in Kiel, Germany, Gustav Neuberg wore a gown sterilized in mercuric chloride. He advocated the use of boots and caps, and segregated clean and dirty cases into separate rooms.[1] Asepsis for the patient and attempts to protect the surgeon or staff date back to Halsted's use of gloves. He initially introduced gloves to protect his scrub nurse's hands against the dermatitis associated with sterilizing instruments in mercuric chloride, and only subsequently proved the value of gloves for sterility.[1] Further evolution of asepsis has involved the development of special air-handling systems in the operating room as well as improvements in surgical attire.

The last 3 to 4 decades have witnessed a philosophical shift in operating room attire, with greater emphasis on reducing the risk of pathogen transmission from the patient to the surgical staff. Although there has been a long-standing risk of disease transmission with a variety of bacterial pathogens (e.g., tuberculosis [TB]) and blood-borne pathogens (e.g., hepatitis B virus [HBV]), fear of infection with the human immunodeficiency virus (HIV) provided the strongest impetus for a resurgent interest in protective surgical wear.

The risk of disease transmission from the patient to the surgical team is a function of the prevalence of infection in the patient population, the frequency and type of exposure, and the risk of infection associated with exposure.[2] The prevalence of infection in the patient population is often beyond the immediate control of the surgical team. The type of exposure is a function of the type of procedure as well as specific surgical techniques. The protective effects of surgical attire have their greatest impact in this area. The types of exposure can be categorized as inhalation, percutaneous, and mucocutaneous. Masks, gloves, and gowns are the respective articles that provide primary protection for each of these types of exposure. Mucocutaneous exposure also can occur on the hands and face, and gloves, masks, and eyewear also should be considered for preventing this occurrence.

The various organisms that pose a risk to the surgical team differ in their characteristics and mechanisms of transmission. These mechanisms define the ideal characteristics of protective attire. The qualities that are necessary to provide effective barriers to these organisms, however, also may compromise the comfort, dexterity, and vision of the surgical team. These problems are elaborated on further as they relate to three of the more common pathogens.

Pathogens

Tuberculosis

Until relatively recently, TB was a major health problem. Physicians caring for patients with TB also were at risk. Spread occurred primarily by inhalation, and surgical masks were an effective barrier against transmission. Improvements in public health plus the development of antibiotics with activity against *Mycobacterium* were extremely effective in nearly eradicating this disease. Unfortunately, TB is undergoing a resurgence. Patients with compromised immune systems appear to be particularly susceptible. Drug-resistant forms present in atypical ways. Physicians caring for these patients must become reacquainted with the possibility of transmission. Conventional surgical attire is effective. Surgeons performing minor procedures, however, such as lymph node biopsy, may not wear masks and other attire and, thus, increase their risk of exposure.

Hepatitis B Virus

The transmission of viral hepatitis from infected patients and health care workers to noninfected patients and health care workers has been a problem for several decades. Surgeons are at greatest risk of acquiring hepatitis B when they are operating on patients who are HBeAg positive. An estimated 40% of American surgeons are infected during surgery at some point during their lifetime; 4% become carriers.[3] Without prophylaxis, the risk may exceed 30% after a single exposure by needle stick or sharp injury to HBeAg-positive blood.[4] There also appears to be a significant risk of acquiring HBV from exposure of skin or mucous membranes to blood from HBeAg-positive carriers. The exact rate of HBV transmission is not known because the infected recipient may not have any symptoms. As many as 5% of health care workers with occupationally acquired HBV subsequently die as a consequence of this infection. There has been additional recent concern about hepatitis C virus, which appears to pose similar risks.

A hepatitis B vaccine derived from recombinant DNA is available. The risk of hepatitis B transmission to a health care worker who has fully been immunized and has shown an immune response after vaccination is virtually nil.[4] Therefore, the most important protection for surgeons is not attire, but immunization.

Human Immunodeficiency Virus

HIV also is a viral, blood-borne pathogen, but its risks of transmission from patient to health care worker are different than those of HBV. The risk of transmission of HIV in the surgical theater remains exceedingly low; however, the universal fatality of HIV infection prompts great concern. In fact, more health care workers die of occupationally acquired HBV than of HIV. Although the mortality rate of HBV is low, its far greater prevalence accounts for the greater number of fatalities.

HIV appears to be transmitted primarily by percutaneous exposure. Initial estimates of the risk of HIV transmission from patients to health care workers and from health care workers to patients were based on assumptions analogous to those of HBV. Experience has brought into question the validity of these assumptions. The reported rates of theoretic seroconversion after a single hollow-needle puncture range from .0003% to .009%.[2] At the end of 1992, however, no seroconversion after an injury from a suture needle or a solid needle used in the operating theater had been reported. Thirty of the 39 cases of definite transmission from a patient to a health care worker have occurred through percutaneous exposure and all have been from hollow-needle injuries. Although the rate of solid (suture)-needle injuries to operating room personnel is relatively high, there is no known case of HIV transmission by this route. The reason may relate to the smaller viral inoculum with solid-needle injuries. The occupational risk of infection with HIV remains unknown. Because of the reported 39.2% incidence of blood–skin contact, however, members of surgical teams feel vulnerable to HIV infection.[5]

Types of surgery that carry an increased risk of HIV transmission include trauma, gynecologic, major abdominal, urologic, vascular, cardiovascular, and orthopedic. Percutaneous injuries or exposure to large amounts of blood are more likely to occur during these operations. Reported rates of surgical glove puncture range from 2.5% to 10%,[6] but this is heavily dependent on the skill of the surgeon, the length of the operation, and the type of surgical procedures performed. It is important to note that intact skin and mucous membranes are an important barrier against HIV, although the risk of mucocutaneous transmission probably is not zero. In 1987, three health care workers who had eczema or dermatitis and who did not observe barrier precautions were exposed to HIV-infected blood and acquired HIV without a sharp injury.[7]

The Role and Development of Specific Attire

Developing protective wear against pathogens with diverse characteristics is a challenge. Impervious materials that are useful in other situations do not allow the dexterity and comfort needed by the surgical team. The development and considerations for each type of attire are considered below.

Gloves

Early gloves were constructed from rubber, making them cumbersome and affected by extremes in temperature. Modern materials and design are directed toward increased comfort and enhancement of tactile sensitivity. In an attempt to furnish these characteristics, glove manufacturers accept a 1.5% manufacture failure rate.[8]

The rate of glove failure is highly dependent on the type of procedure performed, the technique of the operating surgeon, and the length of the operative procedure. Numerous studies report an approximate glove failure rate of 51% for single gloves and 7% for double gloves during invasive procedures.[8] The reported rate of glove failure during minimally invasive procedures (e.g., cardiac catheterization) has been reported to be as high as 17%.[8]

Attempts to define specific mechanisms of exposure have resulted in the conclusions that most glove failures are of unknown etiology and most sharp injuries occur during suturing.[9] Most glove punctures occur on the nondominant hand, and the index finger is injured most frequently.[10] These injuries occur when the nondominant hand is stationary, being used for retraction, and the suture is being placed or passed in and out of the wound. Greater attention to technique and the appropriate use of self-retaining retractors should decrease the incidence of sharp injuries.

The risk of glove failure also is intimately related to the volume of blood with which the surgeon is in contact and the length of the operative procedure. The blood–skin contact rate may exceed 50% in procedures of more than 4 hours' duration.[9] In these cases, double gloving or routinely changing gloves every 1 or 2 hours may be beneficial. In a high-risk patient or one with known viral infection, double gloving, the use of self-retaining retractors, attention to technical details, and routine glove change at set intervals are viable recommendations to prevent glove failure. Most surgeons also find that altering the size of the inner or outer glove compensates for the loss of tactile sensation or numbness that results from double gloving.

Several devices are being tested to alert the surgeon to early glove failure. None has been subjected to a large-scale trial, however, and their effectiveness in reducing blood contact remains unknown.

Gowns

Operative theater gowns were introduced to complete the attire necessary to provide "sterile" technique as early as 1952; however, Beck and Collette noted bacterial passage through wet surgical gowns.[11] Pathogen penetration or "strike through" appears to be retarded only by waterproof materials. These materials have largely been avoided because they cause increased perspiration and heat, making them unbearable for longer procedures. Again, strike through appears to be multifactorial, dependent on pressure and mechanical forces exerted on the gown, the material used, and the length and type of surgery performed.

The surgical gown industry has formulated gown and drape barrier material to withstand bacterial transmission up to a positive pressure differential of 5 psi.[12] Using pressure-sensitive contact film and resistive strain gauge recordings, Altman and colleagues have demonstrated transmural gown pressures in excess of 60 psi. The areas contaminated most frequently are the upper abdomen and forearms of the operating surgeon. Coincidentally, these areas generate such pressures. The next generation of surgical gowns should be reinforced in these areas to withstand higher transmural pressures.

The material used appears to be equally important in determining the incidence of strike through contamination. Early surgical gowns constructed from cotton were noted by Beck and Carlson to allow free two-way "capillary" passage of bacteria through wet areas of the gown.[13] Smith and Nichols tested 11 types of commercially available gowns and once again demonstrated that only those with impervious plastic reinforcement offer complete protection. They also noted the increased incidence of strike through contamination with procedures of more than 2 hours' duration and blood loss exceeding 100 cc.[14] Members of the high-risk surgical specialties should select gowns that provide protection in accordance with the potential threat/risk posed by the patient population and the procedure to be performed.

Gown cuffs are a particular, additional problem. The need for soft, stretchable material often prevents attainment of the barrier effects achieved by the rest of the gown.

No accepted standards exist for measuring gown effectiveness. Each manufacturer may use a different test or criteria. Not surprisingly, manufacturers tend to choose tests that make their product look the best.

Masks/Caps

Masks and caps have long been a part of surgical attire. Newer masks have been formulated with porosity directed at retarding infection from aerosolized pathogens such as TB and particles that may result from the use of a laser or electrocautery. The selection of a mask and cap is directed at coverage of the mouth, nares, scalp, and facial hair. It also is important that men with minor lacerations or dermatitis resulting from shaving protect these areas. Prompt changing of any head and neck garb that becomes obviously contaminated should provide adequate protection. The aerosolization of viral particles with cautery or laser and subsequent inhalation is an unresolved concern. Viral DNA can become aerosolized and inhaled, but whether particles such as HBV or HIV are viable or can produce infection is unknown.[15]

Eyewear

No case of mucocutaneous HIV transmission has occurred in prospective studies of occupational risk; however, the conjunctiva is vulnerable to numerous viral and bacterial pathogens. Although orthopedic, vascular, and cardiothoracic surgery tend to carry the highest risk of facial contamination, such cases represent only 10% of all blood contacts.[16] Recommendations by the U.S. Occupational Safety and Health Administration that "masks in combination with eye protection devices such as goggles or glasses with solid side shields or chin length face shields shall be worn whenever splash, spray, or spatter of droplets of blood or other potentially infectious materials may be generated and eye, nose, or mouth contamination can be reasonably anticipated" are open to interpretation. Blanket statements concerning the use of eyewear will not achieve 100% compliance and are not feasible. The use of eyewear for the protection it affords should be guided by the risk associated with the procedure to be performed.

Footwear and Accessory Recommendations

Although the lower extremity and foot remain unlikely sites of blood–skin contamination, cases that involve voluminous blood loss or copious irrigation may compromise these areas. Conditions such as dermatitis or tinea pedis may compromise skin integrity and provide portals for infective pathogens. We recommend that knee-high shoe covers or Wellington boots be worn in high-risk cases. The gown should be long enough to cover the top of the boot so that fluids running down the gown or spilling from the table are diverted from entering the boot.

Conclusion

As the shift in emphasis from asepsis to protection from patient pathogens begins to dictate the selection of operative theater garb, complete isolation from patients may be neither attainable nor desirable. The risk of disease transmission from patient to surgeon can be minimized, but not avoided entirely. The economic cost of increasing protective wear must be balanced against this risk.

The inadequacies and compromises of current surgical attire often raise questions about alternative strategies to protect the surgical team. Screening of risk factors by history-taking or actual testing (with informed consent) have been considered. Knowledge of a patient's HIV status, however, has serious drawbacks. First, some studies suggest that such knowledge does not reduce the number of blood contacts. Second, a few patients undergo surgery during the interval when they are HIV-infected, but not yet antibody-positive. These "false-negative" patients still pose a risk to the surgical team. Last, testing is not practical in the emergency setting.

Until better strategies emerge, surgeons performing high-risk procedures or working with high-risk patient populations should strongly consider the following guidelines:

1. Meticulous attention to technique and conduct in the operating theater
2. Immunization against hepatitis B
3. Double gloving and routine glove change after 2 hours or visible glove failure
4. Strike through–resistant reinforced gowns
5. Eyewear with side protection
6. Knee-high footwear
7. Immediate change of contaminated head and neck wear

References

1. Williams TG: The history of operating theatre rituals. *Brit J Theater Nurs* 1989; 26:21–24.
2. McKinney WP, Young HJ: The cumulative probability of occupationally acquired HIV infection: The risk of repeated exposures during a surgical career. *Infect Control Hosp Epidemiol* 1990; 11:243–246.
3. Shanson DC: Risk to surgeons and patients from HIV and hepatitis: Guidelines on precautions and management of exposure to blood or body fluid. *BMJ* 1992; 305:1337–1343.
4. Hu DJ: The risk of hepatitis B infection and other blood borne pathogens in health care settings: A review of risk factors and guidelines for prevention. *Bull World Health Organ* 1991; 69:623–630.
5. Popejoy SL, Fry DE: Blood contact and exposure in the operating room. *Surg Gynecol Obstet* 1991; 172:480–483.
6. Brough SV, Hunt TM, Barrie WW: Surgical glove perforations. *Br J Surg* 1988; 75:317.
7. Centers for Disease Control: HIV infection in health care workers exposed to blood of infected patients. *MMWR* 1987; 36:285–289.
8. Quebbeman EJ, Telford GL, Wadsworth K, et al: Double gloving: Protecting surgeons from blood contamination in the operating room. *Arch Surg* 1992; 127:213–217.
9. Wright JG, McGeer AJ, Chyatte D, et al: Mechanism of glove tears and sharp injuries among surgical personnel. *JAMA* 1991; 266:1668–1671.
10. Maha H, Thompson AM, Rainey JB: Does wearing two pair of gloves protect operating theater staff from skin contamination? *BMJ* 1988; 297:597–598.
11. Beck WC, Collette TS: False faith in the surgeons gown and surgical drape. *Am J Surg* 1952; 83:125–126.
12. Altman KW, McElhaney JH, Moylan JA, et al: Transmural surgical gown pressure measurement in the operating theater. *Am J Infect Control* 1991; 19:147–155.

13. Beck WC, Carlson WW: Aseptic barriers. *Arch Surg* 1963; 87:118–126.
14. Smith JW, Nichols RL: Barrier efficiency of surgical gowns: Are we really protected from our patients' pathogens? *Arch Surg* 1991; 126:756–763.
15. Baggish MW, Poiesz BJ, Joret D, et al: Presence of human immunodeficiency virus DNA in laser smoke. *Lasers Surg Med* 1991; 11:197–203.
16. Centers for Disease Control: Surveillance for occupationally acquired HIV infection. U.S. 1981-1992. *MMWR* 1992; 41:823–825.

Minimally Invasive Surgery

Wendy J. Marshall, M.D.

Associate Professor of Surgery, Stritch School of Medicine; Director, Trauma Services, Loyola University Medical Center, Maywood, Illinois

Considerable debate still surrounds the optimal evaluation of patients with blunt or penetrating abdominal trauma.[1] Although many modalities are available, diagnostic peritoneal lavage remains the "gold standard."[2] Peritoneal lavage, which was developed by Root in 1965, revolutionized the diagnosis of intra-abdominal injury and has an accuracy of 97%. It is overly sensitive, however, and leads to nontherapeutic laparotomies in about 25% of cases. Other modalities began appearing in the early 1980s, and abdominal computed tomographic (CT) scanning now has replaced peritoneal lavage in many centers. Studies indicate that peritoneal lavage and abdominal CT scanning are complementary, and that certain injuries not diagnosed by diagnostic peritoneal lavage can be identified by CT scan.[3, 4] The strength of the abdominal CT scan lies in the identification of retroperitoneal injuries and documentation of the extent of solid organ injury. It is of questionable value for the detection of hollow organ, early pancreatic, and diaphragmatic injuries. In addition, abdominal CT takes time and requires a stable patient who must leave the protective environment of the emergency department to go to the radiology suite. Physical examination, which for many years was thought to be reliable in the evaluation of abdominal injury, has an accuracy rate of only 50%. Many patients with abdominal injury have no symptoms and few physical findings. In one recent report, the morbidity of missed injuries or delayed operation approached 42%.[5] Hemoperitoneum initially causes few or no peritoneal findings, and several hours may pass before the abdominal examination becomes positive. Other techniques that have been used for abdominal evaluation include arteriography and magnetic resonance imaging (MRI). These approaches have the disadvantages, however, of being time-consuming and requiring highly trained personnel during a generally tense, acute situation.

Ultrasound and laparoscopy are two recently developed diagnostic tools. Ultrasound has been used extensively in Europe and both techniques are undergoing clinical trials in the United States. Laparoscopy is one of the newer modalities used in trauma and has been extended into the thorax (thoracoscopy) for the evaluation of intrapleural and diaphragmatic injuries.

History

From a historical perspective, laparoscopy has been the tool of gynecologists. Rudick introduced the technique to general surgeons in the 1930s but it did not gain widespread acceptance until the last decade. Laparoscopic cholecystectomy was the turning point for general surgeons, and laparoscopic techniques and equipment now are advancing at a rapid rate. Laparoscopic cholecystectomy is the preferred technique, but herniorrhaphy, colectomy, Nissen fundoplication and other procedures also may be performed laparoscopically rather than by the traditional open technique. George Berci was one of the pioneers in the use of laparoscopic techniques in trauma patients and his initial writings and teachings in the 1980s were not appreciated until recently.[6,7] He expressed concern regarding the high sensitivity but low specificity of peritoneal lavage and the high rate of nontherapeutic laparotomy. He believed that a "quick laparoscopic check" would assess the abdomen more accurately, and maintains this belief today.

Laparoscopy has traditionally been performed in the operating room and has required numerous personnel (e.g., anesthesia agents, nurses, technicians) and expensive and extensive equipment. Because this approach is time-consuming and not particularly economical compared with diagnostic peritoneal lavage, laparoscopy is being studied for use in emergency department evaluation.[8] The initial studies of laparoscopy were performed in the operating room and its accuracy was confirmed at laparotomy. The success of this technique in several centers, led to a reduction in the surgical staff required, and the procedure is now performed under local anesthesia in the emergency department.[8,9]

Livingston prospectively evaluated diagnostic laparotomy before celiotomy in patients with blunt and penetrating injuries.[10] He found the

TABLE 1.
Review of Trauma Laparoscopy*

Primary Author	Year	No. of Patients	Type of Injury
Gazzaniga	1976	37	Mixed
Carnevale	1977	20	Penetrating
Berci	1991	150	Blunt
Sosa	1992	8	Penetrating
Salvino	1993	75	Mixed
Fabian	1993	182	Mixed
Ivatury	1993	100	Penetrating

*From Gadacz T: *Surgical Rounds* 1993; 743. Used by permission.

procedure easy to perform and without complications and noted that laparoscopy decreased the need for celiotomy in selected patients. He did demonstrate technical difficulty in running the small bowel, visualizing the spleen, and evaluating intra-abdominal hemorrhage exceeding 750 cc.

Townsend and colleagues evaluated diagnostic laparoscopy in patients with blunt abdominal trauma.[11] They also found it to be a safe technique, and an effective adjunct to the diagnostic workup.

Salvino prospectively evaluated patients before CT scanning and peritoneal lavage with laparoscopy performed in the emergency department under local anesthesia.[9] He reported that it was safe and relatively pain-free, and that the results changed the treatment plan in 25% of cases.

Several authors have studied and confirmed the value of laparoscopy in penetrating and blunt injuries of the diaphragm.[12, 13] Others have evaluated the role of laparoscopy in defeating flank and retroperitoneal hematomas, with favorable results. Ivatury evaluated laparoscopy for penetrating abdominal wounds and concluded that it was an excellent modality and led to celiotomies for diaphragmatic injuries that otherwise would have been difficult to identify.[14]

Many authors cite the advantages of diagnostic laparoscopy in penetrating abdominal wounds. Although repeated examination or peritoneal lavage is probably the optimal technique for the evaluation of anterior abdominal stab wounds, some controversy surrounds the interpretation of lavage data. Laparoscopy may resolve this question. Laparoscopy performed through a separate incision with closure of the anterior abdominal stab wound may disclose peritoneal penetration or organ injury. If the test is done in the emergency department under local anesthesia, patients may be released and spared a hospital admission.

Early and aggressive nutrition is of paramount importance in trauma patients and the enteral route is preferred. Percutaneous endoscopic gastrostomy has revolutionized the delivery of enteral formulas. Sometimes, however, this is not possible. Laparoscopy provides an alternate approach. Using this technique, a jejunostomy can be placed to allow enteral feedings. This is an example of therapeutic laparoscopy and its use in injured patients.[15, 16]

As part of a multicenter study, Cuschieri compared mini-laparoscopy with peritoneal lavage in blunt abdominal trauma and confirmed that both tests were highly sensitive, with an accuracy rate of 100%.[17] The specificity was 83% for peritoneal lavage and 94% for diagnostic laparoscopy. The predicted value of a positive laparoscopy was 92% compared with 72% for peritoneal lavage. These data are similar to those from studies being performed in the United States.

Although diagnostic laparoscopy is a new technique in the evaluation of abdominal trauma, data support its role in the detection of specific injuries or as an adjunct to either CT scanning or peritoneal lavage. In certain situations, it decreases the incidence of nontherapeutic laparotomy.[18]

Technique

Laparoscopy has traditionally been performed in the operating room. In the operating room, the overall management of the patient is similar to other general surgical cases. If laparoscopy is performed in the emergency department, there are additional considerations. A cooperative patient is needed and, in most cases, intravenous sedation is required. The equipment should be easily accessible on a portable cart with prepackaged instruments. The pneumoperitoneum should be established by either CO_2 or nitrous oxide and back-up tanks should be available. Local anesthesia should be injected at the mini-laparotomy incision or where the Veress needle is to be inserted. Customized packs improve efficiency.

After appropriate skin preparation, gravity is used to position the patient to facilitate visualization. Both insufflation pressures and the patient's vital signs require monitoring. Trocar placement depends on expected injuries, but the surgical technique remains the same regardless of whether general or local anesthesia is used. The approach is either to place a Veress needle or to make an open incision at or just below the umbilicus. Three to 4 L of either CO_2 or nitrous oxide is instilled to create an intra-abdominal pressure of about 15 mm Hg. It is important that the rate of insufflation should be slower in patients who are not under general anesthesia. Either a 10-mL or a 5-mL trocar is inserted through the umbilical opening and a second 5-mL trocar may be placed in an appropriate position for retraction or movement of the bowel. The 5-mL laparoscope may be needed in the subcostal area to improve visualization of the diaphragmatic region and, in some situations, a 30-degree scope may be required. Some authors favor the use of the 10-mL laparoscope through the umbilical opening because visualization is improved.[9] Once the laparoscope and trocars have been placed, a systematic inspection of the abdominal cavity is undertaken. Throughout the procedure, the patient should be monitored by pulse oximetry and vital signs to ensure that respiratory distress is not developing and that an occult diaphragmatic injury does not present as a tension pneumothorax. Movement of the patient on the operating table or stretcher can facilitate visualization of certain areas of the abdominal cavity. In the unanesthetized patient, nasogastric tube decompression and an indwelling Foley catheter will decrease complications and facilitate visualization of the abdominal contents.

Complications

As does any invasive procedure, laparoscopy has potential complications, some of which are specific to the trauma patient. The major problem is tension pneumothorax resulting from an unsuspected diaphragmatic injury. This has been reported by several authors, emphasizing the necessity of careful monitoring.[13] Gas embolization is another potential complication. This has not been described in diagnostic laparoscopy for trauma, but is possible in the presence of either major venous or hepatic injuries. If gas embolization is suspected, the patient should be quickly positioned with the right side up and any air in the heart should be aspirated. Other reported complications include ureteral injury, aortic laceration, and obvious complications from the trocar insertion.[19] Relative contraindications to the use of laparoscopy include patients with previous incisions and pregnancy. Iatrogenic complications increase in these situations.

Laparoscopy in the trauma setting should not be performed by an inexperienced laparoscopist. Familiarity with the equipment and the technique is necessary so the procedure can be performed expeditiously. Throughout the procedure, the patient should be monitored closely for any complications. If laparoscopy is being performed in the emergency department, an operating room should be immediately available.

Gasless Laparoscopy

A gasless laparoscopic system is being studied to determine whether it will reduce complications and facilitate the use of conventional surgical instruments. One of the potential problems with a gasless system is that it requires general anesthesia because of significant peritoneal retraction and, therefore, may not be of value in the emergency department setting. Smith evaluated this system in 58 patients, 27 of whom underwent trauma-related procedures.[20] The 27 cases of abdominal trauma included 11 gunshot wounds, 11 stab wounds, and 5 blunt injuries, and celiotomy was believed to be unnecessary in 20 cases (74%). Smith commented that the exposure was similar to laparoscopy using gas insufflation and reported one major and two minor complications. This system was believed to have other advantages, but further studies are necessary to delineate its role in the overall treatment of patients with abdominal trauma.

Pediatric Laparoscopy

Laparoscopic surgery has been performed widely in adults, but few investigators have discussed its therapeutic or diagnostic use in children. It is being used by some pediatric surgeons in selected cases and appears to be a valuable option in certain situations. Several factors must be taken into consideration when laparoscopy is used in children, particularly those weighing less than 25 kg.[21]

Laparoscopic instruments and technique require modification for pediatric application. A wider selection of smaller-caliber laparoscopes is necessary. Scopes with a caliber of 5 mL are used for laparoscopic hernia repair in children and a combination of 2-mL and 5-mL ports should be considered for the evaluation of pediatric abdominal trauma. Insufflation pressures should be limited to 7 to 8 mL Hg rather than the 14 to 15 mL Hg used in most adults. Most complications associated with laparoscopic procedures in children are related to pneumoperitoneum and intra-abdominal distention. Respiratory physiologic effects of pneumoperitoneum include alterations in the residual capacity and airway pressures. There is a decrease in systemic venous return and the possibility of subcutaneous emphysema. Children are more sensitive to reflux of gastric contents, which would precipitate aspiration with a pneumoperitoneum. Therefore, use of a nasogastric tube is mandatory. Insufflation should be done with either CO_2 or nitrous oxide. CO_2 is preferred because it does not support combustion, is cheaper, and is more readily available. It has a high absorption capacity across the peritoneum, however, and may increase serum HCO_3 and P_{ACO_2} levels, which may precipitate arrhythmias or hypertension. Hypothermia is a well-recognized problem in the injured child and gas insufflation at normal temperatures causes some heat loss. Rapid exchange of the insufflated gas within the peritoneal cavity can lower the core temperature, and a temperature probe should routinely be used.

No data support the role of diagnostic laparoscopy in children with blunt abdominal trauma. As we become more comfortable with the technique in children, however, it should remain a consideration for the future.

Thoracoscopy

The Swedish internist Jacobaeus initially described laparoscopy, and, in 1910, also provided the first description of thoracoscopy.[22] He originally used thoracoscopy for the diagnosis of interpleural abnormalities and then subsequently for the lysis of tuberculous adhesions.[23] Since the 1930s, thoracoscopy has been used with increasing enthusiasm. The indications for this technique have increased dramatically in the last 5 years and have been expanded to the evaluation of thoracic and diaphragmatic injuries. Prospective data now show advantages to a thoracoscopic approach in some traumatic situations. A rigid or flexible bronchoscope was used in the early stages of thoracoscopy, but instruments for evaluating the pleural space have improved. Because of the advances in endoscopic instrumentation, thoracoscopy has been used in the evaluation of thoracic injuries, including persistent air leaks, chylothorax, decortication, and, in particular, diaphragmatic injuries.[24]

Ochsner prospectively evaluated thoracoscopy in the diagnosis of diaphragmatic injuries and found it to be safe and to have extremely high sensitivity and specificity.[25] Thoracoscopy is generally performed in the operating room with the patient intubated, and a biluminal endotracheal tube may be advantageous. The patient is positioned in the right or left lateral decubitus position and the equipment is placed so that visualization of the video monitors is uninterrupted. Standard endoscopy equipment, including a 0-degree and a 30-degree endoscope, should be available, and placement of the trocars is determined by the presumed site of injury. If the thoracoscopic procedure is being undertaken for diagnosis, only a single trocar is necessary. Generally, however, two trocars are placed: one in the third, fourth, or fifth intercostal space along the anterior axillary line, and the second at the seventh or eighth intercostal space in the middle to posterior axillary line. This approach allows the visualization of most of the hemithorax. Insufflation with either CO_2 or nitrous oxide at a pressure of 6 to 10 mL of Hg is usually all that is required. The patient is monitored for hemodynamic instability by vital signs and pulse oximetry. Care must be taken with the use of electrocautery in the thoracic cavity, particularly near nerve structures. Bipolar electrocautery is preferable because the current is better controlled.

Few studies have been conducted on the use of thoracoscopy in the injured patient. It does appear to be useful in the evaluation and perhaps treatment of recurrent pneumothorax,[26] in thoracoscopic decortication, in the evaluation and treatment of chylothorax,[27] in the early evacuation of hemothorax (with prevention of a potential empyema), and in diagnostic evaluation of the mediastinal structures.

Many centers are using thoracoscopy in the initial treatment of recurrent spontaneous pneumothorax, with excellent results.[28] Thoracoscopic decortication is useful because adhesions can be divided, the pleural cavity can be cleaned out with minimal complications, and the lung tissue can be completely reexpanded. Chylothorax, an unusual complication of trauma, can be controlled with either fibrin glue or staple ligation of the thoracic duct.[28]

A persistent hemothorax with incomplete evacuation of the pleural space is a harbinger of empyema, and the treatment options range from early to late decortication. Successful evacuation by early thoracoscopy has been described and is a simpler procedure that provides adequate drainage with fewer complications than thoracotomy.[29]

Diaphragmatic injuries from both blunt and penetrating trauma are difficult to diagnose, and several authors report the successful use of laparoscopy in evaluating the diaphragm from a thoracic approach.[25, 30] Thoracoscopy has several benefits in the injured patient. It is a less invasive procedure that has minimal complications and superior diagnostic capabilities. The improved magnification and visualization through smaller incisions are superior to open procedures. Postoperative recovery is associated with less pain, fewer pulmonary complications, and a shorter hospital stay. The use of laparoscopy in injured patients is relatively new, and randomized clinical trials providing useful data are limited. The thoracic surgical literature is replete with evidence of the usefulness and safety of thoracoscopy, but caution must be exercised in extrapolating these data to the injured patient. Trauma surgeons need to develop thoracoscopic techniques and to improve the available instruments. Thoracoscopy holds great potential in the evaluation and diagnosis of trauma patients, however, and controlled prospective studies are warranted to evaluate its role fully.

Summary

Laparoscopy and thoracoscopy have undergone tremendous change since their introduction in the early 20th century. Dr. George Berci was a pioneer in the development of laparoscopy and deserves credit for his role in introducing this technique. Many authors since his time have developed and performed well-controlled clinical trials to evaluate its role. Laparoscopy is a valuable adjunct in the treatment of patients with blunt abdominal trauma and has expanded from a technique used only in the operating room to a bedside procedure that can be done in the emergency department. Its safety and cost-effectiveness in the present health care climate of cost containment is impressive. Caution must be exercised, however, because emergency laparoscopy should not be performed by the inexperienced and strict surgical principles must be followed to avoid endangering patients for the sake of new technology.

Laparoscopy should move beyond diagnosis in trauma to play a role in therapy. Using currently available instruments, it should prove useful in such procedures as diaphragmatic repair, enterotomy, gastric stapling, and injection of hemostatic agents. Thoracoscopy is a newer technique and requires further clinical evaluation. It also should prove valuable, however, as an adjunct to thoracic CT scanning, and may become the preferred surgical option in selected cases.

References

1. Colucciello SA: Blunt abdominal trauma. *Emerg Med Clin North Am* 1993; 11:107–123.
2. Root HD, Hauser CW, McKinley CR, et al: Diagnostic peritoneal lavage. *Surgery* 1965; 57:633–637.
3. Fabian TC, Mangiante EC, White TJ, et al: A prospective study of 91 patients undergoing both computed tomography and peritoneal lavage following blunt abdominal trauma. *J Trauma* 1986; 26:602–608.
4. Sorkey AJ, Farnell MB, Williams HJ Jr, et al: The complementary roles of diagnostic peritoneal lavage and computed tomography in the evaluation of blunt abdominal trauma. *Surgery* 1989; 106:794–800.
5. Scalea TM, Phillips TF: Injuries missed at operation. *J Trauma* 1986; 26:602–608.
6. Berci G, Sackier JM, Paz-Partlow M, et al: Emergency laparoscopy. *Am J Surg* 1991; 161:332–335.
7. Wood D, Berci G: Mini-laparoscopy in blunt abdominal trauma. *Surg Endosc* 1988; 2:184–189.
8. Sackier JM: Laparoscopy in the emergency setting. *World J Surg* 1992; 16:1083–1088.
9. Salvino C: The role of diagnostic laparoscopy in the management of trauma patients: A preliminary assessment. *J Trauma* 1993; 34:506–513.
10. Livingston DH: The role of laparoscopy in abdominal trauma. *J Trauma* 1992; 33:471–475.

11. Townsend MC, Flancbaum L, Choban PS, et al: Diagnostic laparoscopy as an adjunct to selective conservative management of solid organ injuries after blunt abdominal trauma. *J Trauma* 1993; 35:647–651.
12. Ivatury RR: Laparoscopy in the evaluation of the intrathoracic abdomen after penetrating injury. *J Trauma* 1992; 33:101–108.
13. Gadacz T: Laparoscopy in abdominal trauma. *Surgical Rounds* 1993; 743.
14. Ivatury RR: A critical evaluation of laparoscopy in penetrating abdominal trauma. *J Trauma* 1993; 34:822–827.
15. Sangster W: Laparoscopic-guided feeding jejunostomy. *Surg Endosc* 1993; 7:308–310.
16. Albrink MH: Laparoscopic feeding jejunostomy. *Surg Endosc* 1992; 6:259–260.
17. Cuschieri A: Diagnosis of significant abdominal trauma after road traffic accidents. *Ann R Coll Surg Engl* 1988; 70:153–155.
18. Oza RN: Aortic laceration—a rare complication of laparoscopy. *J Laparoendosc Surg* 1992; 2:235–237.
19. Fabian TC: A prospective analysis of diagnostic laparoscopy in trauma. *Ann Surg* 1993; 217:557–564.
20. Smith RS: Gasless laparoscopy and conventional instruments. *Arch Surg* 1993; 128.1102–1107.
21. Sucker: Surgical laparoscopy, in *Pediatric Laparoscopy*. Quality Medical Publishing, 1993, pp 457–482.
22. Jacobaeus HC: Possibility of the use of a cystoscope for investigation of serous cavities. *Munch Med Wochenschr* 1910; 57:2090–2092.
23. Jacobaeus HC: The practical importance of thoracoscopy in surgery of the chest. *Surg Gynecol Obstet* 1922; 34:289–296.
24. Mack MJ: Present role of thoracoscopy in the diagnosis and treatment of diseases of the chest. *Ann Thorac Surg* 1992; 54:403–409.
25. Ochsner MG: Prospective evaluation of thoracoscopy for diagnosing diaphragmatic injury in thoracoabdominal trauma: A preliminary report. *J Trauma* 1993; 34:704–709.
26. Hazelrigg SR: Thoracoscopic stapled resection for spontaneous pneumothorax. *J Thorac Cardiovasc Surg* 1993; 105:389–393.
27. Fogli L, Gorini P, Belcastro S: Conservative management of traumatic chylothorax—a case report. *Intensive Care Med* 1993; 19:176–177.
28. Shinai T: Thoracoscopic diagnosis and treatment of chylothorax after pneumonectomy. *Ann Thorac Surg* 1991; 52:306–307.
29. Mancini M, Smith LM, Nein A, et al: Early evacuation of clotted blood in hemothorax using thoracoscopy: Case reports. *J Trauma* 1993; 34:144–147.
30. Feliciano DV: The diagnostic and therapeutic approach to chest trauma. *Semin Thorac Cardiovasc Surg* 1992; 4:156–162.

New Directions and Applications for Extracorporeal Cardiopulmonary Support

H. Neal Reynolds, M.D.

Intensivist, Assistant Professor of Medicine, Co-Director, Extracorporeal Lung Assist Program, Department of Critical Care, University of Maryland School of Medicine, R. Adams Cowley Shock Trauma Center, Baltimore, Maryland

Nadar Habashi, M.D.

Intensivist, Assistant Professor of Medicine, Co-Director, Extracorporeal Lung Assist Program, Department of Critical Care, University of Maryland School of Medicine, R. Adams Cowley Shock Trauma Center, Baltimore, Maryland

Ulf Borg, B.S.

Research Associate, Co-Director, Extracorporeal Lung Assist Program, Department of Critical Care, University of Maryland School of Medicine, R. Adams Cowley Shock Trauma Center, Baltimore, Maryland

Recent advances in extracorporeal cardiopulmonary technology and a rapid trend away from high tidal volume, high airway pressure ventilatory support has generated renewed interest in extracorporeal lung assistance. The primary purpose of this chapter is to review and update applications of extracorporeal lung assistance for the traumatized or critically ill patient. The secondary focus is to review other applications, which are generically referred to as extracorporeal support. Such applications include support of patients with cardiogenic shock, hypothermia, refractory cardiac arrest, repair of traumatic aortic rupture, and transplantation. Although the indications vary greatly, the technology is substantially the same. Therefore, with the same skill level and similar equipment, an extracorporeal cardiopulmonary support program could have much wider applicability than a simple "one organ support" approach.

Historical Perspective

Acute Respiratory Failure and Ventilatory Support

Patients with the adult respiratory distress syndrome (ARDS) represent a large percentage of patients who may require extracorporeal lung assistance. According to National Institutes of Health (NIH) estimates,[1] ARDS afflicts about 150,000 individuals annually. The mortality rate has been estimated to range from 30% to 90%,[2,3] with a typical rate of 50%.[4] Although the first formal description of ARDS was provided by Ashbaugh and Petty[5] more than a quarter of a century ago, no specific therapeutic modality has evolved that has a conclusive impact on survival. Traditional management strategy for severe respiratory failure includes ventilatory support adequate to achieve "normal" $Paco_2$, Pao_2, and arterial pH. Despite typical spontaneous tidal volumes of about 7 mL/kg, positive-pressure ventilation has been used with tidal volumes of 10 to 15 mL/kg.[6] In addition, respiratory rates have been adjusted to achieve normocarbia of arterial blood with little regard for resultant high peak airway pressures. There is increasing evidence that "traditional ventilatory support" has deleterious effects on lung parenchyma and function. In 1985, Dreyfuss and colleagues demonstrated that epithelial lesions, hyaline membranes, and protein-rich alveolar fluid developed during relatively high inflation pressure ventilation.[7] In further studies by this group[8] in 1988 and by Bowton and associates[9] in 1989, large tidal volumes were correlated more with alveolar injury than were high airway pressures. Earlier studies by Woo and Hedley-White in 1972 revealed greater lung water accumulation, a fourfold increase in pulmonary macrophages, and intravascular leukocytes during large tidal volume ventilation in a canine model.[10] Others found reduced pulmonary compliance after cyclic lung distention, which was directly related to tidal volume and duration of ventilation.[11,12] Recently, Gattinoni and colleagues demonstrated reduced functional lung tissue in patients with ARDS and further described the remaining lung volume as equivalent to the volume of "baby lungs."[13-15] In effect, using positive pressure–generated tidal volumes of 10 to 15 mL/kg in lungs that may functionally be reduced by half could yield at least a fourfold overdistention of the normal alveoli. If the animal data of Dreyfuss, Woo, and others applies to humans, "traditional" tidal volumes may cause lung lesions pathophysiologically indistinguishable from the underlying ARDS. This implies that traditional tidal volumes alone may cause, amplify, or sustain acute lung injury. This process of large tidal volume–related lung injury has come to be known as "volutrauma."[9]

Oxygenation is maintained by positive end-expiratory pressure (PEEP) and supplemental oxygen. Although it remains controversial, considerable animal data suggest that high concentrations of oxygen may be deleterious. As early as 1783, Lavoisier described inflammatory effects of oxygen, with pulmonary consolidation and congestion.[16] More recently, Hayatdavoudi and associates found perivascular edema, decreased pulmonary compliance, decreased alveolar air volume, and increased alveolar macrophages in rats exposed to 60% oxygen.[17] Adult rats exposed to 100% oxygen tend to die within 2 to 3 days, but may adapt to high concentrations of oxygen if they are exposed to 85% oxygen first.[18, 19] Although the lowest safe level of supplemental oxygen is unknown and there are no conclusive human data about oxygen toxicity. Therefore, high-level oxygen exposure should be minimized whenever possible.[20, 21]

Traditional mechanical ventilation also has complications. Macroscopically visible pulmonary barotrauma occurs in 8% to 88% of mechanically ventilated patients.[22, 23] Specifically, pulmonary interstitial emphysema has been noted in 88% of patients with ARDS, whereas free intrathoracic air was found in 8%. Hepatic blood flow,[24] urinary output, renal blood flow,[25] and cardiac output[26] may all be decreased by positive-pressure ventilation. A less common complication of mechanical ventilation is systemic gas embolism.[27]

Some have suggested a direct etiologic relationship between the development of advanced ventilatory support and the emergence of ARDS.[28] In 1963, Teplitz stated that ". . . ARDS . . . is the result of iatrogenic modifications of the pathology of noncardiogenic pulmonary edema," and that the ". . . pathology of acute respiratory insufficiency . . . had its advent at precisely the same time that blood gases became available for monitoring . . . pulmonary intensive care units were first established . . . (which) dates back to around 1963."[29]

Current goals of ventilatory support are to minimize iatrogenic lung injury, provide respiratory support in a more physiologic manner, and allow "lung rest" when necessary.[30] Options to achieve relative lung rest include permissive hypercapnia. Permissive hypercapnia involves a deliberate effort to limit peak inspiratory pressures and tidal volumes while accepting a compensated hypercapnia as the trade-off.[31, 32] Hickling and associates reported a 16% mortality rate among 50 patients with ARDS who had a predicted mortality rate of 39%.[33] Peak inspiratory pressures were kept at less than 40 cm H_2O and tidal volumes were kept as low as 5 mL/kg, with a resultant mean $Paco_2$ of 62 mm Hg. Others also have questioned the need to achieve "normal" $Paco_2$ if the price is potentially damaging ventilatory support.[34, 35] When permissive hypercapnia fails or acute lung injury is so severe that both oxygen and carbon dioxide exchange are inadequate, it becomes increasingly difficult to avoid ventilator-induced lung injury. Under such circumstances, extracorporeal lung assistance may be indicated.

Extracorporeal Life Support

The historical development of extracorporeal lung assistance has been well described by Bartlett,[36] Lillehei,[37] Gott,[38] Heiss,[39] and others. In review, the ancestor of current extracorporeal lung assistance devices was first developed by John Gibbon and subsequently was used in 1954 as a heart-lung machine during the repair of an atrial secundum defect.[40, 41] Oxygenation of blood was established through direct exposure of blood to gaseous oxygen. The subsequent evolution of the bubble oxygenator by DeWall and Lillehei rapidly accelerated the development of open heart surgery and short-term perfusion.[42] It became evident, however, that sustained support with early heart-lung machines was toxic and perhaps lethal. Lee and associates[43] and Dobell and colleagues[44] demonstrated that the toxic effects of bubble oxygenators resulted from direct blood–gas exposure. The development of the membrane oxygenator in 1956 eliminated or reduced the direct exposure of blood to oxygen, thereby minimizing toxicity.[45] Specifically, Clowes and coworkers used a low-efficiency polyethylene membrane requiring large surface areas to achieve adequate gas exchange. The silicon rubber membrane, developed a year later, was at least ten times more efficient at gas exchange.[46] Within 6 years, Kolobow and others developed blood oxygenators with coiled silicon rubber membranes that completely eliminated direct blood–gas interface.[47] In the early 1970s, White and colleagues published the clinical results of prolonged extracorporeal support in humans.[48] The first adult survivor of extracorporeal membrane oxygenation (ECMO), however, was reported in 1972 by Hill and associates,[49] followed by the first neonatal survivor, who was described by Bartlett and coworkers[50] in 1975. After preliminary studies, the NIH sponsored a multi-institutional comparative trial of ECMO vs. traditional ventilatory management for acute respiratory failure.[51] This study failed to show improved survival with ECMO (9.8% vs. 8.3% with conventional treatment) and severely dampened enthusiasm for extracorporeal lung assistance. The NIH study failed to meet its goal of 300 patients, however, and was discontinued after enrolling only 92 subjects. Nine institutions were involved, several of which had no previous experience with ECMO. Technical problems were a major cause of morbidity and mortality. A national epidemic of influenza was in progress during the study, with more than 50% of the treated patients having an infectious pneumonia. Finally, the patients were subjected to prolonged high-level ventilatory support before the initiation of ECMO and did not have uniform reduction of ventilatory support once they were receiving ECMO.[52] Ultimately, the validity of the ECMO comparative trial, particularly in light of new technology, is in question.

Recent studies by Anderson, Bartlett, and others have shown significantly better patient outcome.[53, 54] Specifically, in a group of patients with an expected 90% mortality, Anderson reported 45% survival. The improved survival appears to be the result of better patient selection, shorter duration of previous ventilatory support, and a veno-venous approach with low-pressure ventilation while receiving ECMO. Most recently, Falke reported survival as high as 80% for patients with ARDS when extracorporeal lung assistance is used as part of a progressive stepped care approach.[55]

In 1978, Kolobow and coworkers demonstrated that total body carbon dioxide production could be removed with only 10% to 30% of the cardiac output and oxygenation could be maintained by the native lungs.[56] In effect, the processes of oxygenation and carbon dioxide removal could be functionally separated. In 1986, Gattinoni and colleagues reported the results of low-frequency positive-pressure ventilation with extracorporeal CO_2 removal in severe acute respiratory failure (LFPPV-ECCO$_2$R).[57] Survival was 48.8% in a group of patients with an expected 90% mortality. Although the Gattinoni report was not controlled, used historical mortality comparisons, and involved only 43 patients, it has served to dramatically redirect the approach of extracorporeal lung assistance. Many reports have appeared since by authors such as Mottaghy and coworkers,[58] Dorrington and associates,[59] and Zobel and colleagues[60] regarding the efficacy of extracorporeal CO_2 removal in animal models. Clinical reports also have appeared demonstrating the efficacy of ECCO$_2$R.[61–63] The largest series of patients treated with ECCO$_2$R was described by Müller and Lennartz and originated from Marburg, Germany. As of 1991, 58 of 114 patients (50.1%) supported with ECCO$_2$R survived despite a predicted mortality of 90% to 100%.[64] There was a trend toward greater survival when heparin-bonded circuitry was used compared to circuitry not treated with heparin (56.2% vs. 46.9%, respectively). Finally, a study funded by the National Heart, Lung and Blood Institute to compare the outcome of patients with ARDS treated with LFPPV-ECCO$_2$R vs. pressure-controlled ventilation was completed in 1991. No difference in outcome was reported with either modality.[65] Reduction in peak airway pressures was documented in only 10 of 22 ECCO$_2$R-treated patients, however, and only for brief periods. Furthermore, the study may suffer from selection bias (40 patients were chosen from 249 candidates) and confounding variables of permissive hypercapnia, computer protocols, traditional ventilatory management, and ECCO$_2$R.

Over the last decade, several significant technical advances have occurred, including the development of high-efficiency microporous membrane lungs, heparin surface bonding technology, and computerized servo-control pump systems. The primary membrane lung for application in ECMO and ECCO$_2$R has been the silicon rubber polymer. Silicon rubber, a lipid, is freely permeable to oxygen, carbon dioxide, and anesthetic gases. According to Zapol and Kolobow, gas is transported through the solid membrane by dissolution into the membrane on the gas phase side, "activated" diffusion through the membrane, and then deabsorption into the blood.[66] Carbon dioxide is many times more soluble than is oxygen (i.e., silicon rubber is "perm-selective"). The silicon membrane lung has a CO_2 transport of about 75 mL/min/m^2.[67] Newer microporous membranes, with heterogenous pore sizes from 0.01 to 1.00 µm, have a carbon dioxide transfer rate of 125 mL/min/m^2.[68] The net effect is equivalent CO_2 clearance with smaller membrane lungs and, therefore, less extracorporeal blood volume. The trade-off in using the microporous membrane lungs is shorter survival of the membrane lungs as a result of plasma leakage.[69]

The recent evolution of heparin surface bonding to cardiopulmonary circuitry and membrane lungs may ultimately reduce bleeding complications during ECMO or ECCO$_2$R.[70–72] Knoch and coworkers noted less blood loss, fewer bleeding complications, and reduced erythrocyte transfusion requirements when heparin-treated systems were used.[73] Others demonstrated successful extracorporeal circulation without systemic heparin when heparin-coated systems were used.[74] Although they are not approved by the U.S. Food and Drug Administration for long-term extracorporeal use, many European centers use the heparin-treated microporous membrane lung for ECMO or $ECCO_2R$.

Mechanically, servo-regulated blood pumps such as the Stöckert computer-aided perfusion system can improve control, reduce circuit complexity, and perhaps ultimately reduce the risks associated with extracorporeal circulation.

In summary, with therapeutic goals redirected toward $ECCO_2R$ and lung rest, the development of veno-venous technology, earlier patient selection, and improvements in technology, interest in extracorporeal life support has been renewed.

Nomenclature for Extracorporeal Life Support

The current nomenclature and collection of acronyms is confusing. The following is offered to define the various modalities and make distinctions. Oxygen delivery is highly flow-dependent, whereas carbon dioxide removal is much less so. Therefore, the real difference between $ECCO_2R$ and ECMO is the flow rate.

ECMO is designed to provide pulmonary or cardiopulmonary support, depending on patient needs and available modalities. ECMO implies relatively high extracorporeal blood flow rates (as much as 80% of cardiac output) to satisfy oxygen needs. ECMO may be accomplished through veno-venous or veno-arterial routes.

$ECCO_2R$ is an extracorporeal pulmonary support modality with the goal of removing all or a substantial portion of the total body CO_2 production while oxygenating through the native lungs. $ECCO_2R$ implies a relatively low blood flow rate (1.0 to 2.5 L/min) and, generally, veno-venous application. Concurrent ventilatory support can greatly be reduced such that minimal CO_2 is removed through the native lungs. At low blood flow rates, extracorporeal oxygen delivery is minimal.

$LFPPV\text{-}ECCO_2R$ initially was described by Gattinoni and emphasizes "lung rest" through the use of very–low-frequency ventilation in conjunction with an extracorporeal circuit for the removal of carbon dioxide. In general usage, the acronym $ECCO_2R$ implies $LFPPV\text{-}ECCO_2R$. In this chapter, $ECCO_2R$ is used as a abbreviation of $LFPPV\text{-}ECCO_2R$.

Partial extracorporeal carbon dioxide removal ($PECO_2R$) involves an extracorporeal circuit used strictly for partial pulmonary assistance in the removal of carbon dioxide. $PECO_2R$ implies low blood flow rates (0.5 to 1.0 L/min), with the goal of removing a fraction of the total body CO_2 production while delivering insignificant amounts of oxygen. $PECO_2R$ requires significant concurrent traditional ventilatory support, complete oxygenation through the native lungs, and substantial clearance in CO_2 through the native lungs. The benefit of $PECO_2R$ is reduction in ventilator airway pressure and barotrauma.

Extracorporeal lung assistance implies lung assistance such as $ECCO_2R$ or partial oxygen support through ECMO using midrange extracorporeal blood flow rates (arbitrary range, 1.0 to 5.0 L/min).

Extracorporeal lung (life) support is a generic term introduced by Bartlett to include all types of extracorporeal support.

Partial heart-lung bypass provides both hemodynamic and pulmonary support. Depending on the indications and equipment available within a particular institution, partial heart-lung bypass may be essentially identical to veno-arterial ECMO.

As indicated in Figure 1, there are two primary distinctions between the various modalities: (1) blood flow rate, and (2) the availability of hemodynamic support. In practice, the clinician determines whether hemodynamic support is indicated. If it is not, a veno-venous approach is adequate. If hemodynamic support is necessary, a veno-arterial approach is required. The blood flow rate is determined by the degree of lung disease and the

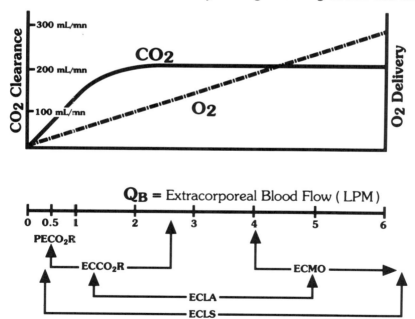

FIG 1.
Relative ranges of extracorporeal life support modalities. Carbon dioxide clearance assumes "sweep gas" is adjusted to keep $Paco_2$ about 40 mm Hg as blood gas (Q_B) is increased. $PECO_2R$ = partial extracorporeal CO_2 removal; $ECCO_2R$ = extracorporeal CO_2 removal; ECLA = extracorporeal lung assistance; ECMO = extracorporeal membrane oxygenation; ECLS = extracorporeal life support; LPM = liters per minute.

ability of the native lungs to supply oxygen partially. The more severe is the lung disease, the less oxygen is supplied through the native lungs and the greater is the extracorporeal blood flow rate.

Patient Selection Criteria and Applications

Respiratory Failure Caused by Diffuse Acute Lung Disease

Selection criteria vary somewhat from institution to institution. The primary criterion is a reasonable chance of reversing the underlying disease causing the respiratory failure. The clinical problem dictates specific selection criteria. If the major clinical problem is inability of the lungs to exchange gas, the National Heart, Lung and Blood Institute study criteria may be adopted[51]: (1) fast entry—Pa_{O_2} <50 mm Hg for more than 2 hours when measured at an FI_{O_2} of 1.0 with PEEP of 5 cm H_2O or more; or (2) slow entry—after 48 hours of maximal medical therapy, Pa_{O_2} <50 mm Hg for more than 12 hours when measured at an FI_{O_2} of 0.6 or greater with a PEEP of 5 cm H_2O or more and a right-to-left shunt exceeding 30%.

Anderson and colleagues used a combination of criteria that screened for patients with failure of gas exchange and risk of ventilator-induced lung injury.[53] Criteria included (1) transpulmonary shunt >30%, (2) Pa_{CO_2} >45 mm Hg after optimal ventilator adjustment and without exceeding a peak inspiratory pressure of 50 cm H_2O, (3) compliance <0.5 mL/kg/cm H_2O, and (4) potential for reversibility as measured by age <60 years and fewer than 6 days of mechanical ventilation. Absolute contraindications include terminal disease, severe neurologic impairment, heparin contraindications, and mechanical ventilation for more than 10 days. Gattinoni used the NIH "ECMO entry" criteria, with the addition that the total static lung compliance must be lower than 30 mL/cm H_2O.[57] Unlike Bartlett and associates, the duration of pulmonary insult and patient age were not considered to be exclusions.

Our criteria include estimates of gas exchange failure and admission criteria based on the potential for high-pressure or high-volume lung injury.

Gas exchange failure criteria include

1. Transpulmonary shunt >30%
2. Compliance <0.5 mL/kg/cm H_2O (ideal weight)
3. NIH ECMO fast entry criteria

The potential for ventilator-induced lung injury is determined by the following:

1. Failure of permissive hypercapnia as defined by inability to limit peak airway pressure to less than 40 cm H_2O despite compensated hyper-

capnia as high as 100 mm Hg. Peak pressures generally are limited by using tidal volumes of 5 to 7 mL/kg or less
2. Sustained peak airway pressure greater than 40 cm H_2O and contraindication to permissive hypercapnia such as intracranial hypertension or renal failure with inadequate renal compensation to hypercarbia (pH <7.20)
3. Significant pulmonary barotrauma to include recurrent pneumothorax, despite peak airway pressures maintained at <30 to 35 cm H_2O

Contraindications to ECMO/ECCO$_2$R include

1. Age >65 years
2. Known terminal disease
3. High-level ventilatory support for more than 7 days
4. Contraindication to heparin (relative contraindication)
5. Immune suppression
6. Inability to achieve adequate vascular access

Other applications of ECMO/ECCO$_2$R are selected based on criteria relevant to the specific disease. The following list of applications is not inclusive, since new indications evolve.

Respiratory Failure Resulting From Status Asthmaticus

At least 2,000 adults die of asthma, every year most in status asthmaticus.[75] If traditional medical therapy fails, mechanical ventilation may be necessary. Complications of mechanical ventilation during status asthmaticus are common and appear significantly more often than with mechanical ventilation for other indications.[76] Specifically, Scoggin and associates noted pneumothorax in 30% of asthma patients, pneumonia in 30%, and hypoventilation in 75%, compared with 5%, 5%, and 10%, respectively, of those receiving mechanical ventilation for other conditions.[76, 77] Patients with status asthmaticus who require mechanical ventilation generally have hyperinflation with markedly elevated airway pressures.[78] Furthermore, during status asthmaticus, carbon dioxide clearance may be reduced whereas arterial oxygenation is maintained. Extracorporeal carbon dioxide removal can achieve lung rest and lower airway pressures while correcting ventilatory insufficiency. Several case reports indicate successful outcomes in cases in which medical therapy failed, mechanical ventilation was complicated, and ECCO$_2$R was used early.[79-81] Smales demonstrated reductions in airway pressure from 85 to 40 cm H_2O and in Paco$_2$ from 88.5 mm Hg (11.8 kPa) to "normal" after the initiation of ECCO$_2$R.[81] Extracorporeal blood flow ranged between 0.8 and 2.0 L/min and, in one case, vascular cannulas as small as 16-F were used. In a related application, Pesenti and coworkers used PECO$_2$R to support a patient with bullous emphysema and recurrent pneumothorax.[82] Extracorporeal blood flow was 0.4 to 0.6 L/min, clearing 22% to 40% of the CO$_2$ production.

No accepted criteria have been established for the use of ECCO$_2$R in status asthmaticus. It seems reasonable to consider $ECCO_2R$ when airway pressures are high, ventilation is inadequate, and deterioration is imminent.

Nonpulmonary Indications for Extracorporeal Support

Rewarming After Accidental Hypothermia

Hypothermia, or central body cooling, generally is defined as a core temperature less than 35° C. Mild hypothermia is defined as a core temperature of 33° C to 35° C, moderate hypothermia as a core temperature of 30° C to 33° C, and severe hypothermia as a core temperature of less than 30° C. The true core temperature must be determined, or a reliable estimate made, because exterior or shell temperature may be as much as 20°C cooler.[83] Therefore, temperature measurement at the rectum or mouth may underestimate significantly the true core temperature. Accurate determinations of core temperature may require the use of esophageal electrodes[84] or deep rectal[83] or urinary bladder probes.[85] The "cardiac fibrillatory threshold is 28° C."[86] Ventricular fibrillation at core temperatures of less than 28° C is the principal cause of death and is usually refractory to cardioversion until the core temperature is elevated.[87, 88] Rewarming of the hypothermic patient may be accomplished by external or internal means. External rewarming is associated with peripheral vasodilatation, hypovolemic shock, and paradoxical acidosis during reperfusion.[89] In addition, the classic "after drop," or further decrease in the core temperature with external heating, may be as large as 2° C to 3° C, further aggravating central hypothermia.[90] Therefore, in cases of profound hypothermia, central reheating is preferable. A variety of core rewarming techniques have evolved, including warm gastric lavage,[91] peritoneal lavage,[92] and warm-water enemas. In the past, accidental hypothermia was associated with a survival rate as low as 20%.[84, 93, 94] Cardiopulmonary bypass (CPB) may have contributed significantly to more recent survival rates of 70% after profound hypothermia.[95]

The first application of CPB for central rewarming was reported in 1967.[96] Many reports of the successful use of this technique in hypothermia have appeared since.[97–100] Although no controlled studies have been done, Hauty and colleagues have concluded that "extracorporeal blood rewarming via cardiopulmonary bypass is THE treatment of choice in cases of severe (<20 degrees) hypothermia." Furthermore, Zell and Kurtz suggested that "in arrested hypothermia, and in the nonarrested but unstable patient, extracorporeal rewarming with cardiovascular support by femoral-femoral bypass is the best technique of central rewarming."[101] Currently, CPB is an accepted procedure for rapid central rewarming.[102] The standard protocol, as adopted from Zell and Kurtz, is shown in Figure 2.[101]

With veno-arterial CPB or ECMO, rewarming rates of 3° C to 10° C per hour can be achieved.[96, 102, 103] Bypass should be continued until the core

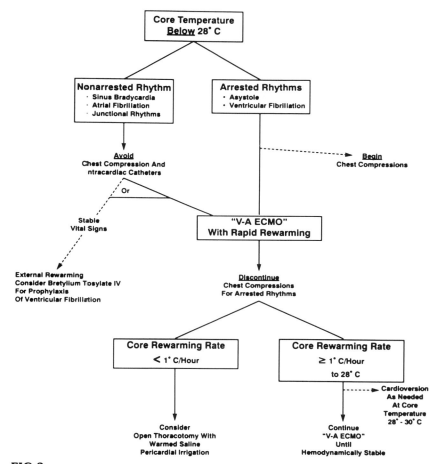

FIG 2.
Protocol for rapid rewarming with partial cardiopulmonary bypass ("V-A ECMO"). (Adapted from Zell SC, Kurtz KJ: Severe exposure hypothermia: A resuscitation protocol. Ann Emerg Med 1985; 14:339–345.)

temperature reaches 30° C to 32° C. In addition to rewarming, CPB can provide hemodynamic support until normal circulation has been restored. For patients with ventricular fibrillation, elective cardioversion can be attempted once the core temperature is well above the fibrillatory threshold.[97, 102]

Repair of Traumatic Rupture of the Aorta

Traumatic rupture of the aorta is common after accidents involving rapid deceleration.[104, 105] As many as 20% of individuals fatally injured in automobile crashes have aortic disruption. Prehospital mortality as high as 85%

has been reported in patients with blunt thoracic aortic disruption.[105] Of those patients who arrive at a medical facility, more than 90% survive long enough to permit diagnostic evaluation.[105] Compared with the heart and aortic arch, the descending aorta is relatively immobile. Distal to the ligamentum arteriosum, the descending aorta is immobilized by intercostal vessels and the pleura. During rapid deceleration, the descending aorta is subject to bending and shearing stresses at the ligamentum arteriosum, resulting in aortic disruption.[106–108]

A dreaded complication of aortic repair is paraplegia. This occurs in 10% to 20% of patients who undergo repair of an aortic disruption. Nine pairs of intercostal arteries arise from the descending aorta that supply branches to the anterior spinal artery.[109] Disruption of the aorta or interruption of flow through the aorta may compromise anterior spinal artery perfusion and lead to paraplegia or paraparesis.

Repair of the aorta generally is accomplished by one of three approaches: (1) cross-clamping of the aorta for proximal and distal control followed by rapid repair without distal aortic perfusion, (2) temporary Gott shunting for distal perfusion,[110] or (3) extracorporeal bypass using a pump and oxygenator.[111, 112] The goal of shunting or bypass is to provide distal perfusion of the abdominal viscera, kidneys, and spinal cord while avoiding proximal hypertension and left ventricular overload. The duration of aortic occlusion, however, usually is shorter with simple aortic cross-clamping.[113] It has been argued that aortic occlusion times less than 30 minutes, which often can be achieved with simple cross-clamping, should minimize the risk of paraplegia.[114] Furthermore, a Gott shunt or extracorporeal bypass may be indicated if a prolonged procedure is anticipated. Despite distal perfusion in these cases, intercostal arteries between clamps would remain underperfused.[115] Fewer neurologic complications have been noted in small series of patients supported with partial bypass.[116] Some investigators have noted improved hemodynamics and less postoperative renal dysfunction when the distal aorta is perfused during cross-clamping.[117] No controlled trial comparing the development of paraplegia with the three modalities has been performed, however.

The Gott shunt may be connected between the ascending aorta, left atrium, or from the left ventricle to the distal aorta. If the patient's native lungs function well, oxygenated blood will be delivered directly into the distal aorta to perfuse the intercostal arteries.

Alternatively, veno-arterial ECMO can rapidly be initiated without prolonging the procedure or increasing surgical exposure. A femoral artery and vein can be cannulated percutaneously using cannulas reinforced with 21-F wire. Extracorporeal blood flow rates of 2.5 to 3.0 L/min are achieved easily. Using veno-arterial ECMO, the distal aorta, intercostal arteries, and, hopefully, anterior spinal artery will be perfused with highly oxygenated blood. With heparin-bonded circuitry, membrane lungs, and "arterial" filters, the use of heparin can be avoided for short perfusion times. Left ventricular afterload can be limited by controlling right ventricular preload, resulting in less hemodynamic instability at the time of aortic clamping and release.

Failure of Cardiopulmonary Resuscitation

Despite the introduction of traditional cardiopulmonary resuscitation (CPR) in 1960,[118] ultimate survival after cardiac arrest remains low. Under optimal conditions, rates of successful resuscitation after brief cardiopulmonary arrest may reach 75%[119] but those after prolonged resuscitation remain dismal. Successful resuscitation and myocardial coronary blood flow both are highly correlated with the coronary perfusion pressure.[120] A coronary perfusion pressure of 15 mm Hg is believed to be the minimal requirement for successful resuscitation in humans.[121] External closed-chest CPR produces low mean arterial pressures and high central venous pressures, resulting in low coronary perfusion pressures.[122, 123] Specifically, Ditchey and colleagues found that ascending aortic pressures and right atrial pressures were "similar," and were associated with minimal coronary blood flow (approximating 1% of the control value before arrest). Open-chest CPR yields improved systemic blood flow,[124] resuscitation,[125] and long-term survival,[126] but may be impractical. With the rapid establishment of partial veno-arterial CPB, however, coronary pressure can be improved, with a mean aortic pressure of 70 mm Hg and a concurrent decrease in the right atrial pressure.[127]

As early as 1976, Mattox and Beall suggested the use of a portable, battery-powered CPB device for resuscitating moribund patients.[128] More recently, using a dog model, Martin and coworkers compared the outcome after prolonged cardiopulmonary arrest resuscitated by traditional CPR vs. CPB.[129] No animal undergoing prolonged CPR survived. All the dogs that received CPB survived, 60% (three of five) without detectable neurologic deficit. Pretto and associates noted similar results, but with less satisfactory neurologic recovery.[130] Others found an additive beneficial effect of epinephrine and CPB.[131]

The outcome in humans after CPB for failed traditional CPR is variable. Overlie and colleagues reported the survival of 6 of 25 patients who underwent portable CPB.[132] They noted improved survival when arrest occurred in the cardiac catheterization laboratory or the intensive care unit. No mention was made of neurologic outcome. In a multicenter study reported by Hill and coworkers involving 187 patients in whom traditional CPR failed, 125 patients underwent CPB.[133] When all causes were included (cardiac and noncardiac), 40 of 187 patients (21.4%) survived. Among the subset of patients with cardiac arrest, 17 (14%) survived more than 30 days. None of those who suffered unwitnessed arrest survived.

CPB may improve the outcome of some patients with witnessed cardiac arrest that occurs under optimal conditions. The necessary skills and equipment for bedside partial CPB and veno-arterial ECMO are essentially identical. Therefore, survival after prolonged CPR may be improved by the assistance of an extracorporeal life support team.

Cardiac Failure and Cardiogenic Shock

When veno-arterial ECMO is applied, substantial blood flow and hemodynamic support can be achieved. When traditional medical therapy or intra-aortic balloon pumping is inadequate for hemodynamic support, veno-arterial ECMO can be instituted rapidly without thoracic incisions. Veno-arterial ECMO, or partial CPB, has the advantage of providing concurrent pulmonary support. There have been many reports of the use of veno-arterial ECMO in the treatment of pediatric cardiac failure[134-136]; these have been reviewed by Zwischenberger and Cox.[137] As of 1992, the pediatric cardiac ECMO registry listed 625 children given cardiac support with ECMO, 47% of whom survived. The most common indication for cardiac support in the pediatric population was inadequate postoperative cardiopulmonary performance. Other indications included cardiomyopathy (4%), cardiac transplantation (4%), and myocarditis (3%). Reedy and associates described 38 adult patients with a mean age of 49 years who were supported with veno-arterial ECMO with an overall survival of 24%.[138] All patients were deemed unresponsive to traditional supportive measures. Initial diagnoses included acute myocardial infarction (12 patients), ischemic coronary disease (15 patients), and cardiomyopathy (7 patients). Blood flow through the ECMO circuit ranged from 2.8 to 6.0 L/min and, once stabilized, averaged about one half the native cardiac output. In addition, McVey and Corke reported successful temporary hemodynamic support after massive propranolol overdose.[139]

Others have suggested that roller pump–driven ECMO increases myocardial wall stress by elevating afterload.[140, 141] Therefore, standard non-pulsatile veno-arterial ECMO may be inappropriate support for the ischemic myocardium. Axelrod and associates suggested that ECMO with "pulsatile blood flow" improves endocardial/epicardial blood flow and myocardial energy metabolism in a dog model.[142] Specifically, a pulsatile blood flow veno-arterial ECMO system designed to create diastolic counterpulsation should be optimal.[143]

The difference between clinical studies and animal studies in regard to the efficacy of veno-arterial ECMO for cardiac support is unclear. Despite conflicting reports, it appears that veno-arterial ECMO may offer an alternative to cardiac support when the underlying process is self-limited or a specific intervention is possible.

Bridge to Transplantation

In general, a patient given ECMO or $ECCO_2R$ for respiratory support should not be concurrently considered for lung transplantation.[144] A commitment to support such a patient given the unpredictable availability of organs is fraught with difficulty. During periods of ECMO or $ECCO_2R$, infections develop, chest tubes are inserted, and vascular access is required, all of which decrease the chances of successful future transplantation. ECMO or $ECCO_2R$ may be beneficial just before transplantation, however, for preoperative correction of an uncompensated respiratory acidosis with an $ECCO_2R$-type focus,[145] or for postoperative support during the "reimplantation response."[146] Many patients who undergo lung transplantation die during the first postoperative week,[147] sometimes as a result of the reimplantation response and not because of rejection. Respiratory failure during the reimplantation response may be profound and refractory to maximal ventilatory support. The reimplantation response, manifested as both functional and radiographic changes, may result from the surgical procedure itself[145] or from reperfusion injury.[148] In either case, the process appears to be reversible; therefore, extracorporeal support is justified for a limited period. Finally, Cooper has suggested a novel application of ECMO in conjunction with transplantation.[144] He states that "ECMO support should be strongly considered for a potential cadaveric donor in whom pulmonary or cardiac status is inadequate . . ." to sustain organ perfusion until organ harvest.

Technique of Extracorporeal Support

Equipment

Details of the technique chosen for extracorporeal support depend on the goals of treatment. If these include hemodynamic support, veno-arterial support with high blood flow rates is necessary. If the goal is minimal oxygen support and primarily CO_2 clearance, low blood flow rates are adequate by the veno-venous route. The hardware used in each case is similar. Institutional techniques have been described in detail elsewhere.[51–53, 57]

No single circuitry is accepted universally. The circuit we use is illustrated schematically in Figure 3. The blood path circuitry is made entirely of polyvinylchloride ⅜-in. internal diameter (I.D.) tubing, with a wall thickness of ⁸⁄₃₂ and Duraflow II heparin surface bonding (Baxter-Bentley, Baxter Healthcare Corporation, Irvine, Calif). All tubing connections are factory-"bonded" to avoid separation. The "raceway" is tygon "Taperflex" (Baxter-Bentley), which allows for tubing diameter transitions from ⅜-in. I.D. to ½-in. I.D. and back to ⅜-in. I.D. without step-up or step-down connectors. A bridge between the drain line and the return line, not shown in the figure, is used for priming and emergencies. During routine operation, the bridge is kept clamped.

A Stöckert-Sorin multiflow roller pump with a Computer-Aided Perfusion System (CAPS); Sorin Biomedical, Irvine, Calif) is used. Blood flow is servo-controlled by the CAPS based on pre-pump and pre-membrane lung pressures. Two Univox gold, 1.8-m², Duraflow II, treated, hollow-fiber membrane lungs (Baxter-Bentley) are arranged in parallel fashion. Before blood is returned to the patient, an in-line device is used as an air trap. During low-flow veno-venous perfusion, a Baxter-Bentley HE-30 cardioplegia "heater" is used; during veno-arterial perfusion, a Baxter-Bentley

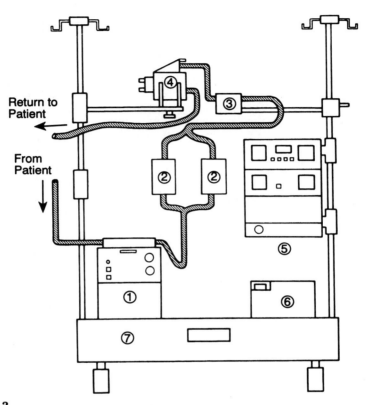

FIG 3.
Extracorporeal cardiopulmonary support *(ECLA)* cart. 1, Multi-speed, servo-controlled roller pump; 2, membrane lungs in parallel geometry; 3, ultrasonic bubble detector; 4, distal air trap or heater; 5, computer-aided perfusion system (CAPS) with pressure, bubble, and level monitors; 6, water heater; and 7, console with battery pack.

AF-1040D adult arterial filter is used. In either case, a bypass around this distal air trap is available to allow component change-out. An attachable ultrasonic bubble monitor and level detector with audible alarms and servo-control of the roller pump is included. Each monitor activates an audible alarm and stops flow in the event of air in the line. The complete perfusion system and console is portable and includes a battery module for 45 minutes of extracorporeal circulatory support.

Each membrane lung has an integral heat exchanger. The heat exchangers are connected in series to a GayMar solid state "T Pump" (Gay-

Mar, Orchard Park, NY) and the blood temperature is continuously monitored and controlled.

"Sweep Gas"

The oxygen supply, or so-called "sweep gas," is temperature-controlled, wall oxygen–delivered through a standard oxygen flow meter. The rate of sweep gas flow is dictated by the patient's arterial Pa_{CO_2} and typically is 2 L/min when the membrane lungs are new and increased incrementally as needed. The blood gases are monitored as shown in Figure 4. The carbon dioxide clearance can be monitored by two techniques. By sampling the blood before and after the membrane lung and applying the Kelman algorithm,[149] CO_2 clearance can be estimated as a function of blood flow, blood temperature, and CO_2 content differences. Alternatively, by monitoring the exhaust gas CO_2 concentration with a mass spectrometer and knowing the gas flow rate, actual CO_2 clearance can be measured. The CO_2 clearance (measured or calculated) may vary widely because of the patient's metabolic state. We expect to achieve 60% to 90% clearance of total CO_2 production, however. As the microporous membrane lung fails, CO_2 clearance tends to drop more rapidly than does oxygenation.

Cannulation

Vascular cannulation is percutaneous using Biomedicus wire-reinforced cannulas with Carmeda bioactive surface treatment (Medtronic Cardiopulmonary, Anaheim, Calif). Drain cannulas are 21-F, 18 cm long, have multiple distal side holes, and generally are placed in a femoral vein. If the siphon pressure is excessively negative, two drain cannulas are inserted and "Y-ed" together. The blood "return" line is placed such that it ends near

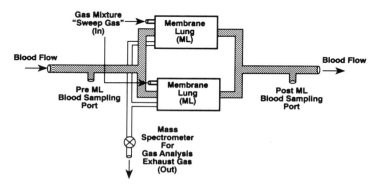

FIG 4.
Monitoring membrane lung CO_2 clearance with mass spectrometer on exhaust gas or by application of the Kelman algorithm to pre- and post-blood P_{CO_2}. Oxygenation monitored by post-membrane lung P_{O_2}.

the right atrium. When the return cannula is placed through the femoral vein, a 21-F, 50-cm cannula is advanced to the level of the diaphragm. When the return cannula is inserted in the internal jugular vein, a 21-F, 18-cm cannula is used. All cannulas are sutured in place, dressed in a sterile fashion, and inspected daily.

Pressure Monitoring

Pressure is continuously monitored in the extracorporeal circuit at four different sites, as shown in Figure 5. The "pre-pump" or "siphon" pressure (P_1) is the only negative pressure in the system and is continuously monitored by the CAPS. Through a servo-regulatory system, the pump rate will slow or stop if the siphon pressure approaches or exceeds a set limit. The negative siphon pressure can be affected by the pump flow rate, hypovolemia, bed height, or obstruction in the drain line. The pump pressure gradient (P_2-P_1) is continuously monitored to observe for "raceway" kinking. The pre-membrane lung pressure (P_2), the highest positive pressure in the system, is not allowed to rise above 400 mm Hg. The pre-membrane lung pressure is monitored continuously by the CAPS and is under servo-control. When the P_2 rises above a set limit, the pump slows or stops completely. The membrane lung pressure gradient (P_2-P_3) is limited to 350 mm Hg. A rise in the membrane lung gradient is assumed to indicate lung clotting. A rise in the pressure gradient (P_3-P_4) indicates clotting in the distal air trap (when bypass is clamped).

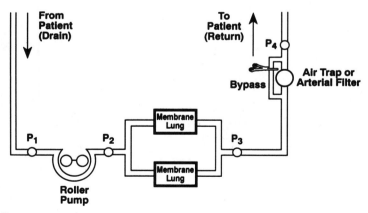

FIG 5.
Blood flow path through extracorporeal circuit. Two membrane lungs arranged in parallel geometry. System pressure monitored at four sites: P_1 (pre-pump), P_2 (pre-membrane lung), P_3 (post-membrane lung), and P_4 ("distal"). P_1 = "siphon pressure" (only negative pressure); P_2 = pre-membrane lung (normally highest system pressure); Δ pump = P_2-P_1; Δ membrane lung = P_2-P_3; Δ air trap = P_3-P_4. (Δ = pressure gradient across a particular system component).

Technical Variations

Many institutions use a "bladder" and "bladder box" on the drain line to act as a buffer against cavitation during accidental drain line occlusion. With the CAPS continuously monitoring the siphon pressure, we have eliminated the bladder and "bladder box" from the circuit.

With the two membrane lungs arranged in a parallel fashion, one membrane lung can be changed at a time without disrupting the blood flow. Because microporous membrane lungs develop plasma leakage and fail within 1 to 6 days, routine change-out is required.

Microporous membrane lungs available include the Baxter-Bentley Univox, the Medtronic Maxima (Medtronic Blood Systems, Inc., Anaheim, Calif) with Carmeda heparin bonding (Carmeda, Stockholm, Sweden), and the Capriox II (Treumo, Inc., Tokyo, Japan). The Maxima and Capriox membrane lungs both have greater priming volumes and, therefore, greater blood requirements for the routine membrane change-outs. Furthermore, the Capriox membrane lung is not heparin surface treated.

The non-microporous Avecor (Avecor Cardiovascular, Inc., Plymouth, Minn) silicon rubber membrane (formerly Sci-Med, Sci-Med Life Systems, Minneapolis, Minn) requires a far greater surface area to achieve gas exchange similar to that of the microporous membranes. As a result, the extracorporeal priming volume is greater. No heparin-treated silicon membranes are available in the United States. Therefore, substantial heparinization is required, with its associated complications. The silicon rubber membranes, however, may last as long as 30 days without change.

Ventilator Management Before and During $ECCO_2R$/ECMO

Permissive hypercapnia is initiated on essentially all ventilator-dependent patients, except those with clear contraindications such as intracranial injury precluding hypercapnia or inadequate renal compensation for hypercapnia. If renal dysfunction is profound, however, continuous dialysis can be performed with bicarbonate dialysate to compensate for the respiratory acidosis. If permissive hypercapnia is adequate to avoid "volutrauma" or barotrauma, the modality is continued. Goals of permissive hypercapnia are to keep the peak airway pressure less than 40 cm H_2O or the tidal volume in the range of 5 to 8 mL/kg, with the arterial pH at 7.20 or greater. Efforts are made to achieve and maintain these tidal volume and airway pressure goals within 72 hours of the initiation of ventilation. If tidal volumes are decreased without other ventilator adjustments, the mean airway pressure and functional residual capacity will decrease, as will oxygenation. Oxygenation has been found to correlate with mean airway pressure.[150-152] Therefore, to maintain oxygenation during tidal volume reduction, either the PEEP or the inspiratory time is increased to maintain mean airway pressure as necessary. If peak airway pressures cannot be reduced to less than 40 cm H_2O or hypoxemia cannot be corrected, the patient is considered to be a candidate for extracorporeal lung assistance (Fig 6).

Once the patient is placed on extracorporeal lung assistance, the ventilator is adjusted to keep peak airway pressures no greater than 35 to 40 cm H_2O using a pressure-driven modality, tidal volumes of 5 mL/kg, and respiratory rates at 2 to 5 breaths per minute. The mean airway pressure is maintained at 20 to 25 cm H_2O with a combination of PEEP and adjustments in the inspiratory times. Oxygen is insufflated through the trachea at 1 to 2 L/min. The inspired fraction of oxygen is decreased to maintain an SaO_2 of at least 85% to 90%.

Anticoagulant Therapy

Heparin remains the current mainstay of anticoagulant therapy. Excellent reviews of the history, pharmacology, use, and complications of heparin are available elsewhere.[153] Most U.S. extracorporeal life support centers use the non–heparin-treated Avecor membrane lung and provide heparinization to maintain the activated clotting time in the range of 180 to 220 seconds. European centers generally use heparin-treated membrane lungs and circuits, and less systemic heparin. The extracorporeal system we use consists of heparin-treated circuitry and membrane lungs. Additional heparin is given at a dosage of 300 to 1,200 U/hr to maintain the partial thromboplastin time at 1½ to 2 times normal. At higher blood flow rates, there are fewer areas of blood stagnation and clotting. Therefore, when higher blood flow rates are necessary and bleeding is a concurrent problem, we may use lower doses of heparin. If bleeding continues to be a major problem even with low-dose heparin, the drug may be discontinued entirely. Some surface clotting is tolerable, since the lungs are routinely changed every 1 to 4 days because of gas exchange failure. Furthermore, the entire extracorporeal circuit is changed every 7 to 10 days of continuous use, clearing small circuit clots.

Because bleeding remains a major complication of CPB, enormous effort has focused on developing alternative ways to avoid bleeding or extracorporeal clotting. Aprotinin, a low–molecular-weight peptide, inhibits trypsin, kallikrein, plasmin,[154, 155] and factor XII.[156] Brunet and colleagues reported complete cessation of heparin-related bleeding during $ECCO_2R$ when aprotinin was infused.[157] Improved hemostasis has been attributed to sustained or preserved adhesive capacity of platelets.[158, 159] Others have noted that aprotinin may reduce complement activation and thereby decrease the "whole body inflammatory response" that is associated with CPB.[160]

Nafamostat mesilate, another protease inhibitor, has been studied in Japan. Nafamostat is a potent synthetic inhibitor of kallikrein, factor X, factor XII, thrombin, and plasmin.[161] When nafamostat was administered by continuous infusion in a dog model, the activated clotting time was prolonged in a smooth, controlled fashion with minimal bleeding.[162] No com-

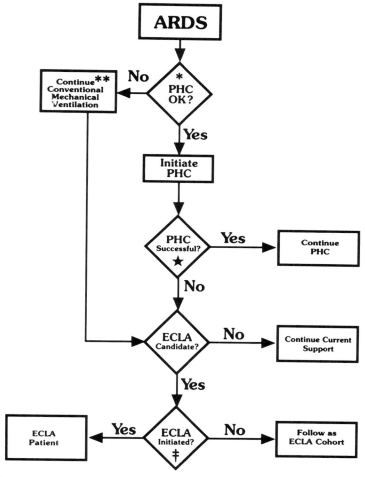

FIG 6.
General algorithm for ventilatory support before progressing to extracorporeal life support. (See manuscript for details.) *PHC = permissive hypercapnia; **PHC = contraindicated in some head injuries; ★PHC = failure (inability to reduce peak airway pressure or minute volume despite significant elevation of Pa_{CO_2}); ‡ECLA = extracorporeal lung assistance (may not be initiated because of lack of family consent, unavailability of equipment, inability to achieve vascular access, etc.); ARDS = adult respiratory distress syndrome.

parative evaluation of anticoagulant treatment of extracorporeal circuits with heparin vs. nafamostat has been performed, however.

Platelets are consumed during extracorporeal life support at least partially as a result of contact with and adherence to foreign surfaces. Activation of the plasminogen-plasmin system also may lead to platelet consumption. Plotz and coworkers noted that tranexamic acid, a plasminogen and plasmin inhibitor, effectively maintained platelet counts during extracorporeal circulation in a rabbit model.[163] When both heparin-treated circuitry and tranexamic acid were used, platelet counts could be maintained, even with complete omission of systemic heparin.

Prostacyclin (Upjohn, Kalamazoo, Mich) and its analogue, iloprost (ZK36374, Berlex Laboratories, Inc., Cedar Knolls, NJ), both inhibit platelet aggregation and release.[164, 165] Prostacyclin was studied by Uziel and associates in combination with heparin during extracorporeal lung assistance.[166] The prostacyclin provided protection against any reduction in the platelet count, whereas the control subjects suffered a 50% reduction in platelets. The platelets regained aggregation capability shortly after the prostacyclin was discontinued. The pharmacology of the synthetic prostaglandin analogue iloprost closely resembles that of prostacyclin. Details regarding iloprost have been extensively reviewed by Grant and Goa.[167] In addition to platelet antiaggregation and vasodilation, iloprost also may possess an undefined cytoprotective effect. In study models of extracorporeal circulation, Cottrell and colleagues found 98% preservation of the platelet count with iloprost vs. 54% in control subjects.[168] Addonizio and coworkers found 85% preservation of platelets vs. 29% in control subjects.[169]

Ultimately, the optimal anticoagulant therapy during extracorporeal circulatory support remains to be determined.

Complications of Extracorporeal Circulatory Support

Bleeding is the most significant complication of extracorporeal cardiopulmonary support. The initial ECMO trial sponsored by the NIH[51] reported a blood product infusion rate of 1,000 to 2,500 mL/day. In the first report of $ECCO_2R$, Gattinoni observed an average blood loss of 1,800 ± 850 mL/day.[57] Major bleeding was noted from the chest tubes and during pulmonary surgery. More recently, Anderson and coworkers used non–heparin-treated circuits and membranes, and systemic heparin to control the activated clotting time to 160 to 180 seconds.[53] Significant bleeding was found in 88% of the 40 patients who were reviewed. The Marburg group, however, used heparin-treated tubing and membrane lungs, and systemic heparin to maintain the activated clotting time at 120 to 150 seconds and antithrombin III infusions to keep those levels near 100%. Blood loss was noted to be 250 to 400 mL/day. Our experience using heparin-treated circuitry and membrane lungs, and low-dose heparin to keep the partial thromboplastin time at 1½ to 2 times normal has been an average blood loss of 200 to 500 mL/day. Most of this loss has been related to change-out of membrane lungs (unpublished data) and not secondary to bleeding. On occasion, heparin has been discontinued completely during surgical procedures and for 48 hours postoperatively, with minimal or no significant postoperative bleeding.

Among neonatal patients receiving ECMO, intracranial hemorrhage is the most significant type of bleeding. Bleeding from locations such as the gastrointestinal tract and cannula insertion sites also is common, however.[170] Weiss and associates recently reported mediastinal hemorrhage during ECMO, which was believed to result from barotrauma.[171] At least one case of retinal hemorrhage has been reported after pediatric ECMO.[172]

A variety of nonhemorrhagic hematologic complications have been noted. Zach and colleagues described a mild reduction in the absolute neutrophil and lymphocyte counts.[173] No relationship to any subsequent infectious complications was noted, however. Hemolysis during extracorporeal circulatory support has long been recognized, occurring in 8% of neonates after any form of extracorporeal support.[174] Hemolysis has been linked to pump type, shear forces, excessive pressure gradients, and highly negative pressures. There appears to be considerable individual and species variation in the susceptibility of erythrocytes to hemolysis.[175] Some have argued that the nearly occlusive roller pump would cause more erythrocyte damage than would the "constrained vortex" pump. Kress, however, was unable to detect any difference in the degree of hemolysis between roller and vortex pumps.[176] In fact, the negative pressures generated before the vortex head may routinely exceed hemolysis thresholds.[177] It may be that the degree of hemolysis is related more closely to the way in which the pump is used than to the nature of the pump itself. Mechanisms other than direct trauma also may cause hemolysis. Steinhorn and associates noted progressively higher plasma free hemoglobin levels as clots began to appear in the extracorporeal circuit.[178] After complete circuit change-out, free plasma hemoglobin returned to normal, implying that circuit thrombosis accounted for the elevated levels of plasma free hemoglobin. Finally, hemolysis is associated with carbon monoxide production and may result in carboxyhemoglobin levels as high as 13%, which are sufficient to interfere with oxygen transport.[179]

When platelets come into contact with foreign, nonbiologic surfaces, some platelets will adhere.[180] During extracorporeal circulation, the platelet count may decrease by 40% to 60%.[181] Hennessy and colleagues noted reductions in the platelet count proportionate to the surface area of the membrane oxygenator.[182] Furthermore, plasma platelet factor (PF) 4 rose and platelet PF4 decreased, suggesting that platelets existed in three conditions: some were unaltered, some had depressed function, and others were essentially nonfunctional. Ultimately, platelet-related hemostatic capability may be overestimated based on the absolute platelet count. When blood comes into direct contact with foreign surfaces, the coagulation cascade is activated. Specifically, thrombin-antithrombin III complexes increase, as do fibrin and fibrinogen degradation products, and the kinin system is activated.[183] Activation of the coagulation cascade may be the motor driving the platelet activation and depletion that is seen during the use of extracorporeal circulation.

The use of extracorporeal circuitry has been associated with the activation of inflammatory mediators.[184, 185] Leukocyte activation mediated by elevated levels of complement may lead to progressive pulmonary dysfunction.[186, 187] Using non–heparin-treated circuitry, Plotz and coworkers noted a 34% increase in C3a associated with a 50% reduction in the leukocyte count immediately after the initiation of extracorporeal life support.[183] There was an associated decline in the clinical pulmonary status. Levels of tumor necrosis factor-α did not change abruptly, and actually declined after 24 hours of continuous extracorporeal support. Others noted C3a levels to increase as high as eight times above baseline after the use of non–heparin-treated circuitry.[188] Recently, heparin-bonded surfaces have been shown to be more biocompatible and to cause less complement activation than do non–heparin-bonded systems.[189] Further advances in membrane lungs and circuitry may continue to improve biocompatibility and to minimize the physiologic insult of extracorporeal support.

A variety of miscellaneous complications also have been reported, including hemodynamic instability after the initiation of extracorporeal support related to transient hypocalcemia.[190]

The Future of Extracorporeal Circulatory Support

The future of extracorporeal circulatory support services is uncertain. There is no indication that the incidence of ARDS is declining. With increasing use of invasive therapeutic and diagnostic modalities and chemotherapy, the incidence of sepsis is rising. Because sepsis is the leading cause of ARDS, it follows that the frequency of ARDS should also increase. In addition, given the trend away from high ventilatory support, other life support techniques must be sought. The list of applications for extracorporeal support is substantial, and good alternatives are not available in many cases. Finally, regionalization of critical care services will promote the development of sophisticated tertiary referral centers with highly advanced life support techniques.

Social change in the form of health care reform, however, may limit the use of expensive therapeutic modalities. A general reduction in research funding may limit scientific advances. The U.S. Food and Drug Administration may continue its stringent policies and requirements, further dampening progress. More optimistically, a cure for ARDS may be found.

From the technical perspective, $ECCO_2R$ is successful in removing CO_2 and providing lung rest in the form of low tidal volumes and reduced airway pressures. The diseased lung also has difficulty with oxygenation, however. Therefore, higher extracorporeal blood flow is required to support oxygenation. In the future, we may be able to continue to keep CO_2 removal separate from the process of oxygenation. To do so will require

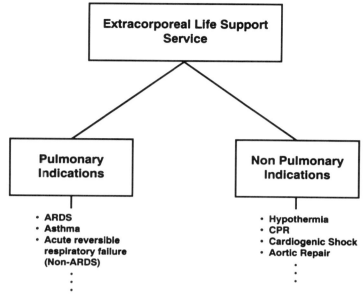

FIG 7.
Structure of extracorporeal life support service, including pulmonary and nonpulmonary capabilities. ARDS = adult respiratory distress syndrome; CPR = cardiopulmonary resuscitation.

efforts to improve oxygen delivery through the native lungs, such as "liquid breathing"[191] or the concurrent use of nitric oxide.[192] In addition, improved automation and servo-control systems, accepted prepackaged circuitry, and improved biocompatibility would be helpful. Progress in the development of membrane lungs is necessary and appears to be imminent. Current silicone rubber membranes are relatively inefficient and microporous membranes have too short a lifespan.

Finally, extracorporeal support programs could be developed that have multiple capabilities, rather than just the support of patients with ARDS (Fig 7). Wider indications for extracorporeal life support should increase its use, maintain operator skills, and expand knowledge more rapidly.

References

1. *Respiratory Diseases: Task Force Report on Problems, Research Approaches, Needs.* Washington, DC, US Government Printing Office, DHEW Publication NO (NIH) 73–432.
2. Fowler AA, Hamman RF, Zerbe GO, et al: Adult respiratory distress syndrome: Prognosis after onset. Am Rev Respir Dis 1985; 132:472–478.
3. Artigas A: Adult respiratory distress syndrome: Changing concepts of clinical evolution and recovery, in Vincent JL (ed): *Update in Intensive Care and*

Emergency Medicine. Berlin, Springer-Verlage, 1988, pp 97–114.
4. Montgomery AB, Stager MA, Carrico CJ, et al: Causes of mortality in patients with the adult respiratory distress syndrome. Am Rev Respir Dis 1985; 132:485–489.
5. Ashbaugh DG, Bigelow DB, Petty TL, et al: Acute respiratory distress in adults. Lancet 1967; 2:319–323.
6. Douglas ME, Downs JB: Respiratory therapy for ventilatory failure, in Shoemaker WC, Thompson WL, Holbrook PR (eds): Textbook of Critical Care. Philadelphia, WB Saunders, 1984, pp 301–310.
7. Dreyfuss D, Basset G, Soler P, et a: Intermittent positive-pressure hyperventilation with high inflation pressures produces pulmonary microvascular injury in rats. Am Rev Respir Dis 1985; 132:880–844.
8. Dreyfuss D, Soler P, Basset G, et al: High inflation pressure pulmonary edema. Respective effects of high airway pressure, high tidal volume, and positive end-expiratory pressure. Am Rev Respir Dis 1988; 137:1159–1164.
9. Bowton DL, Kong DL: High tidal volume ventilation produces increased lung water in oleic acid-injured rabbit lungs. Crit Care Med 1989; 17:908–912.
10. Woo SW, Hedley-White J: Macrophage accumulation and pulmonary edema due to thoracotomy and lung overinflation. J Appl Physiol 1972; 33:14–21.
11. Faridy EE, Permutt S, Riley RL: Effect of ventilation on surface forces in excised dog lungs. J Appl Physiol 1966; 21:1453–1462.
12. McClenahan JB, Urtnowski A: Effect of ventilation on surfactant and its turnover rate. J Appl Physiol 1967; 23:215.
13. Gattinoni L, Pesenti A, Aballi L, et al: Pressure-volume curve of total respiratory system in acute respiratory failure. Am Rev Respir Dis 1987; 136:730–736.
14. Gattinoni L, Pesenti A, Bombino M, et al: Relationships between lung computed tomographic density, gas exchange, and PEEP in acute respiratory failure. Anesthesiology 1988; 69:824–832.
15. Gattinoni L, Pesenti A, Baglioni S, et al: Inflammatory pulmonary edema and positive end expiratory pressure: Correlations between imaging and physiologic studies. J Thorac Imaging 1988; 3:59–64.
16. Lavoisier AL: Memoire sur les alterations qui arruvent a L'air dans plusieurs circonstance ou es trouvent les hommes reunis en societe. Histoire Soc R Med 1785; 5:569–582.
17. Hayatdavoudi G, O'Neil JJ, Barry BE, et al: Pulmonary injury in rats following continuous exposure to 60% O2 for 7 days. J Appl Physiol 1981; 51:1220–1231.
18. Clark JM, Lambersten CJ: Pulmonary oxygen toxicity: A review. Pharmacol Rev 1981; 23:37–133.
19. Crapo JD, Tierney DF: Superoxide dismutase and pulmonary oxygen toxicity. Am J Physiol 1974; 226:1404–1407.
20. Demeke SM, Fanburg BL: Oxygen toxicity of the lung: An update. Br J Anaesth 1982; 54:737–749.
21. Jenkinson SG: Oxygen toxicity. New Horizons 1993; 1:504–511.
22. Petersen GW, Baier H: Incidence of pulmonary barotrauma in a medical ICU. Crit Care Med 1983; 11:67–69.
23. Woodring JH: Pulmonary interstitial emphysema in the adult respiratory distress syndrome. Crit Care Med 1985; 13:786–791.
24. Bonnet F, Richard C, Blaser P, et al: Changes in hepatic flow induced by continuous positive pressure ventilation in critically ill patients. Crit Care Med 1982; 10:703–705.

25. Berry AJ: Respiratory support and renal function. Anesthesiology 1981; 55:655–667.
26. Cassidy SS, Eschenbacher WL, Rovertson CH, et al: Cardiovascular effects of positive pressure ventilation in normal subjects. J Appl Physiol 1979; 47:453–461.
27. Marini JJ, Culver BH: Systemic gas embolism complicating mechanical ventilation in the adult respiratory distress syndrome. Ann Intern Med 1989; 110:699–703.
28. Kolobow T: Acute respiratory failure. On how to injure healthy lungs (and prevent sick lungs from recovering). Trans ASAIO 1988; 34:31–34.
29. Teplitz CC: The core pathobiology and integrated medical science of adult acute respiratory insufficiency. Surg Clin North Am 1976; 56:1091–1133.
30. Slutsky AS, Chairman ACCP Consensus Conference: Mechanical ventilation. Chest 1993; 104:1833–1859.
31. Hickling KG: Ventilatory management of ARDS: Can it affect the outcome? Intensive Care Med 1990; 16:219–226.
32. Kacmerek RM, Hickling KG: Permissive hypercapnia. Respiratory Care 1993; 38:373–387.
33. Hickling KG, Henderson SJ, Jackson R: Low mortality associated with low volume pressure limited ventilation with permissive hypercapnia in severe adult respiratory distress syndrome. Intensive Care Med 1990; 16:372–377.
34. Marini JJ, Kelsen SG: Re-targeting ventilatory objectives in adult respiratory distress syndrome: New treatment prospects—persistent questions (editorial). Am Rev Respir Dis 1992; 146:2–3.
35. Pesenti A: Target blood gases during ARDS ventilatory management (editorial). Intensive Care Med 1990; 16:349–351.
36. Bartlett RH: Extracorporeal life support for cardiopulmonary failure, in Wells SA (ed): Current Problems in Surgery. St Louis, Mosby, 1990, pp 624–705.
37. Lillehei CW: A personalized history of extracorporeal circulation. Trans ASAIO 1982; 28:5–16.
38. Gott VL: Extracorporeal circulation: 1970–1982. Trans ASAIO 1982; 28:17–19.
39. Heiss KF, Bartlett RH: Extracorporeal membrane oxygenation: An experimental protocol becomes a clinical service. Adv Pediatr 1989; 36:117–136.
40. Gibbon JH Jr: Artificial maintenance of circulation during experimental occlusion of the pulmonary artery. Arch Surg 1937; 34:1105.
41. Gibbon JH Jr: Application of a mechanical heart and lung apparatus to cardiac surgery. Minn Med 1954; 37:171.
42. DeWall RA, Warden HE, Read RC, et al: A simple, expendable, artificial oxygenator for open heart surgery. Surg Clin North Am 1956; 36:1025.
43. Lee WH Jr, Krumhaar D, Fonkalsrud EW, et al: Denaturation of plasma proteins as a cause of morbidity and death after intracardiac operations. Surgery 1961; 50 29–39.
44. Dobell ARC, Mitri M, Galva R, et al: Biologic evaluation of blood after prolonged recirculation through film and membrane oxygenator. Ann Surg 1965; 161:617–622.
45. Clowes GHA Jr, Hopkins AL, Neville WE: An artificial lung dependent upon diffusion of oxygen and carbon dioxide through plastic membranes. J Thorac Surg 1956; 32:630–637.
46. Kammermeyer K: Silicone rubber as a selective barrier. Industrial Engineering and Chemistry 1957; 49:1685.

47. Kolobow T, Boloman RH: Construction and evaluation of an alveolar membrane artificial heart-lung. Trans ASAIO 1963; 9:238–243.
48. White JJ, Andrews HG, Risemberg H, et al: Prolonged respiratory support in newborn infants with a membrane oxygenator. Surgery 1971; 70:288.
49. Hill JD, O'Brien TG, Murray JJ, et al: Prolonged extracorporeal oxygenation for acute post-traumatic respiratory failure (shock-lung syndrome). N Engl J Med 1972; 286:629–634.
50. Bartlett RH, Gazzaniga AB, Fong SW, et al: Prolonged extracorporeal cardiopulmonary support in man. J Thorac Cardiovasc Surg 1974; 68:918–932.
51. Zapol WM, Snider MT, Hill JD, et al: Extracorporeal membrane oxygenation in severe acute respiratory failure: A randomized prospective study. JAMA 1979; 242:2193–2196.
52. NHLBI-NIH: *Extracorporeal Support for Respiratory Insufficiency*. Bethesda, Maryland, DHEW Publication.
53. Anderson HL, Delius RE, Sinard JM, et al: Early experience with adult extracorporeal membrane oxygenation in the modern era. Ann Thorac Surg 1992; 53:553–563.
54. Anderson HL, Steimle C, Shapiro M, et al: Extracorporeal life support for adult cardiorespiratory failure. Surgery 1993; 114:161–173.
55. Falke KJ: Reduced mortality rates in severe adult respiratory distress syndrome, in *Proceedings From the Fifth Annual ELSO Meeting, Advances in ECMO, Instructional Course*. Dearborn, Michigan, Extracorporeal Life Support Organization, 1993.
56. Kolobow T, Gattinoni L, Tomlinson T, et al: An alternative to breathing. J Thorac Cardiovasc Surg 1978; 75:261–266.
57. Gattinoni L, Pesenti A, Mascheroni D, et al: Low-frequency positive-pressure ventilation with extracorporeal CO2 removal in severe acute respiratory failure. JAMA 1986; 256:881–886.
58. Mottaghy K, Schaich-Lester D, Lester A, et al: Long-term extracorporeal CO2 removal in sheep for up to 7 days using capillary fiber membrane oxygenators. Trans ASAIO 1987; 33:5654.
59. Dorrington KL, McRae KM, Gardaz J, et al: A randomized comparison of total extracorporeal CO2 removal with conventional mechanical ventilation in experimental hyaline membrane disease. Intensive Care Med 1989; 15:184–191.
60. Zobel G, Pierer G, Dacar D, et al: Extracorporeal CO2 removal in a lung lavage induced respiratory distress syndrome. Int J Artif Organs 1990; 13:430–435.
61. Hickling KG, Downward G, Davis FM, et al: Management of severe ARDS with low frequency positive pressure ventilation and extracorporeal CO2 removal. Anaesth Intensive Care 1986; 14:79–88.
62. Krajewski S, Seitz RJ, Schober R, et al: Prolonged extracorporeal CO2 removal in severe adult respiratory distress syndrome. Intensive Care Med 1987; 13:26–29.
63. Bindslev L, Eklund J, Norlander O, et al: Treatment of acute respiratory failure by extracorporeal carbon dioxide elimination performed with a surface heparinized artificial lung. Anesthesiology 1987; 67:117–120.
64. Muller EE, Lennartz H: The current Marburg management concept, in *Proceedings From the Third Annual ELSO Meetings: Extracorporeal Life Support for Pediatric and Adult Cardiorespiratory Failure, Advanced Techniques in ECLS: Extracorporeal Respiratory Support in Patients With Adult Respira-*

tory Distress Syndrome (ARDS). Ann Arbor, Michigan, Extracorporeal Life Support Organization, 1991.
65. Morris AH, Wallace CJ, Menlove RL, et al: Randomized clinical trial of pressure controlled inverse ratio ventilation with extracorporeal CO_2 removal for adult respiratory distress syndrome. Am J Respir Crit Care Med 1994; 149:295–305.
66. Zapol WM, Kolobow T: Extracorporeal membrane lung gas exchange, in Crystal RG, West JB (eds): The Lung: Scientific Foundation. New York, Raven Press, 1991, 2197–2204.
67. Kolobow T, Bowman RL: Construction and evaluation of an alveolar membrane artificial heart-lung. Trans ASAIO 1963; 9:238–243.
68. Servas FM, Diettrich LJ, Jones K, et al: High efficiency membrane oxygenator. Trans ASAIO 1983; 29:231–236.
69. Mottaghy K, Oedekoven B, Starmans H, et al: Technical aspects of plasma leakage prevention in microporous capillary membrane oxygenators. Trans ASAIO 35:640–643.
70. Tong SD, Rolfs MR, Hsu LC: Evaluation of a randomized comparison of total extracorporeal CO2 removal with conventional mechanical ventilation in experimental hyaline membrane disease. Intensive Care Med 1989; 15: 184–191.
71. Bindslev L, Bohm C, Jolin A, et al: Extracorporeal carbon dioxide removal performed with surface-heparinized equipment in patients with ARDS. Acta Anaesthesiol Scand 1991; 95:125–131.
72. Wilms D, Dembitsky W: Prolonged extracorporeal support for ARDS using surface heparinized equipment. Chest 1992; 102:968–970.
73. Knoch M, Kollen B, Dietrich G, et al: Progress in veno-venous long term bypass techniques for the treatment of ARDS. Controlled clinical trial with the heparin-coated bypass circuit. Int J Artif Organs 1992; 15:103–108.
74. Mottaghy K, Oedekoven B, Poppel K, et al: Heparin coated versus noncoated surfaces for extracorporeal circulation. Int J Artif Organs 1991; 14:721–728.
75. Acute Conditions: Incidence and Associated Disabilities. National Center for Health Statistics Monthly Vital Statistics Report, May 30, 1975.
76. Scoggin CH, Shan SA, Petty TL: Status asthmaticus. JAMA 1977; 238:1158–1162.
77. Zwillich CW, Persons DJ, Creagh CE, et al: Complications of assisted ventilation. Am J Med 1974; 57:161–170.
78. Westerman D, Benatar S, Potgieter P, et al: Identification of the high risk asthmatic patient—experience with patients undergoing ventilation for status asthmaticus. Am J Med 1979; 66:565.
79. MacDonnell KF, Moon HS, Sekar TS, et al: Extracorporeal membrane oxygenator support in a case of severe status asthmaticus. Ann Thorac Surg 1981; 31:171–175.
80. Tamimi K, Kasai T, Nakatani T, et al: Extracorporeal lung assist for patients with hypercapnia due to status asthmaticus. Intensive Care Med 1988; 14:588–589.
81. King D, Smales C, Arnold AG, et al: Extracorporeal membrane oxygenation as emergency treatment for life-threatening acute severe asthma. Postgrad Med J 1986; 62:855–857.
82. Pesenti A, Rossi GP, Pelosi P, et al: Percutaneous extracorporeal CO2 removal in a patient with bullous emphysema with recurrent bilateral pneumo-

thoraces and respiratory failure. *Anesthesiology* 1990; 72:571–573.
83. Lonning PE, Skulberg A, Abyholm F: Accidental hypothermia. Review of the literature. *Acta Anaesthesiol Scand* 1986; 30:601–613.
84. Marin S, Diewold RJ, Cooper KE: Alcohol, respiration, skin and body temperature during cold water immersion. *J Appl Physiol* 1977; 43:211–215.
85. Lilly JK, Boland JP, Zekan S: Urinary bladder temperature monitoring: A new index of body core temperature. *Crit Care Med* 1980; 8:742–744.
86. Fitzgerald FT, Jessop C: Accidental hypothermia: A report of 22 cases and review of the literature, in Stollerman GH (ed): *Advances in Internal Medicine*, vol 27. St Louis, Mosby, Inc, 1982, pp 127–150.
87. DaVee TS, Reineberg EJ: Extreme hypothermia and ventricular fibrillation. *Ann Emerg Med* 1980; 9:100–102.
88. O'Keeffe KM: Accidental hypothermia: A review of 62 cases. *Journal of the American College of Emergency Physicians* 1977; 6:491–496.
89. Lloyd ELL, Mitchell B, Williams JT: The cardiovascular effects of three methods of rewarming sheep from immersion hypothermia. *Resuscitation* 1976; 5:229–233.
90. Savard GK, Cooper KE, Veale WL, et al: Peripheral blood flow during rewarming from mild hypothermia in humans. *J Appl Physiol* 1985; 58:4–13.
91. Harnett RM, Pruitt JR, Sias FR: A review of the literature concerning resuscitation from hypothermia: Part 2. Selected rewarming protocols. *Aviat Space Environ Med* 1983; 54:487–495.
92. Jessen K, Hagelsten JO: Peritoneal dialysis in the treatment of profound accidental hypothermia. *Aviat Space Environ Med* 1978; 49:426–429.
93. Emslie-Smith D: Accidental hypothermia. A common condition with a pathognomonic electrocardiogram. *Lancet* 1958; 2:492–495.
94. Fruehan AE: Accidental hypothermia. Report of eight cases of subnormal body temperature due to exposure. *Arch Intern Med* 1960; 106:218–229.
95. Frank DH, Robson MC: Accidental hypothermia treated without mortality. *Surg Gynecol Obstet* 1980; 151:379–381.
96. Kugelberg J, Schuller H, Berg B, et al: Treatment of accidental hypothermia. *Scand J Thorac Cardiovasc Surg* 1967; 1:142–146.
97. Towne WD, Geiss WP, Yanes HO, et al: Intractable ventricular fibrillation associated with profound accidental hypothermia—successful treatment with partial cardiopulmonary bypass. *N Engl J Med* 1972; 287:1135–1136.
98. Husby P, Andersen KS, Owen-Falkenberg A, et al: Accidental hypothermia with cardiac arrest: Complete recovery after prolonged resuscitation and rewarming by extracorporeal circulation. *Intensive Care Med* 1990; 16:68–72.
99. Althaus U, Aeberhard P, Schupbach P, et al: Management of profound accidental hypothermia with cardiorespiratory arrest. *Ann Surg* 1982; 195: 492–495.
100. Hauty MG, Esrig BC, Hill JG, et al: Prognostic factors in severe accidental hypothermia: Experience from the Mt Hood tragedy. *J Trauma* 1987; 27:1107–1112.
101. Zell SC, Kurtz KJ: Severe exposure hypothermia: A resuscitation protocol. *Ann Emerg Med* 1985; 14:339–345.
102. Davies DM, Miller EJ, Miller JA: Accidental hypothermia treated by extracorporeal warming. *Lancet* 1967; 1:1036–1037.
103. Welton DE: Treatment of profound hypothermia. *JAMA* 1978; 240: 2291–2292.
104. Hartford JM, Fayer RL, Shaver TE, et al: Transection of the thoracic aorta:

Assessment of a trauma system. *Am J Surg* 1986; 151:224.
105. Turney SZ, Attar S, Ayella R, et al: Traumatic rupture of the aorta: A five year experience. *J Thorac Cardiovasc Surg* 1976; 72:727.
106. Parmley LF, Mattingly TW, Marian WC, et al: Non penetrating traumatic injury of the aorta: *Circulation* 1958; 17:1086.
107. Marsh CL, Moore RC: Deceleration trauma. *Am J Surg* 1957; 93:623.
108. Zehnder MA: Delayed post-traumatic rupture of the aorta in a young healthy individual after closed injury: Mechanical-etiological considerations. *Angiology* 1956; 7:252.
109. Culliford AT: Traumatic aortic rupture, in Hood RM, Boyd AD, Culliford AT (eds): *Thoracic Trauma*. Philadelphia, WB Saunders, 1989, 224–244.
110. Gott VL: Heparinized shunts for thoracic vascular operations. *Ann Thorac Surg* 1972; 14:219.
111. Gerbode E, Braimbridge M, Osborn JJ: Traumatic thoracic aneurysms: Treatment by resection and grafting with the use of an extracorporeal bypass. *Surgery* 1957; 42:975.
112. Roberts AJ, Michaels II: The art of bypass techniques and other forms of open protection during thoracic aorta cross clamping, in Bergan JJ, Yao JSI (eds): *Surgery of the Aorta and Its Branches*. New York, Grune & Stratton, 1979.
113. Crawford ES (ed): *Diseases of the Aorta: Including an Atlas of Angiographic Pathology and Surgical Techniques*. Baltimore, Williams & Wilkins, 1984.
114. Laschinger JC, Cunningham JN Jr, Nathan IM, et al: Experimental and clinical assessment of the adequacy of partial bypass in maintenance of spinal cord flow during operations on the thoracic aorta. *Ann Thorac Surg* 1983; 36:417.
115. Crawford ES, Rubio PA: Reappraisal of adjuncts to avoid ischemia in the treatment of aneurysms of the descending thoracic aorta. *J Thorac Cardiovasc Surg* 1973; 66:693.
116. Grosso MA, Brown JM, Moore EE, et al: Repair of the torn descending thoracic aorta using the centrifugal pump with partial left heart bypass: Technical note. *J Trauma* 1991; 31:395–400.
117. Cartier R, Orszulak TA, Pairolero PC, et al: Circulatory support during cross-clamping of the descending thoracic aorta. *J Thorac Cardiovasc Surg* 1990; 99:1033–1047.
118. Kouwenhoven WB, Jude JR, Knickerbocker GG: Closed chest cardiac massage. *JAMA* 1960; 173:1064–1067.
119. Cummins RO, Eisenberg MS, Hallstrom AP, et al: Survival of out-of-hospital cardiac arrest with early initiation of cardiopulmonary resuscitation. *Am J Emerg Med* 1985; 3:114–118.
120. Ralston SH, Voorhees WD, Babbs CF: Intrapulmonary epinephrine during prolonged cardiopulmonary resuscitation. Improved regional blood flow and resuscitation in dogs. *Ann Emerg Med* 1984; 13:79–86.
121. Paradis NA, Martin GB, Rivers EP, et al: Coronary perfusion pressure and the return of spontaneous circulation in human cardiopulmonary resuscitation. *JAMA* 1990; 263:1106–1113.
122. Bircher N, Safar P: Comparison of standard and "new" closed chest CPR and open chest CPR in dogs. *Crit Care Med* 1981; 9:384–385.
123. Ditchey RV, Winkler JV, Rhodes CA: Relative lack of coronary blood flow during closed chest resuscitation in dogs. *Circulation* 1982; 66:297–302.
124. Del Guercio LRM, Feins NR, Cohn JD, et al: Comparison of blood flow dur-

ing external and internal cardiac massage in man. *Circulation* 1965; 31(suppl):1171–1180.
125. Sanders AB, Kern KB, Ewy GA, et al: Improved resuscitation from cardiac arrest with open-chest massage. *Ann Emerg Med* 1984; 13:672–675.
126. Kern KB, Sanders AB, Badylak SF, et al: Long-term survival with open-chest cardiac massage after ineffective closed-chest compression in a canine preparation. *Circulation* 1987; 75:498–503.
127. Shawl FA, Domanski MJ, Punja S, et al: Emergency percutaneous cardiopulmonary (bypass) support in cardiogenic shock (abstract). *J Am Coll Cardiol* 1989; 13:160A.
128. Mattox KL, Beall AC: Resuscitation of the moribund patient using portable cardiopulmonary bypass. *Ann Thorac Surg* 1976; 22:436–442.
129. Martin GB, Nowak RM, Carden DL, et al: Cardiopulmonary bypass vs CPR as treatment for prolonged canine cardiopulmonary arrest. *Ann Emerg Med* 1987; 16:628–636.
130. Pretto E, Safar P, Saito R, et al: Cardiopulmonary bypass after prolonged cardiac arrest in dogs. *Ann Emerg Med* 1987; 16:611–619.
131. Gazmuri RJ, Weil MH, von Planta M, et al: Cardiac resuscitation by extracorporeal circulation after failure of conventional CPR. *J Lab Clin Med* 1991; 118:65–73.
132. Overlie PA, Reichman RT, Smith SC, et al: Emergency use of portable cardiopulmonary bypass in patients with cardiac arrest. *J Am Coll Cardiol* 1989; 13:160A.
133. Hill JG, Bruhn PS, Cohen SE, et al: Emergent applications of cardiopulmonary support: A multiinstitutional experience. *Ann Thorac Surg* 1992; 54:699–704.
134. Rogers AJ, Trento A, Siewers RD, et al: Extracorporeal membrane oxygenation for postcardiotomy cardiogenic shock in children. *Ann Thorac Surg* 1989; 47:903–906.
135. Delius RE, Bove EL, Meliones JN, et al: Use of extracorporeal life support in patients with congenital heart disease. *Crit Care Med* 1992; 20:1216–1222.
136. Bartlett RH, Gazzaniga AB, Fong SW, et al: Extracorporeal membrane oxygenation support for cardiopulmonary failure: Experience in 28 cases. *J Thorac Cardiovasc Surg* 1977; 73:375–386.
137. Zwischenberger JB, Cox CS: ECMO in the management of cardiac failure. *Trans ASAIO* 1992; 38:751–753.
138. Reedy JE, Swartz MT, Raither SC, et al: Mechanical cardiopulmonary support for refractory cardiogenic shock. *Heart Lung* 1990; 19:514–523.
139. McVey FK, Corke CF: Extracorporeal circulation in the management of massive propranolol overdose. *Anaesthesia* 1991; 46:744–746.
140. Bavaria JE, Ratcliffe MB, Gupta KB, et al: Changes in left ventricular systolic wall stress during biventricular circulatory assist. *Ann Thorac Surg* 1988; 45:526.
141. Spencer FC, Wiseman B, Trinkle JK, et al: Assisted circulation for cardiac failure following intracardiac surgery with cardiopulmonary bypass. *J Thorac Cardiovasc Surg* 1965; 49:56.
142. Axelrod HI, Galloway AC, Murphy MS, et al: Percutaneous cardiopulmonary bypass with a synchronous pulsatile pump combines effective unloading with ease of application. *J Thorac Cardiovasc Surg* 1987; 93:358.
143. Axelrod HI, Bauman FG, Galloway AC: Left ventricular stress during extracorporeal membrane oxygenation (letter). *Ann Thorac Surg* 1989; 47:330.

144. Bartlett RH, Kolobow T, Cooper JD, et al: Panel conference, extracorporeal gas exchange, lung transplantation and the artificial lung. Trans ASAIO 1984; 30:679–681.
145. Nelems JM, Duffin J, Glynn MFX, et al: Extracorporeal membrane oxygenator support for human lung transplantation. J Thorac Cardiovasc Surg 1978; 76:28–32.
146. Siegelman SS, Sinha SBP, Vieth FJA: Pulmonary reimplantation response. Ann Surg 1973; 177:30–36.
147. Veith FJ, Koerner SK: The present status of lung transplantation. Arch Surg 1974; 109:734–740.
148. Ichiba S, Okabe K, Date H, et al: Experimental study on veno-venous extracorporeal membrane oxygenation for respiratory failure after lung transplantation. Acta Med Okayama 1992; 46:213–221.
149. Kelman GR: Digital computer procedure for the conversion of PCO_2 into blood CO_2 content. Respir Physiol 1967; 3:111–115.
150. Pesenti A, Marcolin R, Prato P, et al: Mean airway pressure versus positive end-expiratory pressure in mechanical ventilation. Crit Care Med 1985; 13:34–37.
151. Stewart AR, Finer NN, Peters KL: Effect of alterations of inspiratory and expiratory pressures and inspiratory/expiratory ratios on mean airway pressure, blood gases, and intracranial pressure. Pediatrics 1981; 67:474–481.
152. Ciszek TA, Modanlou HD, Owings D, et al: Mean airway pressure—significance during mechanical ventilation in neonates. J Pediatr 1981; 99:121–126.
153. Gravlee GP: Anticoagulation for cardiopulmonary bypass, in Gravlee GP, Davis RF, Utley JR (eds): Cardiopulmonary Bypass, Principles and Practice. Baltimore, Williams & Wilkins, 1993, pp 340–369.
154. Fritz H, Wunderer G: Biochemistry and applications of aprotinin, the kallikrein inhibitor from bovine organs. Drug Res 1983; 33:479–494.
155. Brinkmann T, Schnierer S, Tschesche H: Recombinant aprotinin homologue with new inhibitory specificity for cathepsin. Eur J Biochem 1991; 202:95–99.
156. Laurel M-T P, Ratnoff OD, Everson B: Inhibition of the activation of Hagemann factor (factor XII) by aprotinin. J Lab Clin Med 1992; 119:580–585.
157. Brunet F, Mira JP, Belghith M, et al: Effects of aprotinin on hemorrhagive complications in ARDS patients during prolonged extracorporeal CO_2 removal. Intensive Care Med 1992; 18:364–367.
158. Van Oeveren W, Jansen NJG, Bidstrup BP, et al: Effects of aprotinin on hemostatic mechanisms during cardiopulmonary bypass. Ann Thorac Surg 1987; 44:640–645.
159. Van Oeveren W, Harder MP, Roozendaal KJ, et al: Aprotinin protects platelets against the initial effects of cardiopulmonary bypass. J Thorac Cardiovasc Surg 1990; 99:788–797.
160. Wachtfogel YRT, Kucich U, Hack CE, et al: Aprotinin inhibits the contact, neutrophil, and platelet activation systems during simulated extracorporeal perfusion. J Thorac Cardiovasc Surg 1993; 106:1–9.
161. Aoyama T, Ino Y, Ozeki M, et al: Pharmacological studies of FUT-175, nafamostat mesilate inhibition of protease activity in in-vitro and in-vivo experiments. Jpn J Pharmacol 1984; 35:203–227.
162. Okamoto T, Chung YK, Choi H, et al: Experimental results using nafamostat mesilate as anticoagulant during extracorporeal lung assist for 24 hours in dogs. Artif Organs 1993; 17:30–35.

163. Plotz FB, Van Oeveren W, Alow LS, et al: Prophylactic administration of tranexamic acid preserves platelet numbers during extracorporeal circulation in rabbits. *Trans ASAIO* 1991; 37:M416–M417.
164. Gimson AES, Hughes RD, Mellow P, et al: Prostacycline to prevent platelet activation during charcoal hemoperfusion in fulminant hepatic failure. *Lancet* 1980; 173:1.
165. Turney JH, Fewell MR, Williams RC, et al: Platelet protection and heparin sparing with prostacyclin during regular dialysis therapy. *Lancet* 1980; 219:2.
166. Uziel L, Agostone A, Pirovano E, et al: Effect of PGI2 infusion during long term extracorporeal circulation with membrane lung in sheep. *Int J Artif Organs* 1981; 4:142–145.
167. Grant SM, Goa KL: Iloprost, a review of its pharmacodynamic and pharmacokinetic properties and therapeutic potential in peripheral vascular disease, myocardial ischemia and extracorporeal circulation procedures. *Drugs* 1992; 43:889–918.
168. Cottrell ED, Kappa JR, Stenach N, et al: Temporary inhibition of platelet function with iloprost (ZK36374) preserves canine platelets during extracorporeal membrane oxygenation. *J Thorac Cardiovasc Surg* 1988; 96:535–541.
169. Addonizio VP, Fisher CA, Kappa JR, et al: Prevention of heparin-induced thrombocytopenia during open heart surgery with iloprost (ZK36374). *Surgery* 1987; 102:796–807.
170. Sell LL, Cullen ML, Whittlesey GC, et al: Hemorrhagic complications during extracorporeal membrane oxygenation: Prevention and treatment. *J Pediatr Surg* 1986; 21:1087–1091.
171. Weiss RG, Ball WS, Warner BW, et al: Mediastinal hemorrhage during extracorporeal membrane oxygenation. *J Pediatr Surg* 1989; 24:1115–1117.
172. Sethi SK: Retinal hemorrhages after extra corporeal membranous (sic) oxygenation. *North Carolina Medical Journal* 1990; 51:246.
173. Zach TL, Steinhorn RH, Georgieff MK, et al: Leukopenia associated with extracorporeal membrane oxygenation in newborn infants. *J Pediatr* 1990; 116:440–444.
174. Bartlett RH, Chapman RA, Snedecor S: *Neonatal ECMO Registry Report: National Summary.* Ann Arbor, University of Michigan, 1988.
175. Peirce EC, Corrigan JJ, Kent BB, et al: Comparative trauma to blood in the disc oxygenator and membrane lung. *Trans ASAIO* 1969; 33:33.
176. Kress DC, Cohen DJ, Swanson DK, et al: Pump-induced hemolysis in a rabbit model of neonatal ECMO. *Trans ASAIO* 1987; 33:446.
177. Wielogorski JW, Cross DE, Nwadike EV: The effects of subatmospheric pressure on the haemolysis of blood. *J Biomech* 1975; 8:321–325.
178. Steinhorn RH, Isham-Schopf B, Smith C, et al: Hemolysis during long-term extracorporeal membrane oxygenation. *J Pediatr* 1989; 115:625–630.
179. Subramanian VA, Berger RL: Carbon monoxide accumulation during extracorporeal membrane oxygenation for acute respiratory failure. *Ann Thorac Surg* 1976; 22:195–198.
180. Baier RE, Dutton RC: Initial events in interactions of blood with a foreign surface. *J Biomed Mater Res* 1969; 3:191–206.
181. Lautier A, Awad J, Gille JP, et al: Comparison of platelet deposition between hollow fiber and flat plate membrane oxygenator (MO), in Christel P, Meunier A, Lee AJC (eds): *Biological and Biomechanical Performance of Biomaterials.* Amsterdam, Elsevier Science Publishers, 1986, pp 287–291.

182. Hennessy VL, Hicks RE, Niewiarowski S, et al: Function of human platelets during extracorporeal circulation. *Am J Physiol* 1977; 232:H622–H628.
183. Plotz FB van Oeveren W, Bartlett RH, et al: Blood activation during neonatal extracorporeal life support. *J Thorac Cardiovasc Surg* 1993; 105:823–832.
184. Van Oeveren W, Wildevurr CRH, Kazatchkine MD: Biocompatibility of extracorporeal circuits in heart surgery. *Transfusion Science* 1990; 11:5–33.
185. Westaby S: Organ dysfunction after cardiopulmonary bypass. A systemic inflammatory reaction initiated by the extracorporeal circuit. *Intensive Care Med* 1987; 134:89–95.
186. Stimler NP, Hugli TE, Bloor CM: Pulmonary injury induced by C3a and C5a anaphylatoxins. *Am J Pathol* 1980; 100:327–348.
187. Willinas JJ, Yellin SA, Slotman GJ: Leukocyte aggregation response to quantitative plasma levels of C3a and C5a. *Arch Surg* 1986; 121:305–307.
188. Gardinali M, Cicardi M, Grangi D, et al: Studies of complement activation in ARDS patients treated by long-term extracorporeal CO_2 removal. *Int J Artif Organs* 1985; 8:135–140.
189. Kirschfink M, Kovacs B, Mottaghy K: Extracorporeal circulation: In vivo and in vitro analysis of complement activation by heparin-bonded surfaces. *Circ Shock* 1993; 40:221–226.
190. Meliones JN, Moler FW, Custer JR, et al: Hemodynamic instability after the initiation of extracorporeal membrane oxygenation: Role of ionized calcium. *Crit Care Med* 1991; 19:1247–1251.
191. Fuhrman BP, Hernan LJ, Steinhorn DM: Liquid breathing, in Prough DS, Trytsman RJ (eds): *Critical Care, State of the Art 1993*. Anaheim, Society of Critical Care Medicine, 1993, pp 221–237.
192. Rossaint Rolf, Falke KJ, Lopez F, et al: Inhaled nitric oxide for the adult respiratory distress syndrome *N Engl J Med* 1993; 328:399–405.

Immunomodulation

Richard K. Simons, M.B., B.Chir., F.R.C.S., F.R.C.S.(C)

Assistant Professor of Surgery, Department of Surgery, Division of Trauma, University of California, San Diego School of Medicine, San Diego, California

David B. Hoyt, M.D.

Associate Professor of Surgery, Chief, Division of Trauma, University of California, San Diego School of Medicine, San Diego, California

Death from trauma has been characterized as having a trimodal distribution.[1] The first two peaks occur within minutes to hours of injury, and can be attributed to specific injuries or their immediate complications. The third peak in traumatic death occurs days to weeks after injury and is attributable to delayed complications, commonly sepsis and multiple organ failure.[1-3] These devastating systemic complications are a nonspecific consequence of major injury and are mediated, in part, by perturbations of the host's immune system. In the past few years, interest in the immune response to injury has been increasing. Diverse fields of investigation, including immunology, cell and molecular biology, and genetics, are yielding new insights into this process. We have now reached the point at which therapeutic manipulations of the host's immune response not only are a possibility, but are becoming part of mainstream clinical practice, particularly in the surgical intensive care unit.

This review summarizes host defenses against infection, describes the dysfunctions of the immune system that follow trauma, and summarizes the various ways in which the dysfunctional immune system may be modified in a potentially beneficial way.

Normal Host Defenses

Barriers

The internal milieu of the host is protected from the external environment by barriers that have physical, chemical, and immunologic properties. Skin relies on a relatively inert cornified physical barrier assisted by fatty acids secreted by sebaceous glands and nonpathologic commensal skin flora that, together, protect against invading organisms. The respiratory tract relies on mucociliary function, the protective reflexes of coughing and sneezing, and secreted immunoglobulins to eliminate most microorganisms that gain access to the upper airway.

Perhaps the most threatening environment to the host is its own gastrointestinal tract and its luminal contents. It is a testimony to the integrity of the gastrointestinal barrier that we all are not overwhelmed by this enormous microbiologic threat. The stomach is rendered sterile by the secretion of hydrochloric acid, which effectively kills ingested bacteria. This mechanism also ensures that most of the small intestine remains essentially sterile. The colon, however, (and in minor gastroenterologic disturbances, the small bowel) is a teeming reservoir of pathogenic organisms, predominantly gram-negative aerobes and anaerobes. Their access to the internal milieu is prevented by mucus secretions containing neutralizing IgA antibodies; a metabolically active mucosa that forms a physical barrier; and peristalsis, which prevents prolonged stasis and mechanically removes organisms from the mucosal surface. Mucosal integrity depends not only on anatomic continuity, but on adequate visceral perfusion and several enteral nutrients that are essential to maintain mucosal barrier function. Finally, by a process termed colonization resistance, the balance of microorganisms within the gut inhibit the proliferation of and subsequent invasion by the more pathogenic species. Anaerobes outnumber the more pathogenic aerobes by a factor of 10^4 to 1, and their overwhelming presence in the mucus layer lining the lumen of the intestinal tract assists in preventing access by aerobic gram-negative rods to the internal milieu. Alteration in this favorable balance (e.g., with the use of antibiotics) leads to overgrowth of the more pathogenic aerobic organisms and breakdown of this protective mechanism.

If, for whatever reason, the intestinal barrier fails, then pathogenic gram-negative microorganisms or endotoxin (i.e., lipopolysaccharide [LPS]) can gain access to the portal circulation or the mesenteric lymph nodes by a process called bacterial translocation. This process may have profound effects on the host's immunologic status and result in the development of sepsis and organ failure. This has been termed the *gut origin septic states hypothesis.*

Because these barriers do fail to protect the host completely from microorganisms, many complex adaptive responses, both specific and nonspecific, have evolved in higher organisms to protect the host.

Humoral Mechanisms

Nonspecific humoral mechanisms include the coagulation and complement cascades, both of which become activated with tissue trauma. Coagulation is important in achieving hemostasis and, therefore, in limiting exsanguination and shock. It also assists in limiting access of microorganisms to the general circulation. The complement cascade is activated by tissue trauma, bacteria and their products, and antigen-antibody complexes. Complement activation products (anaphylotoxins) have several immunologic activities in addition to enhancing microbial killing. These include neutrophil

(PMN) chemotaxis, kininlike activities, induction of adherence, and facilitation of phagocytosis. The plasma kallikrein and kinin system is activated in trauma and by LPS, generating bradykinin, a rapidly neutralized proinflammatory peptide. Bradykinin is a potent vasodilator that induces hypotension and increases capillary permeability, resulting in edema and pain. Its metabolic effects include stimulation of cyclic adenosine monophosphate, prostaglandin, and endothelial-derived relaxing factor.

Specific humoral immunity is mediated by antibodies of the various subclasses. Circulatory IgG and IgM, together with the secretory IgA that is present on mucosal surfaces, bind to microorganisms or their toxins, inhibiting growth or toxicity, respectively. This, in combination with complement and the subsequent recruitment of phagocytes, leads to microbial destruction.

Cellular Mechanisms

The macrophage is central to cell-mediated immunity, participating in the phagocytic arm of host defense, both as a participant and as a modulator of PMN function, and in the lymphocyte-mediated immune responses of T cells and B cells, including antigen presentation. In addition, the macrophage is a major secretor of powerful mediators, including a host of recently described cytokines.

PMNs have a relatively high rate of turnover, being released by the bone marrow into the circulation, where they survive for some 6 to 8 hours. They provide a ready pool of phagocytic cells that can be recruited to sites of infection to help localize and neutralize the process. PMN microbicidal activity is mediated by the generation of highly toxic reactive oxygen metabolites, the release of granular enzymes (including proteases), and the production of proinflammatory mediators such as eicosanoids.

Nonphagocytic cell-mediated immunity is a complex process involving macrophages and lymphocytes. Macrophages are required for the handling and presentation of foreign antigen, leading to the activation of helper, suppressor, and regulator T cell populations. Failure in this arm of the immune system is manifested by diminished or absent dermal delayed-type hypersensitivity response to intradermal injection of antigens, a condition termed *anergy*. This condition is associated with an increased risk of infection.

Mediators

Immune system cells are capable of releasing several chemical mediators, including the cytokines. Once released, these mediators interact with receptors on target cells, which may be other immune cells, vascular endothelial cells, or parenchymal cells. This cytokine-receptor interaction signals the immune response to effect changes in the target cells that result in further secretory activity, receptor expression, or structural alterations. The stimuli that initiate this cytokine release are varied, although tissue injury, hemorrhage, infection, and LPS all have been demonstrated to be powerful initiators of this response.

At the local tissue level, the cytokines and other mediators play an important role in modulating, amplifying, and mediating different aspects of the inflammatory response. The principal cytokines responsible for mediating this inflammatory response are tumor necrosis factor (TNF), interleukin-1 (IL-1), interleukin-6 (IL-6), interleukin-8 (IL-8), interferon-γ (IFN-γ), and transforming growth factor-β (TGF-β), in addition to the noncytokine mediators such as platelet activating factor (PAF) and eicosanoids.

Immune Dysfunction After Trauma

Major perturbations of the immune system occur in patients after major injury, placing them at risk for delayed septic mortality. Seventy-five percent of late deaths after trauma and burns result from sepsis.[2,3] The changes in the immune system are significant and global (Table 1). After trauma, there is depression of cell-mediated immunity with decreased expression of HLA-DR receptors on monocytes. These receptors are needed for antigen presentation to T cells.[4] In addition, depressed levels of IL-1, interleukin-2 (IL-2), and IFN-γ have been demonstrated and result in impaired T cell responsiveness to antigen (IL-1, IL-2) and diminished antigen presentation (IFN-γ).[5] Increased circulating levels of immunosuppressive prostaglandin E_2 (PGE$_2$) and shifts in T cell populations with decreased CD3 and CD4 subpopulations also have been demonstrated.[6]

Similar changes have been described after burns involving greater than 40% of total body surface area.[7] Diminished dermal responsiveness to recall antigens; diminished T cell function with increased suppressor cell activity and reversal of the normal helper-suppressor cell ratio function; diminished natural killer cell function and lymphokine-activated killer cells; and a transient depression in B cell numbers and immunoglobulin production all have been demonstrated after major burns. Macrophage function also is altered, with increased suppressor macrophage function associated with increased secretion of PGE$_2$. There are abnormalities in other circulating mediators, such as diminished IL-2 levels, which may be responsible for the T cell functional disturbances. Circulating endotoxin and activated complement, both of which have immunoregulatory properties, are found in the serum of burned patients.

Hemorrhage itself has a major impact on the immunologic system.[8] Phagocytic activity of the reticuloendothelial system is depressed after shock, partially as a result of diminished opsonic activity and fibronectin levels.[9] In addition, the expression of Fc and C3b receptors is decreased in several macrophage populations, leading to decreased clearance of Fc and C3b, and compounding the phagocytic defect.[10] Splenic and peritoneal macrophage cytotoxic activity is impaired after hemorrhage, although Kupffer cells appear to be more active.[11] Significant changes in lymphocyte function also have been demonstrated after trauma and hemorrhage.

TABLE 1.
Immune Dysfunction After Trauma, Burns, and Hemorrhage*

Macrophage
  Decreased Fc and C3b receptor
    expression
  Phagocytic and cytotoxic defects
  Decreased HLA-DR receptor expression
  Impaired antigen presentation
  Increased suppressor macrophage
    function
  Increased production of
    immunosuppressive PGE_2
Lymphocyte
  Loss of recall antigen responses (anergy)
  Depression of B cell and
    immunoglobulin production
  Decreased natural killer and
    lymphokine-activated killer cell activity
  Increased T suppressor activity
  Production of immunosuppressive
    peptides
Neutrophil
  Depressed chemotaxis, phagocytosis,
    chemiluminescence, and intracellular
    killing
Humoral
  Altered cytokine production (increased
    TNF, IL-1, IL-6; decreased IL-2, IL-3,
    IFN-γ)
  Systemic release of other
    immunosuppressive mediators and
    hormones
  Immunosuppressive complement
    activation products
  Decreased serum fibronectin and
    opsonic activity

PGE_2 = prostaglandin E_2; TNF = tumor necrosis factor; IL = interleukin; IFN-γ = interferon-γ.

There is diminished mitogen-induced proliferation[12] and decreased IL-2 production.[13] Diminished interleukin-3 (IL-3) production by lymphocytes may be responsible for the suppressed maturation of both T cells and B cells.[14] Splenocyte IL-6 production is reduced after hemorrhage and may be responsible for the observed defect in B cell maturation and immunoglobulin production.[15] IFN-γ levels also are decreased after hemorrhage, with potential impairment of macrophage activation, cytotoxic T cell activity, and natural killer cell activity.[16]

Other macrophage functions affected by hemorrhage include impaired antigen presentation and altered cytokine production, with increased levels of IL-1, IL-6, and TNF seen early after hemorrhage.[17] Kupffer cells seem to be a predominant source of these cytokines. Levels of IL-1 and IL-6 rise after hemorrhage, peaking at about 2 hours. IL-1 disappears rapidly, although increased IL-6 levels can be sustained for 24 hours.[18, 19] TNF levels peak early, but biologic activity is absent by 24 hours,[20] possibly because of the presence of TNF inhibitors.[21, 22] There also is an increase in cell-associated TNF on Kupffer cells. PGE_2 levels are significantly elevated after hemorrhage, with increased production by Kupffer cells, peritoneal macrophages, and monocytes.[23] PGE_2 has been shown to be a major immunosuppressive mediator. It causes decreased IL-1 and TNF synthesis,[23, 24] decreased expression of the major histocompatibility (MHC) class II antigens,[25] diminished levels of other circulating lymphokines, inhibition of B cell proliferation and immunoglobulin production,[26] and diminished production of IFN-γ. TGF-β, a growth factor with immunosuppressive properties, also is produced in increased amounts by splenic macrophages after hemorrhage.[27]

Alterations in PMN function also have been described after trauma. In a study of 28 patients with the adult respiratory distress syndrome (ARDS), 14 of whom had sustained multisystem trauma, Martin and colleagues were able to demonstrate impaired superoxide production by circulating PMNs in trauma victims compared to control subjects.[28] In addition, PMNs isolated from the airways of patients with ARDS showed profound impairment of both superoxide production and microbial killing. Other investigators have demonstrated a chemotaxis deficit in PMNs isolated from traumatized patients.[29]

The combined effects of these significant changes in macrophage, PMN, and lymphocyte function, together with altered cytokine production, cause a profound immunosuppression of the host after trauma, burns, or hemorrhage, resulting in an increased susceptibility to infection. The underlying mechanism of the immunosuppression appears to be multifactorial.

Mechanisms of Immunosuppression After Trauma

Tissue Injury

Major wounds, such as those caused by burns or devitalizing blunt trauma, pose a double threat to the patient. First, there is a loss of the normal barrier function, which allows pathogens access to the internal milieu. Second, the devitalized tissue itself appears to be responsible for many of the immunosuppressive effects of injury. Early excision and grafting of burn wounds results in more rapid reversal of immunosuppression.[30] Iatrogenic wounds (e.g., surgeries and invasive lines) also represent a breach in barrier protection and may contribute to the traumatic immunosuppression.

Gastrointestinal Tract and Bacterial Translocation

The other major barrier at risk in traumatized patients is the gastrointestinal tract. Shock, severe trauma, endotoxemia, and short-term starvation all have been shown to have a negative effect on the functional integrity of the intestinal mucosa, resulting in the translocation of bacteria or endotoxin into the portal circulation or mesenteric lymph node system.[31] Several authors have suggested that this phenomenon may induce immunosuppression after trauma.[32-35] The reported mechanism for this immunosuppression is believed to be primarily the effects of endotoxin as mediated through macrophage-derived cytokines and other humoral mediators, including eicosanoids. The clinical relevance of bacterial translocation in immunosuppression after trauma, and the subsequent development of systemic sepsis or the systemic inflammatory response syndrome has yet to be clarified.[31]

Stress Hormones

Several endogenous hormones are released after injury, including catecholamines, glucocorticoids, glucagon, and endorphins. This neuroendocrine response may have a significant effect on the immune system. Catecholamines impair T cell proliferation, IL-2 receptor expression, B cell function, and immunoglobulin production, and they diminish phagocytic activity.[36-38] Levels of catecholamines remain elevated only transiently after hemorrhagic shock, but this may be sufficient to initiate immunosuppressive activity.

Glucocorticoids also affect the immune system, causing decreased T cell blastogenesis,[39] reduced IL-2 production,[40] and consequent diminished T cell proliferation. They also impair macrophage function, particularly the expression of 1a and Fc receptors, and reduce IL-1 production.[41] These glucocorticoid-induced changes tend to be short-lived, however, as are the elevations in serum cortisol levels that are seen after hemorrhage, and probably do not explain the sustained immunosuppression that occurs in injured patients.

Endorphins may play a role in immunosuppression after trauma. Levels of β-endorphin are elevated after burn injuries. Exogenously administered opioids modulate both lymphocyte and PMN function.[42]

Mediators

Increased levels of several immunosuppressive humoral mediators are present in the serum of injured patients. Significant amounts of arachidonic acid metabolites are found after trauma. The macrophage appears to be the principal source for these mediators, of which the leukotrienes, thromboxanes, and prostaglandins appear to be the most important. They are produced by the lipoxygenase or cyclooxygenase breakdown of arachidonic acid derived from the phospholipid of cell membranes by the action of phospholipase A_2. The most significant of these immunosuppressive mediators is PGE_2, which is present in significantly increased amounts (eight times normal) after trauma. The presence of PGE_2 has been correlated with decreased IL-1, IFN-γ, and IL-2 production, and with T helper cell numbers.[43] The significance of this effect is illustrated by the total inhibition of these changes when nonsteroidal anti-inflammatory drugs (NSAIDs) or N3 polyunsaturated fatty acids are used to block the production of PGE_2.[44,45]

Other humoral mediators have less clearly defined roles in immunosuppression after trauma. The third complement fragment has been shown to have inhibitory effects on lymphocyte blastogenesis, and PAF in high doses can inhibit lymphocyte proliferation and IL-2 production. These effects are somewhat dose-dependent, and their relevance to the immunosuppression of trauma is unclear.

Suppressor Factors

Christou and Meakins have described an 8-kd peptide identified in the serum of trauma patients that inhibits PMN chemotaxis.[29] Moreover, this chemotaxis inhibition, together with the presence of anergy, was predictive of subsequent septic complications in these patients. If both anergy and impaired chemotaxis were present, the risk of sepsis development was 40%.

Ozkan and others have reported the presence of a serum suppressive factor known as suppressive active peptide in the serum of burn and trauma patients that suppresses T cell and B cell proliferation.[46] The most likely source of this peptide is the degradation products of circulating plasma proteins, particularly fibronectin.[47] Other factors in the range of 10 to 30 kd have been isolated from the serum of trauma patients and have shown suppressive activity on mitogen-induced lymphocyte proliferation.

Soluble receptors to TNF, IL-1, and IL-2 have been isolated in the circulation of trauma patients and are responsible for the inhibition of these cytokine actions. This may be an example of autoregulation of the immune system. Whether these soluble receptors result in pathologic immunosuppression is unknown.

Suppressor Cells

Animal studies have demonstrated increased numbers of circulating CD8+ suppressor T cells 2 hours after hemorrhage.[48] Similar findings have been described after burns and trauma.[49,50] The role of this phenomenon in the immunosuppressive consequences of trauma has not been clarified.

Hypoxia and Ischemia

Relatively short periods of hypotension or hypoxia result in rapid depletion of adenosine triphosphate levels in splenic and peritoneal macrophages.[51] Hypoxia reduces macrophage antigen presentation abilities and is associated with increased production of TNF and PGE_2.[52] Other studies have shown similar effects after hemorrhage, and noted additional suppression of macrophage cytokine production, including IL-1 and IL-6. Splenocyte adenosine triphosphate levels, IL-2 and IL-3 synthesis, and proliferative capacity also were reduced.[53, 54]

Nutritional Deficiency

Severe trauma results in a hypermetabolic state induced by the neuroendocrine response to trauma. Glucagon, epinephrine, and cortisol appear to be chiefly responsible for this phenomenon, which is manifested by hyperglycemia, negative nitrogen balance, and hyperinsulinemia. The combination of this hypermetabolic state and the diminished nutritional intake of acutely injured patients results in a relative protein calorie malnutrition. Nitrogen losses may approach 40 g/day in these patients, and represent a rapid depletion of protein stores. Several studies have documented the importance of aggressive nutritional support in reversing the immunosuppression that occurs after trauma and reducing the incidence of septic complications in seriously injured patients.[55] This suggests that the nutritional deficit imposed by trauma itself is immunosuppressive.

Sepsis and the Systemic Inflammatory Response

As a consequence of the immunosuppression and barrier disruption caused by trauma, there is a high rate of infectious complications such as pneumonia, wound infection, and intra-abdominal abscess. Frequently associated with these complications is a systemic inflammatory response characterized by fever, leukocytosis, hyperdynamic circulation, and, in extreme cases, organ failure and death.[2, 3] This phenomenon, known as sepsis and multiple organ failure, accounts for a large proportion of the delayed mortality seen after trauma. The same response is observed in trauma patients in whom no focus of active infection is found. This is known as the systemic inflammatory response syndrome or the sepsis syndrome.[56] The pathogenesis of both conditions appears to be mediated through the activation of the immune system. Major trauma, shock, and subsequent sepsis are thought to lead to a systemic activation of the immune system, resulting in hemodynamic changes, widespread microvascular injury, and organ failure.

Pivotal in this schema is the macrophage, which appears to mediate many aspects of the systemic inflammatory response to sepsis.[57, 58] The pathologic effects of endotoxin (LPS) are largely mediated by macrophages, which produce various proinflammatory mediators (TNF, IL-1, IL-6, PAF, and eicosanoids). These macrophages also produce additional mediators such as the chemoattractants IL-8 and leukotriene B_4, which activate and recruit PMNs, thus amplifying the inflammatory response. LPS also induces macrophage and endothelial cell procoagulant activity and PAF release, promoting microvascular thrombosis.

LPS and cytokines directly activate PMNs and endothelial cells, resulting in increased expression of adherence molecules and consequent PMN-endothelial cell adherence. PMN-endothelial cell adherence is considered a crucial step in PMN-mediated organ injury, which appears to play an important role in several animal models of shock[59, 60] and reperfusion injury.[61] Endothelial cell injury and subsequent organ failure are thought to be mediated by toxic PMN products, including proteases and oxygen radicals.[62]

The perpetuation of this exaggerated inflammatory response after trauma or sepsis remains the subject of intense investigation and speculation. It appears that the immune system escapes from its autoregulatory control such that the normally protective immunologic mechanisms become injurious to the host. Whether this exaggerated, persistent response is related to the extent of the initial injury, ongoing occult hypoperfusion and tissue ischemia, persistent occult infection, or breakdown of the gastrointestinal barrier leading to translocation is unknown. These and other potential processes, however, may coexist in an injured patient with sepsis.

Immunomodulation

Therapeutic intervention aimed at modifying the immune system is not a new concept. The term *immunomodulation* is being used increasingly to describe some of the new therapeutic interventions targeted at specific aspects of the immune response. Efforts to modify the immune system, however, range from simple interventions designed to restore normal homeostasis with aggressive resuscitation and nutritional support to the latest state-of-the-art manipulations of immune cells, their products, and subcellular processes (Table 2).

Preservation of Normal Defenses

Rapid control of hemorrhage, and early and complete resuscitation with return of tissue oxygenation to all organs is the critical first step in trauma care that can have a favorable effect on the patient's immune system. By limiting hemorrhage, the need for transfusion, and the duration of hypotension, many of the immunosuppressive aspects of trauma can be attenuated. Prompt resuscitation reduces the severity of the global ischemia reperfusion injury that has been demonstrated to be so toxic in animal models of shock.[59, 60]

Early debridement of devitalized wounds, particularly relevant in burn

TABLE 2.
Potential Immunomodulation Strategies in the Trauma Patient

Preservation of normal defenses
   Resuscitation, wound debridement
   Restoration of barriers
   Preservation of gastrointestinal tract function
   Metabolic and nutritional support
Immunologic stimulation
   Immunization
   Biologic response modifiers
   Metabolic stimulation
   Nutritional pharmacotherapy
Immunologic blockade
   Eradication of infection
   Neutralization of endotoxin
   Mediator inhibition
   Nonspecific immunomodulators
   Neutrophil- and endothelium-targeted strategies

injury, has been demonstrated to limit the degree and duration of immunosuppression associated with these wounds, and to limit the duration of the hypermetabolic state.[7, 30] Closure of wounds in the skin integument and mucosal surfaces restores barrier integrity. Restoration of the gastrointestinal tract barrier, however, requires more than merely restoring anatomic continuity. Bacterial translocation will occur unless functional activity also is restored, which requires adequate resuscitation and early institution of enteral feeding.[63]

Prophylaxis against erosive gastritis with histamine$_2$ receptor antagonists may be a double-edged sword in that it abolishes gastric acidity and allows bacterial colonization of the upper gastrointestinal tract. Within 24 hours, the stomach and proximal intestine become colonized with oral microflora, and within 48 hours, colonic organisms begin to predominate. If prophylaxis against erosive gastritis is required, sucralfate may have advantages over acid-neutralizing regimens, in that it provides cytoprotection without the need for alkalinization and, therefore, preserves gastric acidity and sterility. There is some suggestion that this approach results in a reduced incidence of nosocomial pneumonia.[64]

Invasive monitoring lines, Foley catheters, endotracheal tubes, and nasogastric tubes all pose threats to the patient's protective barrier mechanisms and should be used only if specifically indicated.

In addition to restoration of barriers and prompt resuscitation, the other factor that can affect the patient's immune system dramatically is nutritional metabolic support. The hypermetabolic state associated with acute injury imposes a significant strain on the patient's nutritional reserves, with a substantial effect on the immune system. Several studies have demonstrated the efficacy of prompt nutritional support after trauma and burns, as well as a reduced incidence of septic complications.[55] The route and composition of nutritional support seem to be important, with enteral feeding being apparently superior to parenteral nutritional support.[65, 66] Standard formula preparations with high protein and some fiber content appear to be superior to elemental diets.[55, 67, 68] Several specific supplemental nutrients recently have been identified as having specific immunostimulant properties; these are discussed in the next section. It is difficult to estimate accurately the protein calorie requirements of severely stressed patients, and careful nutritional monitoring and modification of dietary regimens is necessary to optimize the level of support.

Immunologic Stimulation

The concept of immunostimulation also is not new, dating from the time of Jenner, who demonstrated the efficacy of active immunization against smallpox with cowpox vaccine.[69] Since that time, many vaccines have been developed against microorganisms or their toxic products, revolutionizing the control of infectious disease. This classic immunization is only one of several mechanisms used to stimulate the immune system.

Immunization

Active and passive immunization against specific organisms in injured patients is essentially limited to the use of antitetanus toxoid and hyperimmune globulin to prevent tetanus, active and passive immunization against rabies, and active immunization against encapsulated organisms after splenectomy. Patients who have undergone splenectomy are at risk for the development of overwhelming postsplenectomy infections, which are associated with significant mortality. The predominant organisms in these infections are encapsulated varieties, particularly pneumococci, *haemophilus influenzae,* and meningococci. Vaccines against these three organisms are available, and have relatively high efficacy and low toxicity. These immunizations should be offered to all patients undergoing splenectomy. Other antibodies, specifically monoclonal antibodies, directed against bacterial products or cytokines are being used to down-regulate the inflammatory response and are discussed in the section regarding immunologic blockade.

Biologic Response Modifiers

Numerous naturally occurring biologic agents stimulate the immune system. Endotoxin, *Corynebacterium parvum* vaccine, bacille Calmette-Guérin, zymosan, and muramyl dipeptide all have demonstrated efficacy in preventing sepsis in animal models. Their clinical use is limited by their unpredictability of action, difficulty in purification, and toxic side effects. Levamisole, an anthelmintic preparation, has been shown to have immunostimulant actions, and in one clinical trial was noted to have efficacy in reducing mortality in patients with intra-abdominal sepsis.[70] Thymopentin has been studied more extensively, and has been shown to reduce postoperative anergy and to increase IL-2 synthesis in patients with burns and those who have undergone cardiac surgery.[6, 71] Neither of these studies, however, demonstrated a reduction in infectious complications or septic mortality.

Many cytokines have immunostimulant properties. TNF, administered intravenously in small doses, results in tolerance to subsequent normally lethal doses of TNF or endotoxin. This effect appears to result from downregulation of TNF messenger RNA production by macrophages and decreased cellular sensitivity to TNF, and is an example of induced tolerance.[72] The clinical application of this effect remains to be determined.

IL-1 increases neutrophil counts and improves survival during experimental *Escherichia coli* infection and endotoxemia in experimental granulocytopenia.[73] This effect has not been studied clinically.

The lymphokine, IL-2, has been studied for its immunostimulant activity and has been used clinically in patients with cancer. The administration of IL-2 has been shown to enhance survival during experimental gram-negative peritoneal infection. It is most effective when it is given at the site of infection and probably acts by stimulating local host defenses.[74, 75] IL-2 has been shown to enhance natural killer cell activity and stimulate the generation of cytotoxic T cells. IL-2 administration has not been studied in injured patients.

IFN-γ is an immunostimulant cytokine. Laboratory studies demonstrate that it increases resistance to intra-abdominal sepsis and improves survival after trauma and hemorrhagic shock.[76] Clinical trials of IFN-γ have shown reversal of trauma-induced suppression of MHC (class II) HLA-DR antigens on macrophages. There was no clear benefit in septic morbidity or mortality in patients given IFN-γ, however.[77, 78] IFN-γ toxicity also limits its usefulness. In a recent note of caution, IFN-γ treatment of normal animals increased the subsequent toxicity of endotoxin.[79] Further clinical studies of this cytokine are needed to define its role as an immunostimulant.

The use of any of these cytokines as immunostimulants, particularly in the trauma patient, must be considered highly speculative and experimental. The major concern is that injudicious stimulation may cause systemic activation of the inflammatory response, with attendant morbidity and mortality from the sepsis syndrome and organ failure.

Colony-stimulating factors of various types have been isolated, including granulocyte colony-stimulating factor, macrophage colony-stimulating factor, granulocyte-macrophage colony-stimulating factor, and IL-3. All are available in recombinant forms and have been used in patients with neutropenia after hematologic cancer, patients with acquired immunodeficiency syndrome, and patients who have undergone bone marrow transplantation. Granulocyte-macrophage colony-stimulating factor also has been given to trauma and burn patients, with improvement of leukocyte counts.[80] A form of insulin-like growth factor reduces gut atrophy and bacterial translocation in rats after major burns (>50% body surface area).[81]

The use of growth factors to stimulate the immune system, increase specific cell lines, and accelerate wound healing is an appealing addition to our armamentarium for stimulating the immune system and healing response. Their use may not be associated with the same risks of systemic inflammation that attend the administration of cytokines.

Metabolic Support, Adenosine Triphosphate-MgCl$_2$

Shock caused by trauma or sepsis results in an energy deficit at the tissue level. This is associated with immunosuppression. Aggressive resuscitation and early nutritional support will limit this defect, but significant energy depletion may persist. Adenosine triphosphate-MgCl$_2$ is an agent aimed at restoring tissue energy levels. Experimentally, it has been shown to restore macrophage antigen-presenting function[53] and splenocyte proliferation[54]; it also decreased levels of TNF and IL-6,[82] and improved survival.[83] Its role in the treatment of patients with septic or traumatic shock has not been determined.

Nutritional Pharmacotherapy

The beneficial effects of early and aggressive nutritional support in the trauma patient have been discussed. Recently, specific nutritional supplements have been found to have immunostimulant properties that go beyond simple metabolic support. Nutrients that have potential or proven pharmacologic effects on the immune system include branched chain amino acids, arginine, glutamine, N3 polyunsaturated fatty acids (N3 PUFAs), RNA, and vitamins A, C, and E.

Branched chain amino acids are the major energy sources for skeletal muscle and the brain during periods of stress and sepsis. In one double-blind study of patients undergoing surgery, nutritional support with increased proportions of branched chain amino acids was shown to improve nitrogen retention, elevate the lymphocyte count, improve plasma transferrin levels, and reverse anergy to skin testing.[84] Nevertheless, this has not translated into improved outcomes, and their use cannot be unequivocally endorsed.[85]

Arginine is a nonessential amino acid that may become essential during stress because of failure of synthetic pathways. Given in pharmacologic doses after injury, it has been shown to have immunostimulant and improved wound healing effects in both humans and experimental animals.[86] At these doses, arginine stimulates pituitary growth hormone, insulin-like growth factor, prolactin, insulin, and other hormones; this has a net positive effect on wound healing and immune function. In addition, L-arginine is a precursor of nitrates, nitrites, and nitric oxide. Nitric oxide has several immunostimulant functions, including improved macrophage killing of bacteria.[87]

Glutamine is a nonessential amino acid that is normally in abundant supply, although levels may fall precipitously during stress. Given in pharmacologic doses, glutamine has beneficial effects on host immunity and decreases septic complications after trauma. At these doses, it improves antimicrobial killing by PMNs and appears to stimulate gut enterocyte function, preserving mucosal integrity and possibly decreasing bacterial translocation, although this has been challenged recently.[68] Mucosal trophism is achieved by either oral or intravenous administration.[88]

Dietary lipid is incorporated into the phospholipids of cell membranes, thereby affecting numerous membrane functions, including membrane receptor expression, cell-to-cell interactions, and signaling.[89] In addition, membrane stimulation (e.g., LPS) leads to the activation of phospholipase A_2, the release of arachidonic acid, and subsequent generation of eicosanoid products. The nature of these arachidonic acid metabolites can dramatically be altered by dietary changes in fat intake. The typical N6-PUFAs found in vegetable oils produce arachidonic acid metabolites that tend to inhibit cell-mediated immune responses by the generation of prostaglandins, notably PGE_2. Immunosuppressive activities of N6-PUFA eicosanoids include inhibition of antibody formation (B cell function), natural killer cell activity, and cytokine release. N3-PUFAs are found primarily in fish oils and generate eicosanoids with less biologic activity than do N6-PUFAs. After the incorporation of N3-PUFAs, macrophages stimulated with LPS show reduced inositol phosphate production, dienoic eicosanoid release, and IL-1/TNF release.[90] In fact, there is some enhancement of cell-mediated immune responses.

Protein synthesis depends on the production of RNA, which itself depends on the precursors purines and pyrimidines. These normally are not essential dietary constituents. In conditions of stress or demonstrated immunosuppression, however, dietary supplementation with nucleotides, particularly uracil, has been demonstrated to reverse aspects of immunosuppression. Uracil has been shown to restore delayed-type hypersensitivity, to stimulate an antigenic proliferative response in T cells, and to reduce abscess formation caused by gram-positive organisms. Dietary nucleotides also may be effective in macrophage activation of the T helper inducer populations.[91] RNAs given to animals receiving low-protein diets restore the immune response and resistance to infection.[92]

The pathogenesis of sepsis and organ injury is thought to be mediated to a great extent by toxic oxygen species. Antioxidants, therefore, have a putative role in limiting the extent of this injury. Vitamins A, C, and particularly E, have antioxidant properties, and have been shown to reduce mortality in animal burn injury studies.[93]

Several of these immunostimulant dietary constituents have been combined into a commercial enteral nutritional formula and subjected to clinical trials,[94–96] the results of which have recently been reviewed.[97] In these studies, a supplemental diet enriched with arginine, N3-PUFAs, RNAs, and selective vitamins resulted in significantly better outcome, decreased septic complications (in particular, wound infections in burned patients) by about

75%, and reduced the hospital stay by about 22%. No effect on mortality was demonstrated.

Immunosuppression after trauma is real and often profound, and the consequences (i.e., septic mortality) are severe. It seems logical, therefore, to attempt to reverse this immunosuppression. Of all the immunostimulant strategies discussed, however, only nutritional pharmacotherapy has been demonstrated to be both efficacious (in terms of outcome and specific immunostimulant activity) and safe. Furthermore, it is unclear which patients are most likely to benefit from this more expensive, enriched nutritional support. Patients with burns over more than 40% of the total body surface area or with equivalent multisystem blunt trauma are likely to fall into that category.

Other potential immunostimulants have not found a place in the treatment of trauma patients. The potential for adverse effects is significant and of real concern. Further laboratory and clinical testing of these agents is required before any recommendations for their use can be made.

Sepsis and Immunologic Blockade

A patient in whom sepsis or the systemic inflammatory response syndrome develops without a proven source of infection is at high risk for the development of progressive multiorgan failure and death. This progressive, often relentless pathologic process appears to be mediated largely by an immune system that has systematically become activated and injurious to the host. Some underlying stimulus, whether it is a persistent septic focus, visceral ischemia, bacterial translocation, or failure of the immune system to autoregulate its response, causes macrophage activation, cytokine release, and secondary changes in PMN and endothelial function, resulting in generalized microvascular injury and organ failure. The therapeutic challenge is to identify and eradicate any underlying process that is fueling the inflammatory response, then to down-regulate those aspects of the immune system that are injurious to the host.

Eradication of Sepsis or Endotoxin

Patients with signs of systemic sepsis require a careful and diligent evaluation for sources of untreated infection. The most common potential sources of unchecked infection and inflammation include major soft-tissue injuries (especially burns), nosocomial infections (particularly pneumonia, line infections, and urinary tract infections), and occult abdominal sepsis from intra-abdominal abscesses, acalculous cholecystitis, or bacterial translocation. In the absence of any obvious source of infection, exploratory laparotomy has been advocated in patients with developing multiple organ failure.[98] This approach no longer prevails, however, in light of the negative operative findings in many of these patients. Nevertheless, an aggressive diagnostic workup, including imaging of the abdomen with ultrasound of the gallbladder and biliary tree and abdominal computed tomography to rule out intra-abdominal abscess, in addition to culture surveillance, may be indicated.

Once a source of sepsis has been identified, every attempt should be made to eradicate it. Burn wounds should be excised and grafted as soon as possible,[7, 30] and devitalized tissue should be debrided.[7] Early fracture fixation and patient mobilization has been shown to reduce the incidence of subsequent organ dysfunction.[99, 100] Any intra-abdominal sepsis must be drained either surgically or by interventional radiologic techniques, and any nosocomial infections should be treated aggressively with appropriate antibiotics (for pneumonia or urinary tract infection), line changes (for line sepsis), or surgical intervention (for wound infections, cholecystitis, or intra-abdominal abscess).

The absence of an identifiable infectious focus is not unusual in septic patients. Meakins and Marshall have suggested that, under these circumstances, the gastrointestinal tract may be the source of sepsis and organ failure by the mechanism of bacterial or endotoxin translocation.[35] The beneficial aspects of early enteral feeding with full formulary diets in preserving gut mucosal integrity may have a major effect on the development of organ failure.

The use of sucralfate rather than histamine$_2$ receptor antagonists also may limit the degree to which the upper gastrointestinal tract becomes colonized with pathogens and, secondarily, may reduce the incidence of nosocomial infection, principally pneumonia.[64] Limiting the use of systemic antibiotics will help to preserve normal gut flora and colonization resistance. Therapeutic augmentation of this effect has been advocated using selective decontamination of the digestive tract as a means of reducing the reservoir of pathogenic organisms. Combinations of orally and parenterally administered antibiotics have been described that lower the colony count of the more pathogenic aerobic gram-negative organisms that populate the intestinal tract and selectively increase the anaerobic population, resulting in the process of selective resistance. Clinical studies using selective decontamination have demonstrated a decreased rate of nosocomial infection, particularly respiratory tract infection, but this has not translated into reductions in the length of hospitalization, ventilator dependence, or mortality, except in small subgroups.[101] Without the identification of a major improvement in outcome or cost benefit, selective decontamination cannot be endorsed unequivocally, and further studies are required.

Immunologic Blockade: Antiendotoxin Strategies

Because most of the deleterious effects of sepsis are thought to be mediated by endotoxin (LPS), several novel approaches to inhibit directly the effects of LPS have been described. Ziegler and colleagues described a series of patients with suspected gram-negative bacteremia who were treated with a human antiserum to the mutant J5 *E. coli* organism.[102] This polyclonal antiserum resulted in a 37% reduction in mortality in the treated patients. The problems associated with human antiserum, however, led to the development of monoclonal antibodies directed at specific LPS antigens. Two subsequent multicenter, double-blind, randomized trials used monoclonal IgM antibodies. One used a murine antibody (E5) directed at an epitope on the lipid A moiety.[103] The second used an IgM human antibody (HA-1A) also directed against lipid A.[104] The subgroup analysis of the E5 study demonstrated improved survival in septic patients who had gram-negative sepsis but were not in septic shock.[103] A subsequent clinical trial using E5, however, failed to confirm this improvement in survival.[105] In addition, IgG antibodies to E5 developed in almost half the patients given this murine product, although the clinical significance of this was not determined.

The experience with HA-1A is somewhat similar. The initial study reported on the use of HA-1A in 543 patients with sepsis. No difference between the treatment and placebo groups was found with respect to overall mortality, but a significant improvement in 28-day survival was seen in patients with gram-negative infections and bacteremia, particularly those with shock.[104] Concerns were raised about the design of this study, the statistical validity of subgroups analysis, and the level of statistical significance obtained.[106] A subsequent randomized, double-blind, multicenter study of HA-1A in patients with gram-negative sepsis and shock failed to demonstrate any benefit and the study was terminated. With inconclusive evidence of efficacy, and given the prohibitive cost ($3,750 per dose) of these agents, neither E5 nor HA-1A has been approved by the U.S. Food and Drug Administration for clinical use in sepsis.[106]

Two other approaches to neutralizing the effects of endotoxin have been described. Bactericidal/permeability increasing protein is a protein with 40% homology with lipid binding protein. Lipid binding protein complexes with LPS to facilitate binding with CD14 cell membrane receptors thought necessary to activate cytokine production by macrophages in response to LPS. Bactericidal/permeability increasing protein appears to exert its effect by a cytotoxic membrane effect on gram-negative organisms, leading to cytolysis, and has been shown experimentally to provide protective capacity against lethal gram-negative bacterial challenge.[107]

Endotoxin neutralizing protein is a recombinant form of a naturally occurring anti-LPS factor produced by the American horseshoe crab *Limulus polyphemus*. Endotoxin neutralizing protein neutralizes LPS toxicity by competing directly with the coagulation zymogens. In animal studies, endotoxin neutralizing protein has been efficacious in improving survival and reducing the degree of organ injury in LPS-mediated sepsis.[108] Clinical trials using bactericidal/permeability increasing protein or endotoxin neutralizing protein are awaited, and these agents do not yet have a role in the clinical arena.

Immunologic Blockade: Mediator Inhibition

Gram-negative sepsis and endotoxin mediate their adverse effects on the host by the elaboration of cytokines and other mediators from host immune cells, particularly macrophages. TNF is thought to be central among the cytokines in mediating the host response to endotoxin, but IL-1, IL-6,

PAF, and eicosanoids also are believed to be important. The interplay between these mediators, their effects on cell receptors, and subsequent cell-to-cell interactions probably are as important as the effects of individual cytokines. Several therapeutic strategies have evolved that target the production, release, or effects of these mediators, either specifically using anticytokine monoclonal antibodies or specific inhibitors, or nonspecifically using immunomodulant drugs such as steroids or NSAIDs to modify the immune response.

Anti-Tumor Necrosis Factor Strategies.—Considerable evidence points to TNF as an important mediator of both gram-negative and gram-positive sepsis. The cytokine appears early after endotoxemia and precedes the appearance of other cytokines. Its appearance is associated with many of the host's responses to sepsis,[109] and the administration of recombinant TNF mimics the septic response to endotoxin.[110] Certain anti-TNF antibody preparations have been shown to be protective in experimental models of sepsis,[111] and concurrent with improved survival, there also is a decreased release of other cytokines, such as IL-1 and IL-6.[112] The results of preliminary clinical studies using anti-TNF monoclonal antibody have been inconclusive, with only transient reductions in serum TNF levels and no survival benefit demonstrated.[113, 114] A recent multicenter trial using anti-TNF monoclonal antibody has reported similar results, with benefit limited to patients with high TNF titers.[115]

Natural inhibitory proteins to TNF are found. Three different types of TNF binding protein have been identified that appear shortly after TNF production and function in an autoregulatory fashion. The natural forms of the binding proteins are not stable and are not useful as clinical agents, although recombinant forms of TNF binding protein are being developed and initial animal studies appear to be promising.[116]

Interleukin-1 Receptor Antagonist.—IL-1 has similarly been associated with the mediation of many of the host's responses to endotoxemia, although the data are less compelling than for TNF. The effects of IL-1 can be blocked by the use of the IL-1 receptor antagonist. This peptide is found in serum after the secretion of IL-1 and appears to be part of the natural feedback control of the immune system. Recombinant forms of this protein given to experimental animals have abrogated many of the effects of IL-1.[117, 118] In phase 2 clinical studies, IL-1 receptor antagonist infusion resulted in a significant decrease in mortality in septic patients. IL-1 receptor antagonist is currently being investigated in a multicenter, double-blind clinical trial.

Interleukin-6 Antibodies.—IL-6 appears later after the onset of endotoxemia or sepsis, but levels appear to be sustained long after levels of TNF and IL-1 have fallen to baseline.[119] A recent multicenter study of septic patients found that increased IL-6 levels, but not TNF levels, were predictive of fatal outcome.[115] Studies in burned patients also suggest that levels of this IL-6 cytokine are more predictive of lethal sepsis after a burn injury than are levels of TNF and IL-1.[120] Clinical trials using antibodies to IL-6 are awaited, although studies in mice have demonstrated the efficacy of anti–IL-6 monoclonal antibody in protecting against lethal E. coli and TNF challenge.[121] In another animal model of sepsis, Il-6 antibodies were able to block TGF-β–mediated splenocyte depression.[122]

Bradykinin Inhibitors.—Vasoactive kinins are released during endotoxic or septic shock. There is no clear relationship between the appearance or concentration of these peptides, however, and the degree of shock or mortality. The specific role that these peptides play in mediating the pathogenesis of shock is unclear. Some of the effects of the kinins are clearly protective in that they stimulate prostacyclin, which is an endothelium-protecting prostanoid, and counteract the effects of vasoconstrictors that appear during shock. Kinin inhibition, therefore, may be a two-edged sword in that it has a tendency to support the hemodynamics during sepsis, but may cause local organ hypoperfusion and other adverse effects.[123] Clinical trials using bradykinin inhibitors are anticipated shortly.

Platelet Activating Factor Antagonists.—PAF, similar to the eicosanoids, is derived from membrane phospholipid by the action of phospholipase A_2 in response to LPS or cytokines. The role of PAF in mediating the pathologic effects of trauma, shock, and sepsis is a complex one involving interaction between PAF, leukocyte proteases, TNF, and other mediators.[124] PAF activity is closely related to eicosanoid production, which it appears to regulate,[125] as well as to TNF and IL-1 release, which it enhances.[126, 127] PAF antagonists inhibit the direct, amplification, and priming effects of PAF and appear to be effective in reducing mortality in experimental models of shock and sepsis. Calcium channel antagonists have anti-PAF actions in addition to restoring transmembrane calcium signals, and have been shown to improve immunologic function, antigen processing, and survival in experimental sepsis.[128] Clinical trials are being conducted to evaluate PAF antagonists.

Immunologic Blockade: Nonspecific Agents

Several pharmacologic agents with significant and potentially therapeutic effects on the immune system have been studied experimentally and clinically, with various results. The best known among these are the glucocorticoids, NSAIDs, and pentoxifylline.

Steroids.—Supranormal levels of endogenous glucocorticoids are part of the normal neuroendocrine response to stress and have been considered to be protective. This finding prompted the administration of pharmacologic doses of steroids to patients with injury, sepsis, and shock. The action of glucocorticoids in stress recently has become better understood; it appears that they function as regulators or dampers of the immune system, acting in an autoregulatory role. Among the immunosuppressive actions of steroids are attenuation of eicosanoid production by macrophages, limitation of complement activation, and stabilization of several cellular and subcellular membranes. In addition, steroids reduce TNF and IL-1 production by macrophages[129, 130] and down-regulate nitric oxide synthase.

With such global suppression of different aspects of the immune system, dramatic changes might be expected in the outcome of patients given pharmacologic doses of these agents. Two recent trials using corticosteroids in sepsis and shock, however, have shown no such benefits.[131, 132] Animal studies that have demonstrated improved survival in sepsis have done so only when glucocorticoids are given early in the course of sepsis, at a point when patients in human clinical trials would not have met inclusion criteria for the studies.[133] It appears that, if steroids are to be effective in the treatment of sepsis and septic shock, they must be given before the onset of severe manifestations of the condition.

Nonsteroidal Anti-Inflammatory Drugs.—Endotoxin, TNF, and IL-1 stimulate phospholipase A_2 activities, resulting in the release of arachidonic acid and other lipid products from membrane phospholipid. Eicosanoids, products of the cyclooxygenase or lipoxygenase degradation of arachidonic acid, participate significantly in the mediation of sepsis and septic shock. The prostaglandins PGF_2, PGE_2, and PGI_2; the thromboxanes; and the leukotrienes are particularly important. PGE_2 has a profound immunosuppressive action, principally on lymphocyte function, whereas PGI_2 has a systemic vasodilative action contributing to the development of systemic hypotension in sepsis. Thromboxane A_2 is a potent platelet aggregator and vasoconstrictor, and contributes to the development of visceral hypoperfusion and pulmonary hypertension in sepsis.

NSAIDs function chiefly by inhibition of the cyclooxygenase pathway, which results in reduced production of these mediators. The NSAID ibuprofen has been studied in several animal models of sepsis and endotoxemia. Ibuprofen decreased levels of PGE_2, improved antigen presentation by macrophages and synthesis of IL-1 and TNF,[134] and maintained lymphocyte IL-2 and IFN-γ synthesis.[135] Its use has been associated with reversal of shock and improvement in pulmonary function, oxygen delivery, and survival.[136, 137] Clinical studies are sparse, although Faist[138] has reported improved cellular immune response and IL-2 production after indomethacin administration in patients undergoing major surgical trauma, and Bernard[139] has demonstrated a significant improvement in hemodynamics and pulmonary function after ibuprofen treatment in patients with sepsis syndrome. In neither of these studies was any significant deterioration in renal function demonstrated as a consequence of NSAID use. This finding was reported in some animal studies and has been proposed as a potential contraindication to NSAID use. Adequate resuscitation appears to be protective against renal dysfunction, which is thought to result from reduced renal blood flow. Thromboxane synthetase inhibitors and thromboxane A_2 receptor antagonists also have been shown to have a beneficial effect on pulmonary function and survival in sepsis in both animals and humans.[140–143] These results, however, have been inconsistent with other studies reporting no benefit.[144, 145]

The role of dietary N3-PUFA incorporation into cell membranes and the subsequent modification of arachidonic acid metabolites produced by cyclooxygenase activity has already been discussed in relation to nutritional pharmacotherapy. It is another way of modifying the eicosanoid response to sepsis or trauma.

Eicosanoids undoubtedly play an important role in the immunosuppression that occurs after trauma and also participate in mediating the septic inflammatory response. Several agents appear to have efficacy in modifying the production of eicosanoids after trauma and sepsis. Their routine clinical use, however, awaits the results of further clinical trials.

Pentoxifylline.—Pentoxifylline is a methylxanthine derivative that acts as a phosphodiesterase inhibitor. In addition to its hemorrheologic actions, pentoxifylline has several effects on the immune system. It has been shown to decrease PMN adherence and aggregation; to reduce PMN superoxide, prostanoid, and protease production; to increase PMN-directed migration; and to decrease cytokine-mediated PMN priming.[146] In addition, pentoxifylline appears to suppress the production of TNF and IL-6, possibly by increasing intracellular cyclic adenosine monophosphate.[147] In various studies, pentoxifylline has been shown to improve hepatic and intestinal blood flow after hemorrhage[148] or bacteremia,[149] to restore cardiac output after hemorrhage[150] or burns,[151] to increase survival,[152, 153] and to reduce the risk of sepsis after hemorrhage.[154, 155] Other phosphodiesterase inhibitors have shown similar properties. Despite these encouraging results, pentoxifylline has yet to find a definite role in the clinical arena.

Immunologic Blockade: Strategies Targeting the Neutrophil and Endothelium

Leukocyte Receptor Antagonist.—Many of the harmful effects of sepsis and shock appear to be mediated through PMN-endothelial cell interactions. This has been demonstrated both on a tissue level[61] and in models of shock and resuscitation.[59, 60] For these interactions to occur, adhesion between PMNs and the endothelium is necessary. This process is mediated by receptors or adhesion molecules expressed on the surface of both PMNs and endothelium. Many of these receptors are up-regulated in the face of endotoxemia or high levels of circulating proinflammatory cytokines such as TNF or IL-1. Blocking PMN-endothelial cell adherence with monoclonal antibodies directed against these receptors ameliorates the harmful effects of ischemia reperfusion in both isolated organs[61] and intact animals subjected to shock.[59, 60] This novel therapeutic approach has not been tested in the clinical arena, and reservations about its indiscriminate use remain. There is some suggestion that down-regulation of PMN-endothelial cell adherence may result in an increased susceptibility to infection.[155]

Oxygen Radical Scavengers.—Phagocytes, principally macrophages and PMNs, mediate tissue injury by elaborating numerous cytotoxic products. Important among these are reactive metabolites of oxygen generated by phagocytes during the respiratory burst. This activity is beneficial when it is directed against ingested microorganisms, but becomes injurious to the host when activated phagocytes release these toxic oxygen species externally, particularly when these cells are tightly adherent to endothelium. The microenvironment created between these cells is relatively inaccessible to endogenous oxygen radical scavengers, and increases the likelihood of tissue injury through the peroxidation of lipid membranes and the denaturation of proteins and other structural elements.[156] This mechanism is thought to be responsible for endothelial injury occurring after leukocyte activation in sepsis and trauma. The use of exogenously administered oxygen radical scavengers could be expected to improve outcome. Some experimental evidence in animals suggests that this may be the case.[157] One study using N-acetylcysteine, however, which boosts the natural glutathione antioxidant system, has demonstrated its ineffectiveness in ameliorating ARDS and other organ failure in septic patients,[158] and a clinical role for antioxidants remains to be established.

Antiproteases.—PMN-derived granular products, in particular proteases, also are thought to have a pathologic role in PMN-mediated injury in sepsis and shock.[159] Antiproteases would be expected to be protective, and have been shown to be protective in in vitro experiments of PMN-mediated tissue injury.[160, 161] A clinical role for their use, however, has yet to be demonstrated.

Nitric Oxide Inhibition.—Nitric oxide has been identified as the endogenously released endothelial-derived relaxing factor that mediates most of the circulatory manifestations of shock and sepsis. This molecule has become the focus of intense investigation in the field of sepsis and septic shock in the last few years. Nitric oxide appears to have a net suppressive effect on lymphocyte responsiveness and leukocyte adherence, but an important microbicidal function.[162] Therefore, the effects of nitric oxide inhibition in sepsis are unpredictable, although one clinical study has reported beneficial effects of nitric oxide synthase inhibitors is septic patients with hypotension.[163] No specific recommendations can be made in regard to the use of nitric oxide inhibitors in sepsis.

Other endothelial-derived vasoactive substances have been isolated, including endothelin, which has vasoconstrictive activities. It is released in increased amounts during sepsis and may have a selective effect on renal and pulmonary vascular beds, affecting renal and pulmonary function adversely and contributing to organ failure.[162, 164] Its role and the potential therapeutic impact of endothelin inhibition remain to be characterized.

Summary

Trauma has a major effect on the immune system that results in generalized immunosuppression involving lymphocyte function, antigen handling, and macrophage activity. This renders the host susceptible to subsequent infection and the development of sepsis and the systemic inflammatory response syndrome. The pathogenesis of sepsis and the systemic inflammatory response syndrome is mediated by unopposed activation of immune cells, the production of cytokines, leukocyte-endothelial cell adherence, and secondary mediator release, which results in microvascular injury, thrombosis, and organ failure. As this inflammatory cascade of events is becoming better understood, opportunities to intervene at various levels in the cascade have been identified. Several of these interventions have been studied extensively in the laboratory, and some have been projected into preliminary clinical trials, with varying results. Only some of these interventions can be recommended unequivocally:

1. Rapid and complete resuscitation with restoration of organ perfusion
2. Early establishment of enteral nutrition with high-calorie, high-protein, full-formula products with consideration of specific nutritional supplements, including arginine, glutamine, RNA, and N3-PUFAs in high-risk patients
3. Aggressive wound debridement, particularly of burn wounds
4. Drainage of any septic focus and adequate use of appropriate antibiotics
5. Restoration of normal mucosal barriers with preservation of gastric acidity

Manipulation of the immune system either to stimulate or to abrogate the immune response using cytokines or growth factors, anticytokine regimens, or nonspecific pharmacologic agents such as steroids or NSAIDs is undergoing intense laboratory and clinical investigation. No single approach has been identified as being unequivocally beneficial in any particular group of patients with trauma or sepsis. Some of these agents, either singly or in combination, may emerge as having major therapeutic potential in the treatment of these patients.

Immunomodulation is a rapidly expanding field that has broken free from the laboratory and is entering everyday clinical practice, particularly in the intensive care unit. The basic scientific fields of immunology, cellular and molecular biology, and medical genetics are increasing our understanding of the host's relationship to injury and sepsis, and are providing clinicians with new therapeutic tools with which to support the host against the ravages of its own immune system and pathogenic microorganisms.

References

1. Trunkey DD: Trauma. *Sci Am* 1983; 249:28–35.
2. Baker CC, Oppenheimer L, Stevens B, et al: Epidemiology of trauma deaths. *Am J Surg* 1980; 140:144.
3. Polk HC: Consensus summary on infection. *J Trauma* 1979; 19:894–896.
4. Hershman MJ, Cheadle WJ, Cuftinec D, et al: An outcome predictive score for sepsis and death following injury. *Injury* 1988; 19:263–266.
5. Faist E, Mewes A, Strasser T, et al: Alteration of monocyte function following major injury. *Arch Surg* 1988; 123:287–292.
6. Faist E, Markewitz A, Fuchs D, et al: Immunomodulatory therapy with thymopentin and indomethacin: Successful restoration of interleukin-2 synthesis in patients undergoing major surgery. *Ann Surg* 1991; 214:264–275.
7. Ninnemann JL: The immune consequences of trauma: An overview, in Faist

E, Ninnemann J, Green D (eds): *Immune Consequences of Trauma, Shock and Sepsis* Berlin, Springer-Verlag, 1989, pp 1–8.
8. Chaudry IH, Ayala A (eds): *Immunologic Aspects of Hemorrhage.* Austin, Tex, Medical Intelligence Unit, RG Landes, 1992, pp 1–129.
9. Saba TM, Lanser ME, Dillon BC: Opsonic fibronectin and phagocytic defense after trauma, in Altura BM, Lefer AM, Shumer W (eds): *Handbook of Shock and Trauma, Volume 1: Basic Science.* New York, Raven Press, 1983, pp 167–181.
10. Ayala A, Perrin MM, Wagner MA, et al: Enhanced susceptibility to sepsis following simple hemorrhage: Depression of Fc and C3b receptor mediated phagocytosis. *Arch Surg* 1990; 125:70–75.
11. Ayala A, Perrin MM, Wang P, et al: Hemorrhage induces enhanced Kupffer cell cytotoxicity while decreasing peritoneal or splenic macrophage capacity: Involvement of cell associated TNF and reactive nitrogen. *J Immunol* 1991; 147:4147–4154.
12. Abraham E, Chang Y-H: The effects of hemorrhage on mitogen-induced lymphocyte proliferation. *Circ Shock* 1985; 15:141–149.
13. Abraham E, Lee RJ, Chang Y-H: The role of interleukin 2 in hemorrhage-induced abnormalities of lymphocyte proliferation. *Circ Shock* 1986; 18:205–213.
14. Miyajima A, Miyatake S, Schreurs J, et al: Coordinate regulation of immune responses by T-cell derived lymphokines. *FASEB J* 1988; 2:2462–2473.
15. Abbas AK: A reassessment of the mechanisms of antigen-specific T-cell dependent B-cell activation. *Immunol Today* 1988; 9:89–94.
16. Livingston DH, Apel SH, Welhausen SR, et al: Depressed interferon-gamma production in monocyte HLA-DR expression after severe injury. *Arch Surg* 1988; 123:1309–1312.
17. Ayala A, Perrin MM, Chaudry IH: Defective macrophage antigen presentation following hemorrhage is associated with the loss of MHC class II (Ia) antigens. *Immunology* 1990; 70:33–39.
18. Abraham E, Richmond JN, Chang YH: Effects of hemorrhage on interleukin 1 production. *Circ Shock* 1988; 25:33–40.
19. Ayala A, Perrin MM, Ertel W, et al: Differential effects of hemorrhage on Kupffer cells: Decreased antigen presentation despite increased inflammatory cytokines (IL-1, IL-6 and TNF) release. *Cytokine* 1992; 4:66–75.
20. Ayala A, Perrin MM, Meldrum DR, et al: Hemorrhage induces an increase in serum TNF which is not associated with elevated levels of endotoxin. *Cytokine* 1990; 2:170–174.
21. Ertel W, Morrison MH, Ayala A, et al: Anti-TNF monoclonal antibodies prevent hemorrhage induced suppression of Kupffer cell antigen presentation and MHC class II antigen expression. *Immunology* 1991; 74:290–297.
22. Porteu F, Nathan C: Shedding of tumor necrosis factor receptors by activated human neutrophils. *J Exp Med* 1990; 172:599–607.
23. Ertel W, Morrison MH, Ayala A, et al: Blockade of prostaglandin production increases cachectin synthesis and prevents depression of macrophage functions following hemorrhagic shock. *Ann Surg* 1991; 213:265–271.
24. Kunkel SL, Spengler M, May MA, et al: Prostaglandin E_2 regulates macrophage-derived tumor necrosis factor gene expression. *J Biol Chem* 1988; 263:5380–5384.
25. Zlotnik A, Shimonkevitz R, Kappler J, et al: Effect of prostaglandin E_2 on in-

terferon gamma induction of antigen presenting ability of P38 D1 cells and on IL-2 production by T-cell hybridoma. *Cell Immunol* 1985; 90:154–166.
26. Knapp W, Baumgartner G: Monocyte-mediated suppression of human B lymphocyte differentiation in vitro. *J Immunol* 1978; 121:1177–1183.
27. Ayala A, Meldrum DR, Perrin MM, et al: The release of transforming growth factor-beta following hemorrhage: Its role as a mediator of host immunosuppression (abstract). *FASEB J* 1992; 6:A1604.
28. Martin TR, Pistorese BP, Hudson LD, et al: The function of lung and blood neutrophils in patients with the adult respiratory distress syndrome. *Am Rev Respir Dis* 1991; 14:254–262.
29. Christou MV, Meakins JL: Partial analysis and purification of polymorphonuclear neutrophil chemotactic inhibitors in serum from anergic patients. *Arch Surg* 1983; 18:156–160.
30. Echinard CE, Sasail-Sulkowska E, Burke PA: The beneficial effect of early excision on clinical response and thymic activity after burn injury. *J Trauma* 1982; 22:560–565.
31. Napolitano LM, Baker CC: Bacterial translocation: Fact or fancy, in Maull KE, Cleveland DV, et al (eds): *Advances in Trauma and Critical Care*, vol 7. St Louis, Mosby, 1992, pp 79–96.
32. Border JR, Hasset J, LaDuca J, et al: The gut origin septic states in blunt multiple trauma [ISS = 40] in the ICU. *Ann Surg* 1987; 206:427–448.
33. Deitch EA, Ma W-J, Ma L, et al: Endotoxin induces bacterial translocation: A study of mechanisms. *Surgery* 1989; 160:292–300.
34. Rush BF, Sori AJ, Murphy TF, et al: Endotoxemia and bacteremia during hemorrhagic shock. The link between trauma and sepsis? *Ann Surg* 1988; 207:549–554.
35. Meakins JL, Marshall JC: The gastrointestinal tract: The motor of MOF. *Arch Surg* 1986; 121:197–201.
36. Crary B, Borysenko M, Sutherland DC, et al: Decrease in mitogen responsiveness of mononuclear cells from peripheral blood after epinephrine administration in humans. *J Immunol* 1983; 130:694–697.
37. Feldman RD, Hunninghake GW, McArdle WL: Beta adrenergic receptor-mediated suppression of interleukin 2 receptors in human lymphocytes. *J Immunol* 1987; 139:3355–3359.
38. Loegering DJ, Commins LM: Effect of beta receptor stimulation on Kupffer cell complement receptor clearance function. *Circ Shock* 1988; 25:325–332.
39. Clayman HN: Corticosteroid and lymphoid cells. *N Engl J Med* 1972; 287:388–397.
40. Gillis S, Crabtree GR, Smith KA: Glucocorticoid-induced inhibition of T-cell growth factor production: The effect on mitogen induced lymphocyte proliferation. *J Immunol* 1979; 123:1624–1631.
41. Snyder DS, Unanue ER: Corticosteroids inhibit murine macrophage Ia expression and interleukin production. *J Immunol* 1982; 129:1803–1805.
42. Deitch EA, Xu D, Bridges RM: Opioids modulate human neutrophil and lymphocyte function: Thermal injury alters plasma beta endorphiln levels. *Surgery* 1988; 104:41–48.
43. Faist E, Mewes A, Baker CC, et al: Prostaglandin E_2 dependent suppression of interleukin 2 production in patients with major trauma. *J Trauma* 1987; 27:837–848.
44. Ertel W, Morrison MH, Ayala A, et al: Blockade of prostaglandin production increases cachectin synthesis and prevents depression of macrophage functions following hemorrhagic shock. *Ann Surg* 1991; 213:265–271.

45. Magrum LJ, Johnston PV: Modulation of prostaglandin synthesis in rat peritoneal macrophages with omega 3 fatty acids. *Lipids* 1983; 18:514–521.
46. Ozkan AN, Ninnemann JL: Circulating mediators in thermal injuries: Isolation and characterization of a burn injury induced immunosuppressive serum component. *J Burn Care Rehabil* 1985; 6:147–151.
47. Hoyt DB, Ozkan AN, Easter DW: Isolation of an immunosuppressor trauma peptide and its relationship to fibronectin. *J Trauma* 1988; 28:907–913.
48. Abraham E, Chang YH: Generation of functionally active suppressor cells by hemorrhage and hemorrhagic serum. *Clin Exp Immunol* 1988; 72:238–242.
49. Antonacci A, Reaves L, Calvano S, et al: Flow cytometric analysis of lymphocyte subpopulations after thermal injury in human beings. *Surg Gynecol Obstet* 1984; 159:1–8.
50. Wang BS, Heacock EH, Wu AV, et al: Generation of suppressor cells in mice after surgical trauma. *J Clin Invest* 1980; 66:200–209.
51. Chaudry IH, Sayeed MM, Vaue AE: Differences in the altered energy metabolism of hemorrhagic shock and hypoxemia. *Can J Physiol Pharmacol* 1976; 54:750–756.
52. Morrison MH, Ertel W, Ayala A, et al: Depressed antigen presentation of peritoneal macrophage following hypoxia is associated with altered release of inflammatory mediators. *FASEB J* 1992; 6:A1614.
53. Meldrum DR, Ayala A, Chaudry IH: Energetics of defective macrophage antigen presentation following hemorrhage as determined by ultraresolution 31P nuclear magnetic resonance spectrometry: Restoration with ATP-MgCl$_2$. *Surgery* 1992; 112:150–158.
54. Meldrum DR, Ayala A, Wang P, et al: Association between decreased splenic ATP levels and immunodepression: Amelioration with ATP-MgCl$_2$. *Am J Physiol* 1991; 261:R351–R357.
55. Alexander JW, McMillan BG, Stinnett JD, et al: Beneficial effects of progressive protein feeding in severely burned children. *Ann Surg* 1980; 192:505–517.
56. Bone RC, Balk RA, Cerra FB, et al: Definitions for sepsis and organ failure and guidelines for the use of innovative therapies in sepsis. *Chest* 1992; 101:1644–1655.
57. Lowry SF: Cytokine mediators of immunity and inflammation. *Arch Surg* 1993; 128:1235–1241.
58. Molloy RG, Mannick JA, Roderick ML: Cytokines, sepsis and immunomodulation. *Br J Surg* 1993; 80:289–297.
59. Vedder NB, Winn RK, Rice CL, et al: A monoclonal antibody to the adherence-promoting leukocyte glycoprotein, CD18, reduces organ injury and improves survival from hemorrhagic shock and resuscitation in rabbits. *J Clin Invest* 1988; 31:939–944.
60. Mileski WJ, Winn RK, Vedder NB, et al: Inhibition of CD18-dependent neutrophil adherence reduces organ injury after hemorrhagic shock in primates. *Surgery* 1990; 108:206–212.
61. Vedder NB, Winn RK, Rice CL, et al: Inhibition of leukocyte adherence by anti-CD18 monoclonal antibody attenuates reperfusion injury in the rabbit ear. *Proc Natl Acad Sci U S A* 1990; 87:2643–2646.
62. Anderson BO, Brown JN, Harken AL: Mechanisms of neutrophil mediated tissue injury. *J Surg Res* 1991; 51:170–179.
63. Daly J, Bonau R, Stofberg P, et al: Immediate post operative jejunostomy feeding. *Am J Surg* 1987; 153:198–206.

64. Driks MR, Craven DE, Celli BR, et al: Nosocomial pneumonia in intubated patients given sucralfate as compared to antiacids or histamine type 2 blockers. *N Engl J Med* 1987; 317:1376–1382.
65. Moore FA, Moore EE, Jones TN, et al: TEN vs. TPN following major abdominal trauma-reduced septic morbidity. *J Trauma* 1989; 29:916–923.
66. Alverdey JC, Aoys E, Moss GS: Total parenteral nutrition promotes bacterial translocation from the gut. *Surgery* 1988; 104:185–190.
67. Mainous M, Xu D, Liu Q, et al: Oral TPN induced bacterial translocation and impaired immune defenses are reversed by refeeding. *Surgery* 1991; 110:277–284.
68. Xu D, Qi L, Thirstrup C, et al: Elemental diet induced bacterial translocation and immunosuppression is not reversed by glutamine. *J Trauma* 1993; 35:821–825.
69. Jenner E: *An Inquiry Into the Causes and Effects of the Variolae Vaccinae, a Disease.* London, Sampson Low, 1798.
70. Meakins JL, Christou NV, Shizgal HM, et al: Therapeutic approaches to anergy in surgical patients. *Ann Surg* 1979; 190:286.
71. Waymack JP, Jenkins M, Wardon GD, et al: A prospective study of thymopentin in severely burned patients. *Surg Gynecol Obstet* 1987; 164:423–430.
72. Sheppard BC, Fraker DL, Norton JA: Prevention and treatment of endotoxin and sepsis lethality with recombinant human tumor necrosis factor. *Surgery* 1989; 106:156.
73. Van der Meer JW, Barza M, Wolff SM, et al: A low dose of recombinant interleukin-1 protects granulocytopenic mice from lethal gram-negative infection. *Proc Natl Acad Sci U S A* 1988; 85:1620.
74. Weyand C, Goronzy J, Fathman CG, et al: Administration of in vivo recombinant interleukin-2 protects mice against septic death. *J Clin Invest* 1987; 79:1756.
75. Chong KT: Prophylactic administration of interleukin-2 protects mice from lethal challenge with gram-negative bacteria. *Infect Immun* 1987; 55:668.
76. Livingston DH, Malangoni MA: Interferon-gamma restores immune competence after hemorrhagic shock. *J Surg Res* 1988; 45:37–43.
77. Hershman MJ, Apple SH, Wellhausen SR, et al: Interferon gamma treatment increases HLA-DR expression on monocytes in severely injured patients. *Clin Exp Immunol* 1989; 77:67.
78. Polk HC, Cheadle WG, Livingston DH, et al: A randomized prospective clinical trial to determine the efficacy of interferon gamma in severely injured patients. *Am J Surg* 1992; 163:191–196.
79. Jurkovich GJ, Mileski WJ, Maier RV, et al: Interferon gamma increases sensitivity to endotoxin. *J Surg Res* 1991; 51:197–203.
80. Cioffi WG Jr, Burleson DG, Jordan BS, et al: Effects of granulocyte-macrophage colony-stimulating factor in burn patients. *Arch Surg* 1991; 126:74–79.
81. Huang KF, Chung DH, Herndon DN: Insulin like growth factor 1 reduces gut atrophy and bacterial translocation after severe burn injury. *Arch Surg* 1993; 128:47–54.
82. Wang P, Ba ZF, Morrison MH, et al: Mechanism of beneficial effects of ATP-MgCl2 following trauma, hemorrhage, and resuscitation: Down-regulation of inflammatory cytokine (TNF, IL-6). *J Surg Res* 1992; 52:364–371.

83. Harkemah AM, Chaudry IH: Magnesium-adenosine triphosphate in the treatment cf shock, ischemia and sepsis. *Crit Care Med* 1992; 20:263–275.
84. Cerra FB, Mazuski JE, Chute E, et al: Branched chain metabolic support: A prospective randomized double blind trial in surgical stress. *Ann Surg* 1984; 199:286–291.
85. Brennan M, Cerra FB, Daly JM, et al: Report of a research workshop: Branched chain amino-acid in stress and injury. *JPEN J Parenter Enteral Nutr* 1986; 10:446–452.
86. Daly JM, Reynolds J, Sigal RK, et al: Effect of dietary protein in amino acids on immune function. *Crit Care Med* 1990; 18:S86–S93.
87. Kierk SJ, Barbul A: Role of arginine in trauma, sepsis, and immunity. *JPEN J Parenter Enteral Nutr* 1990; 14:226S–229S.
88. Hwang TL, O'Dwyer ST, Smith RJ, et al: Preservation of small bowel mucosa using glutamine enriched parenteral nutrition. *Surg Forum* 1986; 56:58.
89. Kinsella JE, Lokesh B, Broughton S: Dietary polyunsaturated fatty acids and eicosanoids: Potential effects on the modulation of inflammatory and immune cells: An overview. *Nutrition* 1990; 6:24–45.
90. Billiar TR, Bankey PE, Svingen BA, et al: Fatty acid intake and Kupffer cell function: Fish oil alters eicosanoid and monokine production to endotoxin stimulation. *Surgery* 1988; 104:343–348.
91. Cerra FP: Nutrient modulation of inflammatory and immune function. *Am J Surg* 1991; 161:230–234.
92. Van Buren CT, Rudolph FB, Kulkarni A, et al: Reversal of immunosuppression induced by protein-free diet: Comparison of nucleotides, fish oil and arginine *Crit Care Med* 1990; 18:S114–S117.
93. Fang C, Peck MD, Alexander JW, et al: The effect of free radical scavengers on outcome after infection in burned mice. *J Trauma* 1990; 30:453–456.
94. Alexander JW, Gottschlich MM: Nutritional immunomodulators in burn patients. *J Crit Care Med* 1990; 18:S149–S153.
95. Daly JM, Lieberman MD, Goldfine J, et al: Enteral nutrition with supplemental arginine, RNA, and omega 3 fatty acids in patients after operation: Immunologic metabolic and clinical outcome. *Surgery* 1992; 112:56–67.
96. Bower RH, Lavin PT, LiCari JJ, et al: A modified enteral formula reduces hospital length of stay (LOS) in patients in intensive care units (ICU). Presented at the 14th European Society of Parenteral and Enteral Nutrition Congress on Clinical Nutrition and Metabolism, Vienna, Sept 1992.
97. Alexander JW: Immunoenhancement via enteral nutrition. *Arch Surg* 1993; 128:1242–1245.
98. Polk HC, Shields CL: Remote organ failure: A valid sign of occult intraabdominal infection. *Surgery* 1977; 81:310–313.
99. Border J, LaDuca J, Siebel R: Priorities in the management of the patient with polytrauma. *Prog Surg* 1975; 14:84–120.
100. Johnson KD, Cadambi A, Seibert GB: Incidence of ARDS in patients with multiple musculoskeletal injuries: Effect of early operative stabilization of fractures. *J Trauma* 1985; 25:375–384.
101. Goris RJA, Vandalen R: Selective decontamination in the intensive care unit, in Maull KI, Cleveland HC, Feliciano DV, et al (eds): *Advances in Trauma and Critical Care,* vol 7. St Louis, Mosby, 1992, pp 61–78.
102. Ziegler EJ, McCutchan JA, Fierer J, et al: Treatment of gram-negative bacteremia in shock with human antiserum to a mutant *Escherichia coli. N Engl J Med* 1982; 307:1225–1230.
103. Greenman RL, Schein RMH, Martin MA, et al: A controlled clinical trial of E5

murine monoclonal IgM antibody to endotoxin in the treatment of gram-negative sepsis. *JAMA* 1991; 266:1097–1102.
104. Ziegler EJ, Fisher CJ, Sprung CL, et al: Treatment of gram-negative bacteremia and septic shock with HA-1A human monoclonal antibody against endotoxin. *N Engl J Med* 1991; 324:429–436.
105. Wenzel R, Bone R, Fein A, et al: Results of a second double blind randomized control trial of anti-endotoxin antibody E5 in gram-negative sepsis (abstract), in *Program and Abstracts of the 31st Interscience Conference on Antimicrobial Agents and Chemotherapy.* Chicago, American Society for Microbiology, 1991, p 294.
106. Luce JM: Introduction of new technology into critical care practice: A history of HA-1A human monoclonal antibody against endotoxin. *Crit Care Med* 1993; 21:1233–1241.
107. Marra M, Wilde C, Collins M, et al: The role of bactericidal/permeability increasing protein as a natural inhibitor of bacterial endotoxin. *J Immunol* 1992; 148:532–537.
108. Fletcher MA, McKenna TN, Quance JL, et al: Lipopolysaccharide detoxification by endotoxin neutralizing protein. *J Surg Res* 1993; 55:147–154.
109. Michie HR, Manogue KR, Spriggs DR, et al: Detection of circulating tumor necrosis factor after endotoxin administration. *N Engl J Med* 1988; 318:1481–1486.
110. Tracey KJ, Beutler B, Lowry SF, et al: Shock and tissue injury induced by recombinant human cachectin. *Science* 1986; 234:470–474.
111. Tracey KJ, Fong Y, Hesse DG, et al: Anti-cachectin/TNF monoclonal antibodies prevent septic shock during lethal bacteremia. *Nature* 1987; 330:662–666.
112. Fong Y, Tracey KJ, Moldawer LL, et al: Antibodies to cachectin/tumor necrosis factor reduced interleukin 1 and interleukin 6 appearance during lethal bacteremia. *J Exp Med* 1989; 170:1627–1633.
113. Exely A, Cohen J, Buurman W, et al: Monoclonal antibody to TNF and severe septic shock. *Lancet* 1990; 335:1275–1277.
114. Vincent J, Bakker J, Mareçaux G, et al: Administration of anti-TNF antibody improves left ventricular function in septic shock patients. *Chest* 1992; 101:810–815.
115. Fisher CJ, Opal SM, Dhainaut J-F, et al: Influence of an anti-tumor necrosis factor monoclonal antibody on cytokine levels in patients with sepsis. *Crit Care Med* 1993; 21:318–327.
116. Peppel K, Crawford D, Beutler B: A tumor necrosis factor (TNF) receptor-IgG heavy chain chimeric protein as a bivalent antagonist of TNF activity. *J Exp Med* 1991; 174:1483–1489.
117. Ohlsson K, Bjork P, Bergenfeldt M, et al: Interleukin 1 receptor antagonist reduces mortality from endotoxic shock. *Nature* 1990; 348:550–552.
118. Wackabayashi G, Gelfand JA, Burke JF, et al: A specific receptor antagonist for interleukin 1 prevents *Escherichia coli*-induced shock. *FASEB J* 1991; 5:338–343.
119. Damas P, Ledoux D, Nys M, et al: Cytokine serum level during severe sepsis in human IL-6 as a marker of severity. *Ann Surg* 1992; 215:356–362.
120. Schluter B, Konig B, Bergmann U, et al: Interleukin 6—a potential mediator of lethal sepsis after major thermal trauma: Evidence for increased IL-6 production by peripheral blood mononuclear cells. *J Trauma* 1991; 31:1663–1670.

121. Starnes HF, Pearce MK, Tewari A, et al: Anti-IL-6 monoclonal antibodies protect against lethal *Escherichia coli* infection and lethal tumor necrosis factor alpha challenge in mice. *J Immunol* 1990; 145:4185–4191.
122. Ayala A, Knotts JB, Ertel W, et al: Role of interleukin 6 and transforming growth factor-β in the induction of depressed splenocyte response following sepsis. *Arch Surg* 1993; 128:89–95.
123. Bonner G: Kalikrinin systems in shock, in Neugebauer AE, Holaday JW (eds): *Handbook of Mediators in Septic Shock.* Boca Raton, Fla, CRC Press, 1993, pp 167–192.
124. Hosford D, Koltai M, Paubert-Braquet M, et al: Analysis of platelet-activating factor in endotoxic shock and sepsis using a probability matrix. A critique of meta-analysis, in Neugebauer AE, Holaday JW (eds): *Handbook of Mediators in Septic Shock.* Boca Raton, Fla, CRC Press, 1993, pp 439–456.
125. Fletcher JR, DiSimone G, Earnest MA: Platelet activating factor receptor antagonist improves survival and attenuates eicosanoid release in severe endotoxemia. *Ann Surg* 1990; 211:312–316.
126. Olson NC, Joyce PB, Fleisler LN: Role of platelet-activating factor and eicosanoids during endotoxin-induced lung injury in pigs (pt 2). *Am J Physiol* 1990; 258:H1674.
127. Christman BW, Lefferts PL, Blair IA, et al: Effect of platelet activating factor receptor antagonism on endotoxin-induced lung dysfunction in awake sheep (pt 1). *Am Rev Respir Dis* 1990; 142:1272.
128. Meldrum DR, Ayala R, Perrin MM, et al: Diltiazem restores susceptibility to sepsis following hemorrhage. *J Surg Res* 1991; 51:158–164.
129. Beutler B, Korchin N, Milsark IW, et al: Control of cachectin/tumor necrosis factor synthesis: Mechanisms of endotoxin resistance. *Science* 1986; 232:977.
130. Snyder DS, Unanue ER: Corticosteroids inhibit murine macrophage Ia expression and interleukin 1 production. *J Immunol* 1982; 129:1803.
131. Bone RC, Fisher CJ Jr, Clemmer TP, et al: A controlled clinical trial of high-dose methylprednisolone in the treatment of severe sepsis and septic shock. *N Engl J Med* 1987; 317:658.
132. Hinshaw LB, Veteran's Administration Systemic Sepsis Cooperative Study Group: Effect of high dose glucocorticoid therapy on mortality in patients with clinical signs of systemic sepsis. *N Engl J Med* 1987; 317:659–666.
133. Hinshaw LB, Archer LT, Beller-Todd BK, et al: Survival in primates in LD_{100} septic shock following steroid/antibiotic therapy. *J Surg Res* 1980; 28:151.
134. Ertel W, Morrison MH, Ayala A, et al: Blockade of prostaglandin production increases cachectin synthesis and prevents depression of macrophage functions after hemorrhagic shock. *Ann Surg* 1991; 213:265–271.
135. Ertel W, Morrison MH, Meldrum DR, et al: Ibuprofen restores cellular immunity and decreases susceptibility to sepsis following hemorrhage. *J Surg Res* 1992; 53:55–61.
136. Hubbard JD, Janssen HF: Increased microvascular permeability in canine endotoxic shock: Protective effects of ibuprofen. *Circ Shock* 1988; 26:169.
137. Butler RR, Wise WC, Halushka PV, et al: Gentamicin and indomethacin, the treatment of septic shock: Effects on prostacyclin and thromboxane A_2 production. *J Pharmacol Exp Ther* 1983; 225:94.
138. Faist E, Ertel W, Cohnert T, et al: Immune protective effects of cyclooxygenase inhibition in patients with major surgical trauma. *J Trauma* 1990; 30:8–18.

139. Bernard GR, Reines HD, Halushka PV, et al: Prostacyclin and thromboxane A_2 formation is increased in human sepsis syndrome. Am Rev Respir Dis 1991; 144:1095.
140. Svartholm E, Bergquist D, Hadner U, et al: Thromboxane A_2-receptor blockade and prostacyclin in porcine Escherichia coli shock. Arch Surg 1989; 142:669.
141. Fukumoto S, Tanaka K: Protective effects of thromboxane A_2 synthetase inhibitors on endotoxin shock. Prostaglandins and Leukotrienes in Medicine 1983; 11:179.
142. Taneyama C, Sasao J, Senna S, et al: Protective effects of ONO 3708 in new thromboxane A_2 receptor antagonists during experimental endotoxin shock. Circ Shock 1989; 28:69.
143. Slotman GJ, Burchard KW, D'Arezzo A, et al: Ketoconazole prevents acute respiratory failure in critically ill surgical patients. J Trauma 1988; 28:648–654.
144. Fletcher JR, Short BL, Casey LC, et al: Thromboxane inhibition in gram-negative sepsis fails to improve survival, in Samuelsson B, Paoletti R, Ramwell PW (eds): Advances in Prostaglandins, Thromboxanes, and Leukotriene Research. New York, Raven Press, 1983, p 12.
145. Furman BL, McKechnie K, Parratt JR: Failure of drugs that selectively inhibit thromboxane synthesis to modify endotoxin shock in conscious rats. Br J Pharmacol 1984; 82:289.
146. Mandell GL: ARDS, neutrophils and pentoxifylline. Am Rev Respir Dis 1988; 138:1103–1105.
147. Wang P, Ba ZF, Morrison MH, et al: Mechanism of beneficial effects of pentoxifylline and hepatocellular function after trauma, hemorrhage, and resuscitation. Surgery 1992; 112:451–458.
148. Flynn WJ, Cryer HG, Garrison RN: Pentoxifylline restores intestinal microvascular blood flow during resuscitated hemorrhagic shock. Surgery 1991; 110:350–356.
149. Steeb GD, Wilson MA, Garrison RN: Pentoxifylline preserves small-intestine microvascular blood flow during bacteremia. Surgery 1992; 112:756–764.
150. Wang P, Ba ZF, Zhou MD, et al: Pentoxifylline restores cardiac output in tissue perfusion after trauma-hemorrhage and decreases susceptibility to sepsis. Surgery 1993; 114:352–359.
151. Vaughan WG, Horton JW, White DJ: Burn induced cardiac dysfunctions reduced by pentoxifylline. Surg Gynecol Obstet 1993; 176:459–468.
152. Coccia MT, Waxman K, Solliman MH, et al: Pentoxifylline improves survival following hemorrhagic shock. Crit Care Med 1989; 17:36–38.
153. Barroso HA, Schmidt-Schonbein GW: Pentoxifylline pretreatment decreases the pool of circulating activated neutrophils, in vivo adhesion to endothelium and improves survival from hemorrhagic shock. Biorheology 1990; 27:401–418.
154. Waxman K, Clark L, Soliman MH, et al: Pentoxifylline in resuscitation of experimental hemorrhagic shock. Crit Care Med 1991; 19:728–732.
155. Sharar SR, Winn RK, Murry CE, et al: A CD18 monoclonal antibody increases the instance and severity of subcutaneous abscess formation after high-dose Staphylococcus aureus injection in rabbits. Surgery 1991; 110:213–220.
156. Reilly PM, Schiller HJ, Bulkley GB: Pharmacologic approach to tissue injury mediated by free radicals and other reactive oxygen metabolites. Am J Surg 1991; 161:488–503.

157. Bernard GR, Lucht WD, Niedermeyer ME, et al: Effect of N-acetylcysteine on the pulmonary response to endotoxin in the awake sheep and upon in vitro granulocyte function. *J Clin Invest* 1984; 73:1772–1784.
158. Jepsen S, Herlevsen P, Knudsen P, et al: Antioxidant treatment with N-acetylcysteine during adult respiratory distress syndrome: A prospective, randomized, placebo-controlled study. *Crit Care Med* 1992; 20:918–923.
159. Anderson BO, Brown JM, Harken AH: Mechanisms of neutrophil mediated tissue injury. *J Surg Res* 1991; 51:170–179.
160. Smedley LA, Tonnesen MG, Sandhaus RA, et al: Neutrophil mediated injury to endothelial cells. Enhancement by endotoxin and the essential role of neutrophil elastase. *J Clin Invest* 1986; 77:1233.
161. Baird BR, Cheronis JC, Sandhaus RA: O_2 metabolites and neutrophil elastase synergistically cause edematous injury in isolated rat lungs. *J Appl Physiol* 1986; 61:2224.
162. Parratt JR, Stoclet JC, Furman BL: Substances mainly derived from vascular endothelium as chemical mediators in sepsis and endotoxemia, in Neugebauer EA, Holaday JW (eds): *Handbook of Mediators in Septic Shock.* Boca Raton, Fla, CRC Press, 1993, pp 381–394.
163. Petros A, Bennett D, Vallance P: Effect of nitric oxide synthase inhibitors on hypotension in patients with septic shock. *Lancet* 1991; 338:1557.
164. Masaki T: The discovery, the present state, and the future prospects of endothelin. *J Cardiovasc Pharmacol* 1989; 13:S1.

Treatment of the Pediatric Patient in an Adult Trauma Center

John B. Fortune, M.D.
Associate Professor of Surgery, Department of Surgery, Albany Medical Center, Albany, New York

David H. Kuehler, M.D.
Assistant Professor of Surgery, Department of Surgery, Albany Medical Center, Albany, New York

Traumatic injury during childhood is a tremendous problem in America, not only in its magnitude and social implications, but also in the potential ability of the medical community to provide optimal care for injured children. Each year, nearly 1.5 million injuries occur to children younger than 15 years; as a result of these injuries, there are about 500,000 hospitalizations and between 15,000 and 20,000 deaths.[1–4] Of all the trauma that occurs in America, children are the victims in about 25% of cases.[5]

Almost all authorities have shown, and pediatricians have emphasized, that the medical treatment of pediatric patients differs in numerous ways from that of adults. This also is true of trauma management, because many aspects of the mechanisms and magnitude of injury, the physiologic response to injury, and the nature of therapeutic interventions distinguish trauma problems among age groups. Given these obvious differences, there has been some concern that trauma centers that provide care primarily for adults are less capable of managing trauma in younger patients.[6–9] With the availability of pediatric specialists based in children's hospitals, numerous "pediatric trauma centers" have been developed that are devoted specifically to the care of injured children and have the specially trained personnel, equipment, and facilities that presumably best meet the needs of these patients.

As with all trauma, however, the geographic distribution of trauma in childhood is ubiquitous. Because centers designed specifically and solely for the treatment of pediatric patients usually are located in high-density urban areas,[8–10] not all injured children can be transferred expeditiously to a "pediatric trauma center." Therefore, some, diagnostic and therapeutic interventions for some injured children must be provided in centers that are not designed exclusively to treat these patients.

The goal of this chapter is to define some of the differences in care that may arise in pediatric trauma and to present paradigms for the optimal care of injured children in trauma centers that treat adults most often. Although the term "adult trauma center" often is used to refer to nonspecialized trauma centers that provide care to injured children, the term "comprehensive trauma center" is used in this chapter to represent those centers that treat traumatic injury primarily in adults, but also have a special commitment to a "pediatric trauma program" for the care of injured children.

In addition, planning for the management of pediatric trauma does not focus only on the trauma center. The concept of a "trauma system" is extremely important in defining the total care of the pediatric patient from the time of injury through the acute hospital course and into the rehabilitation period. Therefore, some attention is directed toward the development of a systems approach to pediatric trauma care in which the trauma center is a vital, but not the sole, component.

Adult and Pediatric Trauma

Demographics and Injury Types

About 25% of all cases of traumatic injury in America involve a child younger than 15 years.[5] Extrapolating some detailed statewide data analyses to the national experience, the annual rate of serious injury in children can be calculated at about 11.6 cases per 100,000 population.[11] Compared with adult series, the per capita death rate for children is about 20% of that for adults. These mortality figures belie the actual impact of pediatric trauma, however, because the rate of hospitalization for trauma in children can be as high as 56% of that in adults.[11] In general, the lower incidence of trauma events combined with the fact that children younger than 15 years constitute only 28% of the population explains the greater number of *adult trauma centers*.

Examination of the demographic and injury pattern differences between adult and pediatric trauma is difficult, because few series contain both categories of patients. Therefore, it may be useful to compare the mechanism and magnitude of injury between adults and children from two large data bases that have been developed for each group. For analysis of adult data, the results of the Major Trauma Outcome Study (MTOS) developed by Champion and colleagues provide the most comprehensive national data base.[12] Data on more than 80,000 trauma patients, of which less than 10% were children, from 139 institutions in the United States and Canada were analyzed between 1982 and 1987. These data can be compared with the most comprehensive data registry for children, the National Pediatric Trauma Registry managed by DiScala and associates.[13] This data registry now includes information on more than 32,000 cases from nearly 62 pediatric and comprehensive trauma centers that submitted data between 1987 and 1993. Although a comparison of these two registries will not provide information regarding the overall prevalence of trauma in the two different age groups, some inferences concerning the mechanism and severity of trauma can be made.

Figures 1 and 2 show some results of a comparison between these two registries. In all components of these figures, adult and pediatric trauma are directly contrasted for each category. Figure 1 shows that the sex distribution in both age categories is similar, with males sustaining major injury about twice as often as females. In regard to the type of injury, children sustain penetrating injuries less than half as often as do adults, although

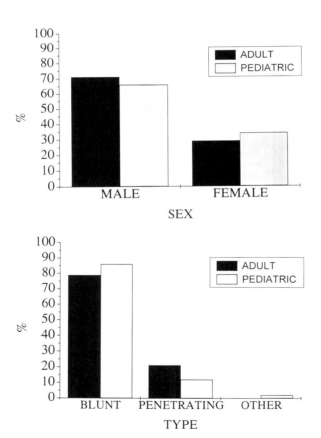

FIG 1.
A comparison of adult and pediatric trauma from large registries shows that the sex distribution is fairly similar between the two age groups. With respect to the broad categorization of the type of injury, it appears that adults sustain penetrating injuries more commonly than do children.

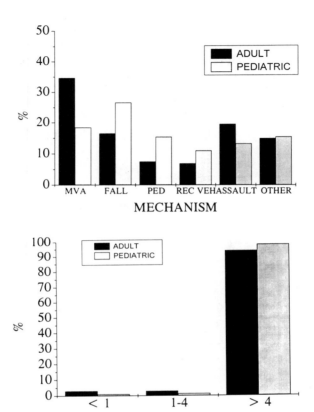

FIG 2.
A comparison of the mechanism of injury between children and adults shows that motor vehicle accidents are most common among adults, whereas falls resulting in serious injury are most common among children. A comparison of the Revised Trauma Score between the two age groups reveals that, in both groups, the incidence of extremely serious injury reported to the registry is small. MVA = motor vehicle accident; PED = pedestrian accident; REC VEH = injury associated with a recreational vehicle (i.e., motorcycles, bicycles, all-terrain vehicles, etc.).

recent data have shown that the magnitude of penetrating injuries is increasing, particularly in young teenagers.[14] Figure 2 shows a comparison of the mechanism of injury between the two age groups. Falls and pedestrian-type accidents are more likely to occur among children, whereas motor vehicle accidents and assaults are more common among adults. Falls resulting in serious injury are more common among children, but also represent a fairly large proportion of injuries in adults. Attempting to compare the severity of injury between adults and children is more difficult. Both major trauma data bases categorize injuries in terms of Injury Severity Score (ISS); however, the analyses generally have been performed using different break points along the ISS continuum, making direct comparison difficult. Physiologic derangement can be compared between these two large populations by examining the Revised Trauma Score in Figure 2. According to most authorities, a Revised Trauma Score of 4 or less, which is seen rarely in either population, signifies a tremendously severe injury. Scores of 5 or greater, in most cases, represent injuries from which the patient generally *could* survive. In both trauma data bases, it is evident that most of the individuals entered into the registries sustain survivable injuries. Further analysis shows that, as in the adult population, when death occurs in children, it usually happens shortly after the injury—sometime between the time of the incident and arrival at the emergency department.[7, 11, 15] Unfortunately, many of these children die of a preventable cause.[7, 15]

This comparison of trauma registries actually highlights the *similarities* between pediatric and adult patients with respect to mechanism and severity of injury. In general, although trauma centers are more likely to treat adults involved in motor vehicle accidents and children involved in pedestrian accidents and falls, these comparisons do not show a significantly different injury pattern between the age groups.

An evaluation of specific body sites injured reveals that the pediatric population sustains a greater proportion of head injuries; nearly 50% of all trauma deaths among children result from head injury.[16] Although head injury also predominates in adults, many more chest and abdominal injuries contribute to mortality when compared to the pediatric population.

Special Aspects of Pediatric Trauma

Before the various system approaches to pediatric trauma are discussed, it is important to review some special aspects of pediatric trauma and to introduce some ideas that affect the treatment of injured children in various types of trauma centers. A summary of these differences is provided in Figure 3. This is not intended to be a comprehensive outline of the physiologic differences between adults and children, nor is it a complete guide to the treatment of pediatric patients. Excellent reviews of these topics can be found elsewhere.[17–19]

Physiologic Differences of the Injured Child

A child's habitus contributes to the spectrum of injuries that are seen most commonly in this age group. With a relatively small body area, forces are distributed over less mass, and multisystem injuries are slightly more frequent than in adults.[17] The amount of force that may cause a relatively focal injury in an adult when applied to the chest, for example, will probably result in injuries to several organ systems in a child, and may be more

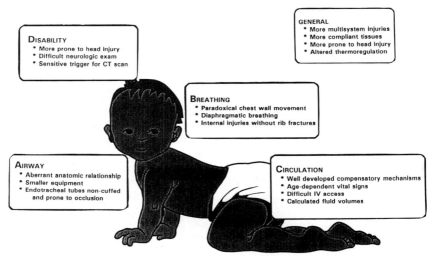

FIG 3.
A representation of some special aspects of pediatric trauma related to the initial assessment phase of the management of these patients. Although this is not a comprehensive list, some of the major differences that distinguish pediatric trauma are noted. CT = computed tomography; IV = intravenous.

life-threatening. In a child, tissues tend to be more elastic and the bony integrity is not as well defined. The normally rigid chest cavity of an adult tends to fracture, whereas that of a child tends to bend, resulting in less external injury, but more contusion to the lungs and mediastinum. More energy may be transmitted to internal structures without significant external evidence of injury. On the other hand, the presence of a rib fracture in a child may suggest extremely severe internal injuries because of the force necessary to cause the fracture.[20]

Because of the relative disproportion of children's heads to their bodies and the loose ligaments of their cervical spines, children are more prone to head injury.[17] In addition, because younger children have a more prominent occiput, the neck actually may be flexed when the child is lying supine. To maintain "in-line stabilization" for possible cervical spine injuries, a small towel may have to be placed under the shoulders to create a neutral position.

Thermal homeostasis also is a serious concern in the treatment of a young trauma victim. An increased ratio of body surface area to weight in children results in a rapid loss of heat compared to adults. Attention should be paid to maintaining a warm environment and providing heated intravenous fluids for a child with trauma.

Airway

Teenagers have the same airway configuration as do adults, but gaining and maintaining a stable airway can present problems in younger children.

Achieving an airway proved difficult in 25% of the pediatric patients in a study by Nakayama and coworkers that was conducted in the prehospital setting.[21] In most of these cases, the lack of an adequate airway was deemed life-threatening. When this entire study group was analyzed, 42% of all attempts to secure an airway at the accident scene were unsuccessful. Compared with adults, in whom successful maintenance of an airway in the field can be expected in about 80% to 90% of cases, pediatric airway management is more difficult.[21]

Aberrant anatomic structures and relationships often complicate airway maintenance in young children. An infant has a small oral cavity with a large tongue that makes visualization of the vocal cords difficult. The larynx is more cephalad and anterior, and the vocal cords are shorter, precluding easy visualization. The airway below the larynx is smaller and easily occluded by blood, vomitus, or other secretions.[22]

Emergency airway maintenance in a child involves the use of artificial airways that must be inserted somewhat differently than in adults because of the relatively large tongue. Artificial airways are usually inserted by moving the tongue out of the way with a tongue depressor and advancing the device along the radius of the pharynx.[23] Caution must be exercised, because an excessively large oropharyngeal airway may actually obstruct the pharynx. Ventilation may be assisted with a bag-valve mask device, although care must be taken to avoid aspiration because of the gastric distention that frequently is seen in pediatric patients.

Endotracheal intubation involves much smaller tubes and laryngoscopes, and the use of appropriately sized equipment is vitally important. Because of the child's short trachea, it is essential that the appropriate length of tube be placed past the larynx to avoid right mainstem bronchial intubation. While intubation is being performed, the use of pulse oximetry is helpful to avoid hypoxic episodes.

Much attention has been paid recently to rapid-sequence intubation using appropriate sedatives and paralytics. In general, the same relative drug doses are used in children as in adults, including pretreatment with 0.01 mg/kg of pancuronium or vecuronium (to avoid subsequent fasciculations with succinylcholine), midazolam (0.5 mg/kg), and succinylcholine (2 mg/kg in infants; 1 mg/kg in children). In the pediatric population, the circulation time required for the drugs to become effective may be somewhat less than in adults, varying between 15 and 20 seconds in infants, 30 and 40 seconds in children, and 60 and 70 seconds in adolescents.[17]

Once the patient is intubated, the ventilator is set for tidal volumes of 10 to 12 mL/kg with ventilatory rate appropriate to maintain the desired P_{CO_2}. If sudden deterioration occurs, several possibilities should be considered, including misplacement of the tube, endotracheal or bronchial obstruction, and tension pneumothorax.

Breathing

The chest wall of a young child may be so compliant that the mechanics of respiration are markedly altered. The movement of the diaphragm to initiate inspiration may cause a "paradoxical" movement of the chest wall, which in turn may reduce the effective tidal volume. Any limitation of chest wall or abdominal expansion may significantly impair the efficiency of ventilation and gas exchange. In addition, because of the limited reserve in a child, pain from chest wall contusion may seriously limit the effectiveness of the breathing pattern, further reducing breathing volumes.

One of the major concerns in injured children, and one that often is overlooked in adults as well, is the presence of gastric distention. Children tend to swallow air during periods of stress, and the addition of air from mask ventilation can cause gastric dilatation severe enough to limit diaphragmatic excursion. In any child with abdominal distention, the early initiation of nasogastric drainage should be considered to improve ventilatory function. Oral-gastric intubation should be used in neonates and infants, because children in this age group are obligate nose-breathers.

Circulation

The treatment of shock may be one of the most important management differences between adult and pediatric patients. In general, younger children have a greater tolerance for blood loss because of a greater reserve of compensatory mechanisms. As in the adult, the child's cardiovascular system compensates for blood loss by increasing the heart rate and systemic vascular resistance until losses exceed 25%. Because of the child's smaller size and absolute blood volumes compared to the adult, however, the amount of blood that can be lost before an irreversible shock state occurs is much lower. As in an adult, the initial evaluation of a child for signs of shock should include an examination for activity of any compensatory mechanism, such as a narrow pulse pressure and the loss of brisk capillary refill.[17]

Because a child's vital signs vary somewhat from those of an adult, identification of abnormalities requires an appreciation of normal pediatric values. Table 1 lists the pulse, blood pressure, and respiratory rates that can be expected in children of different age groups. Younger children normally have much higher pulse rates and correspondingly lower blood pressures than are expected in adults. A common rule of thumb for calculating the lower limits of systolic blood pressure is to use the following formula: systolic blood pressure = $70 + 2\times$ (age).

Control of hemorrhage is the key therapeutic intervention to prevent the onset of shock. Because blood volumes are so small in young children, all external bleeding should be controlled as quickly and completely as possible. Signs of internal bleeding into the chest or abdomen also should be heeded and early operative intervention may be necessary to stop any ongoing hemorrhage. Fortunately, massive cavitary bleeding is less common in children than in adults, so good clinical judgment is necessary to determine when early operative intervention is required.

Intravenous access must be obtained rapidly to begin crystalloid resuscitation in any child with impending signs of shock. Younger children, how-

TABLE 1.
Expected Normal Vital Signs in Children*

Age (yr)	Respirations (breaths/min)	Pulse (bpm)	Systolic Blood Pressure (mm Hg)
<1	30–45	120–150	60–80
2–4	20–30	100–110	80–100
5–8	15–20	90–100	90–100
8–11	12–20	85–100	100–110
>12	12–16	60–90	100–120

*This provides a baseline from which comparisons can be made for the individual patient to determine whether the child is in shock or respiratory distress.

ever, have poor peripheral intravenous access sites, and the presence of increased systemic vascular resistance makes peripheral intravenous access even more difficult. If peripheral sites cannot be obtained in children, cutdown over the saphenous vein should be quickly initiated. Once the saphenous vein has been isolated, the largest possible intravenous cannula should be inserted to allow rapid flow of fluids to replenish losses. In infants, when intravenous access cannot be achieved in less than 90 seconds, interosseous access should be attempted. A small incision is made in the skin 2 cm distal to the tibial tuberosity on the flattened medial aspect of the tibia and the interosseous needle is directed slightly downward. The only contraindications to this approach include possible proximal vascular disruption or fracture of the tibia. Because the needle penetrates the sinusoids of the marrow cavity, flow rates as high as 100 mL/min can be obtained safely.

Central lines are rarely used in children, primarily because they are difficult to insert as a result of the small size of the veins relative to the intravenous catheters. In older children, subclavian or jugular access can be obtained, and large-bore intravenous catheters should be used in these positions to allow rapid intravenous infusion. The Seldinger technique frequently facilitates the use of central lines, because the wire can act as a convenient guide over which large resuscitation catheters can be placed.

Once intravenous access has been obtained, as many as three boluses of crystalloid, using a volume of 20 mL/kg, can be given. If the hemorrhagic shock state has not been reversed after the third or fourth bolus and other causes (e.g., spinal cord injury, pneumothorax, or cardiac tamponade) are not present, blood should be administered rapidly with a bolus of 10 to 20 mL/kg. If there is still no response, sites of cavitary bleeding should be sought and surgical intervention initiated.

The response to resuscitation in children is assessed similarly to the way it is in adults. The compensatory mechanisms should be reversed, with stabilization of the blood pressure and heart rate. Early in the resuscitation attempt, the arterial pH and lactate levels should be measured to assess the metabolic consequences of the shock state. Adequate resuscitation is reflected by improvement in these values toward normal ranges.

Disability

Head injury in a child is diagnosed in much the same fashion as in an adult, although a good neurologic examination may be difficult to obtain in younger children because of extreme anxiety and uncooperativeness of the patient. The hallmark of a head injury is a decrease in the level of consciousness and responsiveness that can be determined by examination, preferably before the child is sedated or paralyzed. Any evidence of an altered mental status, even if the child is thrashing about, should be pursued with a cranial computed tomography (CT) scan. Any child who has extreme depression in mental status should be considered for early intubation to maintain appropriate levels of oxygenation and to provide a means by which hyperventilation can be accomplished.[17, 18] Minimum criteria for obtaining a CT scan have not been defined, although any child with a Glasgow Coma Scale of 12 or less should be examined. Vomiting more than twice, facial fracture, severe bruising about the head, and significant multiple trauma are potential indications for further radiologic evaluation.[24] The mechanism of injury, including a fall from a relatively low height (i.e., from furniture or playground equipment), in younger children also should be included in protocols that define which patients should undergo cranial CT. Outcome from a particular level of disability after injury is usually better in children than in adults. Therefore, even with an extremely low Glasgow Coma Scale score on hospital admission, full neurologic resuscitation should be undertaken and continued vigorously to avoid secondary head injury. Aggressive therapy should be continued unless signs of brain death or massive, irreversible cerebral damage are evident.

Abdominal Injuries

One of the major differences in the surgical treatment of pediatric and adult trauma involves the diagnosis and management of abdominal injuries. Historically, a small amount of blood in the abdomen (about 30 mL in an adult) detected by diagnostic peritoneal lavage was judged sufficient to warrant exploratory laparotomy. More recently, it has been shown by several groups that *expectant management* of splenic and hepatic injuries in children, and in some adults, may be warranted to avoid operation. Therefore, in multiple studies from different centers, the use of abdominal CT scanning is considered relatively safe for the initial diagnosis of abdominal injuries.[25, 26] The presence of a splenic or hepatic injury in an otherwise hemodynamically stable child with no peritoneal signs can be followed up with frequent physical examination and observation for falling hematocrit levels. Exploratory laparotomy is generally not undertaken until the child requires about 40 mL/kg of transfused blood (which suggests massive blood loss or continued oozing from the ruptured viscus) or experiences severe peritoneal irritation. This may be one area in which the therapeutic techniques developed in children have been applied to adults, although there appears to be a higher frequency of delayed operation for ongoing bleeding in adult patients.

The Ideal Pediatric Trauma Center

Standards for Pediatric Trauma Centers

Because of the differences in potential diagnostic and treatment protocols for pediatric and adult patients, specialty centers for the treatment of pediatric trauma should prove advantageous. Several definitions of "optimal pediatric trauma care" have been proposed by various surgical and pediatric organizations. The Committee on Trauma of the American College of Surgeons (ACS) has established optimal trauma care standards defining minimal standards for pediatric trauma centers in the appendix of the *Minimal Standards of Trauma Care* document.[5] Figure 4 outlines the personnel who may be involved in the resuscitation of an injured child according to these guidelines.

The commitment required for a pediatric trauma center usually is found only in full service pediatric hospitals. Recommendations from the ACS state that a pediatric surgeon "is expected to be the director of the pediatric trauma service," and that "all surgical and medical pediatric specialists may be involved in the care of the injured child."[5] Facilities that should be available in a pediatric trauma center include a specifically designed emergency department for the treatment of pediatric trauma, a separate and distinct pediatric intensive care unit, and ancillary facilities that are staffed specifically for the pediatric patient. Other personnel involved in the pediatric team should include pediatric trauma nurses, pediatric intensive care unit nurses, respiratory therapists, physical therapists, and other specialists in technical areas, who have specific training in pediatric trauma.

In another position paper, this one from the American Pediatric Surgical Association,[6] it is suggested that pediatric trauma be managed by a fully organized, identifiable, and functioning pediatric trauma service that is under the direction of a pediatric surgeon. Although these guidelines do not mandate that separate areas of the hospital be designated for pediatric trauma care, they do state that the pediatric component of a trauma center should be separate and identifiable.

The Problem With Pediatric Trauma Centers

Pediatric trauma centers provide a committed level of care with a focus on injured children, but are too few and far between to handle effectively *all*

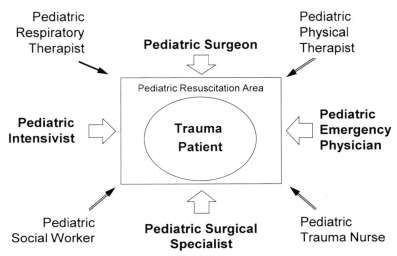

FIG 4.
A diagram of personnel involved in the resuscitation of a pediatric trauma patient at a "pediatric trauma center." Because these centers are usually based in full-service pediatric hospitals, all individuals participating in the resuscitation can be expected to be pediatric specialists from various areas of pediatric surgery and medicine. Unfortunately, this concentration of specialists is found in only a few centers throughout the country.

of the pediatric trauma that occurs in this country. Fewer than 30 pediatric trauma centers exist in only 21 states.[27] Even in the more populous states, there are usually only 2 or 3 of these institutions to serve the entire population. Although the involvement of pediatric surgeons in the management of pediatric trauma is desirable, the relative shortage of these specialty surgeons poses a problem for the adequate staffing of pediatric trauma centers. Only 22 programs in the United States currently offer fellowships in pediatric surgery, with a total enrollment of 37 fellows.[28, 29] According to the American Board of Surgery, 35 surgeons became certified in pediatric surgery in 1992 after successfully completing the biennial certifying examination.[29] Since 1976, 595 surgeons have been certified as having special qualifications in pediatric surgery.[30] There are 454 members of the American Pediatric Surgical Association in the United States, not all of whom are devoted to the treatment of pediatric trauma.[31] These figures reveal the relative shortage of the specially trained surgeons who have been proposed to direct the teams that will care for the nearly 25% of all trauma cases in the United States that involve children. Although treatment in a specialty pediatric trauma center is desirable, the reality is that most injured children in the United States will be cared for in adult trauma centers that may or may not have a special commitment to pediatric patients.

Treatment of the Pediatric Patient in a Comprehensive Adult Trauma Center

A comprehensive trauma center is an institution that is classified primarily as an adult center with a special commitment to pediatric care. For the purposes of definition, this center also may be the equivalent of a level II pediatric trauma center as defined by the Committee on Trauma of the ACS.[5] In these centers, the care of injured children must be integrated into the available resources of the entire trauma center. As a result, specific facilities, specialists, and ancillary medical personnel may not be specifically designated for the treatment of pediatric patients, and care may be provided by a team comprised of pediatricians and surgeons with primary training in *adult* trauma (Fig 5). Because of the nature of geography and population distribution, however, these institutions are called on to provide a substantial amount of care for injured children. For such programs to be successful, adherence to the following principles may be helpful.

Commitment and Scope

Any trauma center that proposes to care for pediatric patients must make a specific commitment to provide the services necessary to treat children. A particular specialist whose only responsibility is the injured child is not required, but a qualified team of professionals must be designated. These individuals comprise the "pediatric trauma program" within the full-service hospital and may be a subset of the adult trauma team. The hospital administration must make a special commitment to provide appropriate case management resources to the pediatric trauma program so that designated nurse coordinators are available to organize the care of pediatric patients. The pediatric trauma program must be recognized by the hospital as a specific, independent program within the institution. The program must be represented at the highest level of hospital government so that its needs can be considered appropriately among the many demands on hospital resources.

Once the organization of the pediatric trauma program within the hospital has been established, it is necessary to describe both the scope of the program and the service area from which patients will be referred. The scope of the program basically is defined by the type of patients that the program members feel qualified to treat. For instance, if no one in the pediatric trauma program is trained to manage pediatric head trauma, a child with such an injury should be referred to the closest facility that can provide such care. Pediatric trauma programs within comprehensive trauma centers generally should be capable of handling most injuries, except perhaps burns, spinal cord injuries, and cardiovascular injuries. Patients with these injuries may be stabilized within the regional pediatric trauma program and then transferred to the nearest level I pediatric trauma center. Certain programs may lack a particular pediatric specialist, such as a pediatric urologist, a pediatric neurosurgeon, or a pediatric plastic surgeon; a

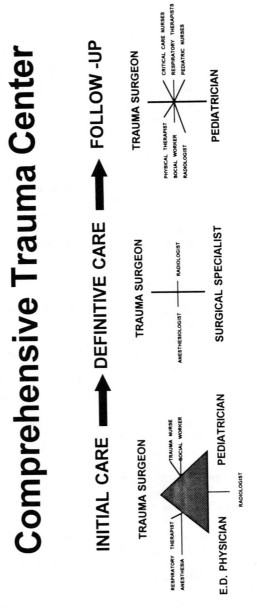

FIG 5.
A paradigm for treatment in the "comprehensive trauma center" where specialists trained primarily in adult surgery care for pediatric patients. This diagram outlines the team concept that is necessary for optimal care and shows that any pediatric specialists who are available should be involved in the treatment of injured children. At different phases in the child's care, the composition of the team may change, but the trauma surgeon always should direct the overall therapy. *ED* = emergency department.

child requiring these services may have to be transferred to a pediatric trauma program with such a specialist.

The next step is to define the geographic boundaries from which patients will be referred to a comprehensive trauma center with a pediatric trauma program. If the hospital lies within the traditional service area for an established pediatric trauma center, there should be no competition for these patients and arrangements should be made to send all of them to the pediatric trauma center from the scene of the injury. If no pediatric trauma center is nearby, however, the referral pattern for children will most likely be the same as for adults. If other level II adult trauma centers in the region are incapable of providing care for the pediatric patient, the level I comprehensive trauma center may have a larger service area for children than for adults. These regional referral patterns should be negotiated with other trauma centers in the region so that the prehospital providers have a clear protocol for the transportation of injured children that can be used as a reference for triage.

Commitment to pediatric care extends beyond the confines of the trauma center. Trauma care must include a *systems approach* to the trauma patient, and any trauma center committed to pediatric trauma care must work with the regional emergency medical service organization in the areas of education and protocol development. If no pediatric trauma center lies within the region, the trauma center with a pediatric trauma program must take the lead in stimulating appropriate educational opportunities for prehospital providers in the optimal treatment of the injured child. In addition, pediatric trauma programs must cooperate fully with emergency medical service agencies to establish appropriate prehospital protocols defining optimal therapy in regard to airway, breathing, circulation, and resuscitation of the child in the field. Medical control, if possible for the prehospital treatment of the pediatric trauma patient, should be assumed by a trauma center with a defined pediatric trauma program.

Composition of the Pediatric Trauma Team

Figure 5 illustrates the potential composition of the pediatric trauma team at the various stages of therapy for an injured child after arrival at the trauma center. Because pediatric surgeons may not be available, the team leader may be an adult trauma surgeon with a special interest in pediatric trauma care. This surgeon should be well acquainted with the principles of pediatric trauma management and should have successfully completed a Pediatric Advanced Life Support (PALS) course. The hallmark of a successful pediatric trauma team, however, is the participation of a pediatrician with a commitment to or interest in trauma care at all appropriate phases of resuscitation and follow-up care. There are some areas in the treatment of injured children for which a pediatrician can provide valuable expertise, such as intravenous access, ventilator management, fluid and electrolyte management, and accurate dosing of appropriate medications. If a pediatric intensivist is available, this individual should participate in the resuscitative phase as well as the intensive-care phase of patient care. If an individual with intensive-care training is not available, a pediatrician with an interest in pediatric critical care or pediatric trauma should be a member of the pediatric trauma team.

Emergency medicine physicians with an interest in pediatric care who have completed a PALS course may be involved in the initial resuscitation of a child, along with appropriate emergency department nurses and specially trained pediatric nurses who may be called from the pediatric intensive care unit or pediatric surgical units. The trauma team also should contain therapists with some advanced or special training in the application of their field of expertise to the pediatric patient. Respiratory therapists involved in the care of injured children from the initiation of the resuscitation should be knowledgeable regarding the use of pediatric ventilators and appropriate inhalation therapies for children. Physical therapists and social workers should understand the specific medical needs of children, as well as their social and psychological needs as progress is made through the follow-up and rehabilitative phases of the child's care.

During the definitive care or operative phase of the child's treatment, anesthesiologists with special training in pediatric anesthesia should be called on. The support of operating room nurses with special qualifications and skills in the provision of appropriate care to the pediatric patient during surgery also should be enlisted.

Facilities

Specific pediatric resuscitation areas are not available in most trauma centers. Trauma resuscitation of the injured child usually is undertaken in an adult resuscitation area that has been reconfigured to manage pediatric trauma. Because children require specific instrumentation for invasive resuscitation, the use of a pediatric resuscitation cart that is brought to the resuscitation room has become popular. Table 2 lists possible components of such a cart, which can be wheeled from a permanent storage place into any area of the emergency department where pediatric resuscitation is undertaken.

Typically, this is a standard mobile cart that has been converted for use for medical instrumentation. Each drawer may contain a specific set of instruments or medications that can be used for certain aspects of pediatric resuscitation. Prominently displayed on the cart should be a table of guidelines indicating typical instrument sizes and medication dosages for children of different ages and weights. This could be provided by a Broselow Pediatric Tape, or standard programs could be available in the emergency department computer to generate specific drug dosages and tube sizes for children of specific weights. An example of one such computer printout is provided in Figure 6 for a child who weighs 20 kg and is 3 years old. Only the child's name, weight, and age are required to generate this computer printout, which can be obtained in less than 30 seconds.

One area of the pediatric trauma cart should contain instrument packs for performing specific procedures, such as the insertion of a chest tube,

TABLE 2.
Components of a Pediatric Trauma Cart

Top
   Laryngoscopes and blades (0, 1, 2, 3, 4)
   Magill forceps
   Bag-valve masks (infant, child, adult)
   Endotracheal tubes (2.5–5.5 uncuffed, 6.0–9.0 cuffed)
   Stylets, topical anesthetic, lubricant, cuff syringes, tongue blades
   Oral airways (0–5), nasal airways (12–30 French)
   CO_2 indicator
First drawer
   Resuscitation drugs metered to appropriate doses
   Dosage reference system
Second and third drawers
   Suction catheters (5–18 French)
   Yankauer catheter
   Foley catheters (8–16 French)
   Nasogastric tubes (10–18 French, 5 French infant tube)
   Intravenous catheter (12–25 gauge)
   Microdrip and macrodrip intravenous tubing
   Interosseous needle
   Stopcocks, needles, syringes
   Pediatric blood pressure cuffs
Fourth drawer
   Pediatric cutdown tray
   Pediatric thoracostomy tray
   Pediatric diagnostic peritoneal lavage (DPL) tray
   Chest tubes (10–32 French)
   Pediatric splints
   Pediatric collars

peritoneal lavage, venous cutdown, and open thoracotomy. The instruments should be appropriate for use in children and the contents of each pack should be familiar to all members of the pediatric trauma team. In some cases, this pediatric trauma cart can follow the patient throughout the hospital stay so that the equipment is always available in the event emergency resuscitation is necessary later in the patient's hospital course.

```
TOMMY SMITH                    AGE:  3.0 YRS      WEIGHT: 20.00 KG              DATE: 02/15/94
THE PEDIATRIC INTENSIVE/PROGRESSIVE CARE UNITS OF THE CHILDREN'S HOSPITAL AT ALBANY MEDICAL CENTER

    ETT SIZE: 5.0    DEFIB. START DOSE (JOULES): 40          B.S.A. (SQ. M.) 0.79
    *************** ACLS DRUGS ***************    MAINTENANCE FLUID PER HOUR   (1800 ML/SQ. M./DAY)  59 ML
                                                  INSENSIBLE FLUID LOSS PER HOUR (300 ML/SQ. M./DAY)  9 ML
        DRUG        STRENGTH    DOSE/KG    MG      CC
  EPI. SYRINGE      1:10,000    .01 MG/KG  0.20   2.0    ********* NEUROMUSCULAR BLOCKADE AND ANESTHETICS *********
  BICARBONATE       1 MEQ/CC    1 MEQ/KG   20     20     ** FOR INTUBATION IN PRESENCE OF ANESTHESIOLOGY OR PICU ATTENDING **
  ATROPINE SRNGE    0.1 MG/CC   .02 MG/KG  0.40   4.00
  Ca Cl             10%         10 MG/KG   200    2.0    DRUG            STRENGTH   DOSE/KG      MG        CC
  LIDOCAINE         2%          1 MG/KG    20     1.00   PAVULON         1 MG/CC    .1 MG/KG     2.00     2.00
                                                         SUCCINYLCHOLINE 20 MG/CC   1.5 MG/KG    30.00    1.50
                                                         THIOPENTAL      25 MG/CC   5 MG/KG      100.00   4.00
                                                         FENTANYL        50 MCG/CC  5MCG/KG      0.100    2.00
  ********** CONTINUOUS DRUG INFUSIONS **********        KETAMINE (IV)   10 MG/CC   1 MG/KG      20.0     2.00
                                                         ATRACURIUM      10 MG/CC   0.7MG/KG     14.00    1.40

                                          ADD TO 100 ML  *************** MISCELLANEOUS DRUGS ***************

1 CC/HR = .05 MCG/KG/MIN                  6.00 MG        DRUG            STRENGTH   DOSE/KG       MG        CC
E.G.: EPI, NOREPI, ISUPREL, PGE1                         NARCAN          .4 MG/CC   .1 MG/KG      2.0     5.0
                                                         DEXTROSE        25%        .5 GM/KG      10000    40
1 CC/HR = .5 MCG/KG/MIN                   60.0 MG        LORAZEPAM       2 MG/CC    .05 MG/KG     1.0     0.50
E.G.: NITROPRUSSIDE, NITROGLYCERINE                      MIDAZOLAM       5 MG/CC    .05 MG/KG     1.0     0.20
                                                         MANNITOL        25%        .25 GM/KG     5000    20
1 CC/HR = 2 MCG/KG/MIN                    240 MG         DECADRON(SHOCK) 4 MG/CC    4 MG/KG       80      20
E.G.: DOPAMINE, DOBUTAMINE
                                                              MILLIGRAMS OF HYDROCORTISONE = 40 x DECADRON
1 CC/HR = 10 MCG/KG/MIN                   1200 MG                "         " METHYLPREDNISOLONE = 8 x DECADRON
E.G.: LIDOCAINE

1 CC/HR = 1 MCG/KG/HOUR                   2000 MICROGRAMS  ******** DIGITALIZATION ********
E.G.: FENTANYL                                             * DIGITALIZING ** IV ** Q8H (MICROGRAMS) ** MAX TDD = 1000 **
                                                           *    TOTAL/KG  (TOTAL)    DOSE 1   DOSE 2   DOSE 3
1 CC/HR = .05 MG/KG/HOUR                  100 MG           *       20   (  400  )     200      100      100
E.G.: MIDAZOLAM                                            *
                                                           * MAINTENANCE ** IV ** Q12H (MICROGRAMS) ** MAX = .125/D ***
1 CC/HR = .0005 UNITS/KG/HOUR             1.00 UNITS       *    TOTAL/KG/DAY  (TOTAL/DAY)     A.M.    P.M.
E.G.: VASOPRESSIN                                          *        5       (  78  )         39       39

1 CC/HR = .025 UNITS/KG/HOUR              50.0 UNITS
E.G.: INSULIN
```

FIG 6.
A printout of a computer-generated guideline sheet that helps in the determination of equipment requirements and drug doses for the resuscitation of a child. This is a comprehensive sheet that is useful not only for resuscitation, but also for medical problems. It has been generated from a simple computer program and requires the input of only the child's name, age, and weight. A printout such as this can be available in less than 30 seconds after the input of information.

Follow-up Care/Rehabilitation/Psychosocial Care

Once the child has been stabilized through either adequate resuscitation or operative intervention, transfer to the appropriate unit within the hospital is necessary. Members of the pediatric trauma team should continue to direct the patient's care within these units.

If possible, the seriously injured patient should be transferred to a pediatric intensive care unit in which the facilities and personnel are devoted to the care of children. In this setting, a pediatric intensivist or a pediatrician with expertise in intensive care works with the trauma team to monitor the child and provide appropriate intervention as deemed necessary. The nursing staff should be trained in the principles of pediatric critical care as applied to ventilator and intravenous fluid management. An individual with expertise in pediatric critical care always should be in the hospital to address any alteration in hemodynamics or gas exchange that may require immediate intervention.

If no pediatric intensive care unit is available, the child will be admitted to a critical care unit that provides care primarily for adults. In much the same fashion that an injured child is resuscitated in an adult emergency department, the care provided in an adult critical care unit must involve interventions and equipment appropriate for children. Of crucial importance is the availability of a team of specially trained nurses who have a specific interest and expertise in the critical care of children. Special advanced training for these nurses should be coordinated with the pediatrician so that the potential problems of children are recognized. The differences between adults and children with respect to physiology, diagnosis, and therapy may be even greater in the critical care setting than in the resuscitation area.

As in the initial evaluation, particular attention must be paid to airway maintenance during the period spent in the critical care unit. The endotracheal tubes used in smaller children do not have a cuff; as a result, an air leak will occur with each positive-pressure inspiration. Therefore, special attention must be paid continually to the adequacy of the inspiratory tidal volumes. Because the smaller tubes tend to become occluded more easily, recognition of airway obstruction is a key issue in pediatric intensive care. Pressure-controlled ventilators are used more commonly in children and must be monitored for the adequacy of the tidal volume.

Because children have less reserve than do adults, recognition of appropriate vital signs and neurologic function in children of different ages is important. In trying to achieve normal hemodynamics, it must be remembered that blood pressures tend to be lower and pulse rates higher in children. Inserting intravenous lines, drawing blood, and maintaining an appropriate fluid balance have special nuances in the pediatric population. Fluid volumes must be customized to the weight of each child and the ongoing disease process. Recognizing pain levels in infants who are not able to express a pain response adequately also is important. Abnormalities of the vital signs, such as unexpected tachycardia, tachypnea, or grunting, may suggest pain that requires small doses of narcotics. Finally, the psychosocial differences between children and adults must be understood. The importance of parental visitation and its calming effect on the child's demeanor may require that visiting hours be expanded for children who are being treated in an adult intensive care unit. The involvement of social workers to address family problems brought on by the injury is even more important in the care of a child than that of an adult. The needs of parents, who may have other children and job responsibilities, or who may have traveled long distances to be near the child in the trauma center, should be accommodated as much as possible to enhance the child's psychological support.

If an injured child is to be treated in an adult critical care unit, all members of the critical care team need to remain aware of potential situations in which the needs of the child may exceed the resources of the facility. In such cases, it is important that all providers be honest and realistic about their capabilities, so that appropriate decisions regarding transfer of the child to a higher level of care can be made if necessary.

Once the child's condition has stabilized and he or she has been moved out of the intensive care unit, early intervention with respect to rehabilitation or home health care needs is necessary. Physical therapy and occupational therapy consultations should be obtained early in the patient's course, as soon as the child can benefit. Early transfer to rehabilitation facilities may promote a more rapid and complete recovery of neurologic and ambulatory function. Preventive splinting and early joint mobilization for children with head injuries may prevent potential complications such as contractures and decubitus that may impair adequate rehabilitation. Rehabilitation specialists in this field should have some understanding of the particular problems of pediatric patients with respect to the effect of injury and impairment of growth and development.

Evaluation of a Pediatric Trauma Program in an Adult Trauma Center

Once different levels of pediatric trauma care have been identified, outcomes from institutions with different approaches to such care should be compared. For this purpose, the TRISS methodology is used (Table 3).[12, 32] For each patient, the Revised Trauma Score (which usually is measured at the time of admission to the trauma center) and the ISS are calculated. Using results obtained from the MTOS, a predicted survival can be calculated for each patient according to national norms. A Z-score then is calculated by determining the difference between the actual and the predicted number of survivors, and dividing this by a scale factor proportional to the standard error of difference between the observed and the predicted proportion surviving. The Z-score may be positive or negative depending on whether the survival rate at a particular institution is greater or less than that predicted by the baseline probability function for the comparison set of the MTOS. Absolute values of Z exceeding 1.96 establish a statistically

TABLE 3.
TRISS Methodology From the Multiple Trauma Outcome Study (MTOS)*

1. For each patient:
   Calculate Revised Trauma Score (RTS)
   Calculate Injury Severity Score (ISS)
   Determine age $<$ or $\geq$ 55 yr (AGE)
2. Determine probability of survival:
   $P_s = 1/(1 + e^{-b})$
   where $b = b_0 + b_1$ (RTS) $+ b_2$ (ISS) $+ b_3$ (AGE)
   $b_0 = -1.2470$
   $b_1 = 0.9544$
   $b_2 = -0.0768$
   $b_3 = -1.9052$
3. Compare outcome with MTOS norm:
   Determine actual survivors: (A)
   Calculate expected survivors: $E = \Sigma P_s$
   Determine difference: $A - E$
4. Calculate Z:
   $Z = (A-E)/S$
   where $S = \sqrt{\Sigma P_i \cdot (1-P_i)}$
   $P_i = P_s$ of the ith patient

*Once a probability of survival (P_s) for each patient has been determined, these can be compared to actual outcomes to arrive at a Z-score for the institution. Although a direct comparison of Z-scores from different institutions is not statistically valid, trends with respect to quality of care can be determined. Wide variations in the Z-score from one institution to another may suggest outcome differences.

different outcome ($P < .05$) between the experience of a particular institution and the national experience. An M-score is calculated, which demonstrates how closely the study population reflects the injury severity of the MTOS population. An M-score of greater than 90% suggests good correlation.

The applicability of trauma scores and TRISS methodology to pediatric patients has been demonstrated in several studies.[33] In published reports from pediatric trauma centers, the Z-score has always been greater than zero, and often has been greater than the threshold (1.96), predicting a statistically significant improvement in outcome over the MTOS (Table 4). Other studies predicting survival demonstrate that care in a pediatric trauma center may result in a shorter length of stay, better psychosocial outcome, and improved overall outcome as measured by return to normal function.

Attempting to define the outcome of pediatric trauma care in trauma centers that are not designed specifically for children is difficult. It is important to determine outcome variables in this situation, however, to answer the following question: Is it important at all costs to transfer a patient to a specialized pediatric trauma center, or can care be provided safely at a comprehensive trauma center in situations where access to pediatric trauma centers is limited?

Table 4 shows the Z-scores from different nonpediatric trauma centers for comparison with those from pediatric trauma centers. In the study from San Francisco by Knudsen and associates,[34] the results of pediatric trauma care in a large urban area were evaluated. This study examined the records of 353 injured children younger than 18 years who were treated at

TABLE 4.
TRISS Z-Scores and Mortality Rates From Pediatric and Adult Trauma Centers*

Author	Number of Patients	Z-Score	M-Score†	Mortality (%)
Pediatric trauma centers				
Kaufmann et al.[33]	346	1.85	NR	6.9
Eichelberger et al.[37]	1,562	2.93‡	NR	2.8
Eichelberger et al.[38]	594	1.21‡	NR	2.7
Nakayama et al.[39]	603	0.32	NR	3.2
Peclet et al.[40]	2,234	2.87	NR	2.2
Kauffman et al.[41]	376	1.35	0.93	7.2
Eichelberger et al.[42]	1,009	1.95‡	0.91	2.8
Nakayama[36]	1,881	3.90	NR	4.1
Adult trauma centers				
Knudson et al.[34]	353	1.88	0.96	6.0
Fortune et al.[35]	303	1.64	0.94	4.2
Nakayama et al.[36]				
Urban	1,293	3.33	NR	4.1
Rural	1,441	1.12	NR	6.2
Bensard et al.[27]	410	0.47	0.87	2.0

*In general, the Z-scores do not define any consistent major differences between the two types of institutions.
†NR = not reported.
‡Blunt trauma.

a trauma center where pediatric surgeons were not involved directly in most of the management decisions. About 33% of the injuries were penetrating and most of the children were older than 14 years. The resultant Z-score of 1.88 led the authors to conclude that the outcome of children admitted to an adult trauma center with experience in pediatric care compares favorably with national standards. A critique of this report questioned the inclusion of many older adolescents with penetrating injuries in the study, suggesting that this may not reflect the typical pediatric trauma population seen at most trauma centers.

A study from Albany Medical Center examined 4 years of experience treating 303 severely injured children using a model in which adult trauma surgeons worked closely with pediatric intensivists.[35] Initial resuscitation and definitive intervention were provided under the control of the surgical staff, after which the patient was treated in the pediatric intensive care unit jointly by the pediatric intensivists and the trauma team. The Z-score in this series was 1.64, resulting in the conclusion that a committed relationship between adult trauma surgeons and pediatric intensivists will yield favorable results in a trauma center when pediatric surgeons are not available.

Another study highlights the experience of Lehigh Valley Hospital in Pennsylvania, in which the practice model involved the treatment of pediatric patients by the adult trauma service with a mandatory consultation with a pediatrician.[43] The patients were cared for in the adult intensive care unit by the adult trauma team with some help from the pediatrician, although there was little involvement by pediatric surgeons. External and internal peer review of this program showed that no deaths were preventable. The Z-score was not available to describe the entire group, although Z-scores for individual segments of the study population were not different from those of adults.

In another report, Bensard and colleagues documented the pediatric trauma experience at Denver General Hospital.[27] In this program, trauma surgeons treated all pediatric patients throughout their hospital stay. Children were placed in the pediatric intensive care unit or on the general pediatric floor, depending on their needs. Pediatric consultation was provided by in-house pediatric residents, attending physicians, intensivists, anesthesiologists, and neonatologists. For the 410 children treated in this program, the mortality rate was 2%, with no documented preventable deaths. The Z-score for children from this series was 0.47. A direct comparison of outcome statistics from this center and those from a prominent pediatric trauma center showed few differences.

More recently, Nakayama used the trauma registry of the Pennsylvania Trauma Systems Foundation to study outcome differences between pediatric and nonpediatric trauma centers.[36] In this study, the experience of pediatric trauma centers in large urban areas was compared to the outcome of injured children cared for in nonpediatric trauma centers throughout the rest of the state. Most of the children were treated in nonpediatric centers, although, on an institutional basis, the rate of pediatric trauma admissions was higher at the pediatric trauma centers.

The comparative results showed that the mortality was highest in the rural nonpediatric centers, but the death rate in the urban nonpediatric centers compared favorably with that in the pediatric centers (4.1%). Using TRISS methodology, the Z-scores for the pediatric centers and the urban nonpediatric centers were similar and showed an improvement over the national experience statistically. The rural trauma centers had a lower Z-score overall, but when the probability of survival was stratified, no statistical significance with respect to survival existed. The authors concluded that regional differences in pediatric trauma care did exist, and that the higher mortality in the rural centers may be a result of lack of access to prehospital care.

In comparing all the reports on this topic, little documented difference is seen between outcome in pediatric centers and nonpediatric centers when all variables can be appropriately adjusted. There is no question that certain aspects of care may require the special training and resources available in a pediatric trauma center, although these may not be measurable by mortality rates. Cost-effectiveness, resource utilization, and patient satisfaction, as well as other nuances of optimal pediatric surgical care, have not been included as variables in studies examining this topic.

Decision Tree for Triage of the Pediatric Patient

After each trauma center determines its level of commitment to and degree of involvement in pediatric trauma care, a formal protocol should be developed to determine which children will be treated in the facility and at what point a decision will be made to transfer a child to a pediatric trauma center. Protocol development should involve all members of the pediatric trauma team and the hospital administration so that the appropriate decision paradigm can be invoked immediately to avoid unnecessary delay in patient care. Figure 7 illustrates a general protocol for determining where a child should be treated; important decisions are made during the prehospital, resuscitation, and follow-up phases of care.

The first decision that must be made either by protocol or by medical control of the prehospital care providers, is the initial destination of the injured child. Several triage scores can be used in children, the most important being the Revised Trauma Score and the Pediatric Trauma Score (Tables 5 and 6). The Revised Trauma Score has been proven to be effective for the triage of adults and involves an assessment of the neurologic status, blood pressure, and the respiratory rate. In general, a trauma score less than 8 indicates that the patient should be taken directly to a level I or level II trauma center.

The Pediatric Trauma Score addresses the triage of a child more specifically. It involves scoring parameters that include the size of the child as well as the more descriptive components of airway patency particularly intended for infants. Survival rates of nearly 100% are seen in children with Pediatric Trauma Scores of greater than 8.[44] At scores less than 8, however, survival

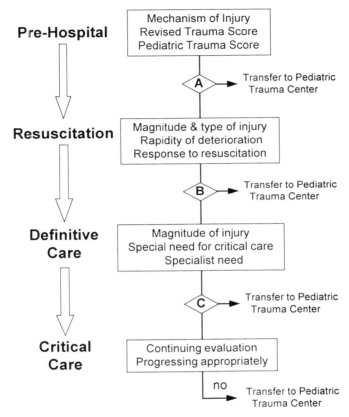

FIG 7.
A decision tree outlining the factors that determine whether a patient should be transferred to a higher level of pediatric trauma care. *Triangles* denote decisions, and *points* and *rectangles* provide potential reasons why transfer would be considered.

decreases rapidly; therefore, it is imperative that children with low pediatric trauma scores be taken directly to institutions with dedicated pediatric trauma programs. As indicated by the National Pediatric Trauma Registry, this probably includes only about 4% to 5% of all injured children. The mechanism of injury also is important in triage decisions made early after an accident. In most cases, the mechanism of injury guidelines proposed by the ACS apply to children, except that the distance for falls should be appropriately adjusted. A rule of thumb is that, if a child falls from an elevation more than two times his or her own height, the possibility of serious injury should be considered and care in a pediatric trauma center is appropriate.

TABLE 5.
The Revised Trauma Score

Component	Coded Value				
	4	3	2	1	0
Glasgow Coma Scale score	13–15	9–12	6–8	4–5	3
Systolic blood pressure (mm Hg)	>89	76–89	50–75	1–49	0
Respiratory rate (breaths/min)	10–29	>29	6–9	1–5	0

Hemodynamic and respiratory stability must be taken into account in determining the first facility to which the child should be taken. A rapidly deteriorating blood pressure or inability to gain an airway may necessitate transportation to the nearest hospital for rapid stabilization. For these reasons, hospitals interested in providing pediatric trauma care should maintain continuing education programs, such as PALS, with community hospitals. Continuing instruction in the rapid, early stabilization of injured children is important for all facilities who may be called to provide such care. In addition, the educational process must emphasize the fact that decisions regarding transfer must be made *early* after the child arrives at the hospital. The prehospital care provider must remain close to the resuscitation so that immediate transportation to the next level of pediatric trauma care can be arranged. Unnecessary evaluation or delay in arranging transportation to or acceptance at a facility caring for pediatric injuries must be avoided to ensure rapid, definitive care.

The next decision in treatment triage arises at the time of initial resuscitation. In each institution with a pediatric trauma program, there may be inadequacies, such as in the treatment of burns or spinal injuries, or in cardiovascular surgery. If, during the resuscitation of the child, injuries are discovered in anatomic systems that cannot be treated in the pediatric trauma program, immediate transfer to an institution with these special facilities should be considered. At this point, judgments must be made regarding the existence of any life-threatening injuries (e.g., abdominal bleeding) that require treatment before transfer. All efforts should be made to stabilize the child before any transportation is considered. Providing intubation and adequate intravenous access before transport may be very important to maintain the stability of the child until the next level of care is reached. If an airway is provided, the transferring medical personnel must have sufficient experience in airway management and be able to insert a new airway if patency is lost.

TABLE 6.
The Pediatric Trauma Score

Component	Category		
	+2	+1	-1
Size (kg)	>20	10-20	<10
Airway	Normal	Able to be maintained	Unable to be maintained
Systolic blood pressure (mm Hg)*	>90	50-90	<50
Central nervous system	Awake	Obtunded level of consciousness	Coma/decerebrate
Skeletal	None	Closed fracture	Open/multiple fractures
Cutaneous	None	Minor	Major/penetrating

*If proper size blood pressure cuff is not available, blood pressure can be assessed by assigning +2 = pulse palpable at wrist, +1 = pulse palpable at groin, and -1 = no pulse palpable.

The final triage decision is made after the child is stabilized, at which time it must be determined whether the critical care facilities in the pediatric trauma program are adequate to provide appropriate care for the child. This may be particularly apparent in the case of an injured infant or neonate who may have required initial stabilization and operative treatment at a facility that has only an adult intensive care unit. The lack of appropriate ventilators, airway expertise, and nursing protocol necessitates transfer to an institution with a formal pediatric intensive care unit. Anticipation of prolonged hospitalization, for which a pediatric social worker or other resources of a pediatric unit may be helpful, also may suggest the advisability of transfer. The need for specialized services for a particular injury, such as a complex fracture, neurologic trauma, or massive soft-tissue trauma that would require repeated operations or specialized monitoring, also may mandate transfer.

The staff of the pediatric trauma program must be comfortable with their ability to care for the injured child. Not only should these issues be discussed within the pediatric multidisciplinary conferences, but strong liaisons should be established with the nearest pediatric trauma center so that appropriate, mutually acceptable guidelines can be established. To solidify these discussions, formal transfer agreements should be developed and agreed on by both the potential transferring and accepting institutions. The pediatric trauma center, in turn, should use the services of the pediatric trauma program in a comprehensive trauma center for follow-up care, if necessary, so that the final aspects of the child's care may be provided closer to home.

Conclusion

The magnitude and demographics of pediatric trauma in the United States require a coordinated approach to trauma care provided by facilities with different levels of resources necessary to treat injured children. Although the pediatric trauma center with its team of specialists particularly trained to care for injured children is the ideal model for pediatric trauma care, the relative scarcity of these facilities requires the involvement of other institutions in this problem.

Several studies have shown that an *adult* trauma center that has a special commitment to the treatment of pediatric trauma can provide adequate care to injured children. Because there are many differences between the care of injured children and adults, however, special consideration must be given to the development of a pediatric trauma program within the adult trauma center. If an adult trauma center is to care for injured children, a special commitment must be made so that appropriate medical staff, equipment, and hospital resources can be allocated to meet the special needs of these patients. In addition, institutions with pediatric trauma programs must take a leadership role in developing a trauma system to ensure appropriate triage and prehospital care of the pediatric patient. Ongoing quality assurance programs must be initiated to confirm that the outcome of care in adult trauma centers with pediatric trauma programs remains satisfactory and within the standards established by similar institutions and pediatric trauma centers.

The serious problem of childhood injury can be addressed through a coordinated effort between pediatric trauma centers and adult trauma centers with pediatric trauma programs. As in all trauma, each institution must be involved not only in providing medical care, but also epidemiologic and preventive programs to reduce this problem in American society.

References

1. Haller JA, Beaver BL: Overview of pediatric trauma, in Touloukian RJ (ed): *Pediatric Trauma*. St Louis, Mosby, 1990, pp 3–13.
2. McCarthy DL, Surpure JS: Pediatric trauma: Initial evaluation and stabilization. *Pediatr Ann* 1990; 19:584–596.
3. Ramenofsky ML: Emergency medical services for children and pediatric trauma system components. *J Pediatr Surg* 1989; 24:153–155.
4. Ribbeck B, Runge JW, Thomason MH, et al: Injury surveillance: A method for recording codes for injured emergency department patients. *Ann Emerg Med* 1992; 21:37–40.
5. American College of Surgeons, Committee on Trauma: *Resources for Optimal Care of the Injured Patient*. Chicago, American College of Surgeons, 1990.
6. Harris BH, Barlow B, Ballantine TV, et al: American Pediatric Surgical Association Principles of Trauma Care. *J Pediatr Surg* 1992; 27:423–426.
7. Harris BH: Creating pediatric trauma systems. *J Pediatr Surg* 1989; 24:149–152.

8. Haller JA, Shorter N, Miller D, et al: Organization and function of a regional pediatric trauma center: Does a system of management improve outcome? *J Trauma* 1983; 23:691–696.
9. Ramenofsky M, Luterman A, Quindlen E, et al: Maximum survival in pediatric trauma: The ideal system. *J Trauma* 1984; 24:818–823.
10. Eichelberger MR, Bowman LM, Sacco WJ, et al: Trauma scores vs. revised trauma score in TRISS to predict outcome in children with blunt trauma. *Ann Emerg Med* 1989; 18:939–942.
11. Cooper A, Barlow B, Davidson L, et al: Epidemiology of pediatric trauma: Importance of population-based statistics. *J Pediatr Surg* 1992; 27:149–154.
12. Champion HR, Copes WS, Sacco WJ, et al: The major trauma outcome study: Establishing national norms for trauma care. *J Trauma* 1990; 30:1356.
13. DiScala C: *National Pediatric Trauma Registry—Phase 2: Quarterly Report.* Boston, National Institute on Disability and Rehabilitation Research, Tufts New England Medical Center, 1993.
14. Schwab CW: Violence: America's uncivil war. *J Trauma* 1993; 35:657–665.
15. Vane D, Shedd FG, Grosfeld JL, et al: An analysis of pediatric trauma deaths in Indiana. *J Pediatr Surg* 1990; 25:955.
16. Centers for Disease Control, Division of Injury Control, Center for Environmental Health and Injury Control: Childhood injuries in the United States. *Am J Dis Child* 1990; 144:627–646.
17. Schafermeyer R: Pediatric trauma. *Emerg Med Clin North Am* 1993; 11:187–205.
18. Inaba AS, Seward PN: An approach to pediatric trauma, unique anatomic and pathophysiologic aspects of the pediatric patient. *Emerg Med Clin North Am* 1991; 9:523–548.
19. Eichelberger MR (ed): *Pediatric Trauma.* St Louis, Mosby, 1993.
20. Garcia VF, Gotschall CS: Rib fractures in children: A marker of severe trauma. *J Trauma* 1990; 30:695.
21. Nakayama DK, Gardner MJ, Rowe MI: Emergency endotracheal intubation in pediatric trauma. *Ann Surg* 1990; 211:218–223.
22. Chameides L (ed): *Pediatric Advanced Life Support.* Dallas, American Heart Association, 1990.
23. American College of Surgeons, Committee on Trauma: *Advanced Trauma Life Support Course for Physicians.* Chicago, American College of Surgeons, 1993.
24. Rivara F, Tanaguchi D, Parish RA: Poor prediction of positive computed tomographic scans by clinical criteria in symptomatic pediatric head trauma. *Pediatrics* 1987; 80:579–583.
25. Newman KD, Eichelberger MR, Randolph JG: Abdominal injury, in Eichelberger MR, Pratsch GS (eds): *Pediatric Trauma Care.* Rockville, Md, Aspen Publishers, 1988, pp 101–104.
26. Tepas JJ: Abdominal trauma, in Ehrlich FE, Heldrich FJ, Tepas JJ (eds): *Pediatric Emergency Medicine.* Rockville, Md, Aspen Publishers, 1987, pp 229–237.
27. Bensard DD, McIntyre RC, Moore EE, et al: A critical analysis of acutely injured children managed in an adult level I trauma center. *J Pediatr Surg* 1994; 29:11–18.
28. Karnell LH: Residency manpower trends. *Am Coll Surgeons Bull* 1991; 76:26–27.
29. Copeland EM: Report of the American Board of Surgery. *Am Coll Surgeons Bull* 1990; 75:37–40.

30. Shuck JM: Report of the American Board of Surgery. *Am Coll Surgeons Bull* 1993; 78:52–55.
31. American Pediatric Surgical Association: *Membership Director.* Covina, Calif, APSA, 1991.
32. Boyd CR, Tolson MA, Copes WS: Evaluating trauma care: The TRISS method. *J Trauma* 1987; 27:370.
33. Kaufmann CR, Maier RV, Kaufmann EJ, et al: Validity of applying adult TRISS analysis to injured children. *J Trauma* 1991; 31:691.
34. Knudson MM, Shagoury C, Lewis FR: Can adult trauma surgeons care for pediatric trauma. *J Trauma* 1991; 32:729–739.
35. Fortune JB, Sanchez J, Feustel PJ, et al: A pediatric trauma center without a pediatric surgeon: A four-year outcome analysis. *J Trauma* 1992; 33:130–139.
36. Nakayama DK, Copes WS, Sacco W: Difference in trauma care among pediatric and non-pediatric trauma centers. *J Pediatr Surg* 1992; 27:427–431.
37. Eichelberger MR, Bowman LM, Sacco WJ, et al: Trauma score versus revised trauma score in TRISS to predict outcome in children with blunt trauma. *Ann Emerg Med* 1989; 18:939.
38. Eichelberger MR, Mangubat EA, Sacco WJ, et al: Comparative outcomes of children and adults suffering blunt trauma. *J Trauma* 1988; 28:430–434.
39. Nakayama DK, Saitz EW, Gardner MJ, et al: Quality assessment in the pediatric trauma care system. *J Pediatr Surg* 1989; 24:156–158.
40. Peclet MH, Newman KD, Eichelberger MR, et al: Patterns of injury in children. *J Pediatr Surg* 1990; 25:85.
41. Kauffman CR, Rivara F, Maier RV: Pediatric trauma: Need for surgical management. *J Trauma* 1989; 29:1120.
42. Eichelberger MR, Mangubat EA, Sacco WJ, et al: Outcome analysis of blunt injury in children. *J Trauma* 1988; 28:1109.
43. Rhodes M, Smith S, Boorse D: Pediatric trauma patients in an "adult" trauma center. *J Trauma* 1993; 35:384–393.
44. Jubelirer RA, Agarwal NN, Beyer FC, et al: Pediatric trauma triage: Review of 1,307 cases. *J Trauma* 1990; 30:1544.

Pelvic Fractures

Roger E. Huckfeldt, M.D.

Instructor, Trauma Fellow, Division of General Surgery, Oregon Health Sciences University, Portland, Oregon

Richard J. Mullins, M.D.

Associate Professor, Director, Trauma Service, Division of General Surgery, Oregon Health Sciences University, Portland, Oregon

Donald D. Trunkey, M.D.

Professor, Chairman, Department of Surgery, Division of General Surgery, Oregon Health Sciences University, Portland, Oregon

Pelvic fractures are a common injury in our high-speed society and represent an immediate threat to life as well as potential long-term disability in those who survive the initial insult. A successful outcome depends on rapid diagnosis and effective treatment of associated pelvic injuries, life-threatening hemorrhage, and injuries remote from the fracture site. The treatment plan also must prevent systemic inflammation and sepsis complications, and achieve optimal bony stabilization to reduce long-term morbidity. Pelvic fractures are arguably the most difficult injuries to treat and exemplify the need for a multidisciplinary approach to trauma care. Although the trauma surgeon directs the initial phase of resuscitation and stabilization, a team approach including orthopaedic surgeons, radiologists, and blood bank personnel is important in limiting mortality and morbidity from pelvic injuries. This chapter outlines the comprehensive care of the trauma patient with pelvic injury.

Incidence

All surgeons who are involved in the care of seriously injured patients will face the challenges of pelvic injury at some point. It is estimated that pelvic fractures account for 3% of all fractures[1] and 1 of every 1,000 hospital admissions,[2] and are the third most frequent documented injuries in motor vehicle crashes.[3] Gilliland reported a 14% incidence of pelvic fracture in hospital admissions for trauma over a 1-year period.[4]

The mechanism of injury remains relatively constant throughout most reported series. Motor vehicle accidents are responsible in 57% to 73% of cases, auto-pedestrian incidences in 11% to 18%, motorcycle accidents in 5% to 10%, crush injuries in 4% to 8%, and falls in 6% to 11%.[5–10] Mortality in patients with pelvic fractures is high and attributed to initial hemorrhage, delayed sepsis, and associated injuries. Moreno and colleagues stratified mortality rates by mechanism of injury in a review of 538 patients with pelvic fracture. In this series, mortality was 5% in injuries resulting from motor vehicle accidents, 12% in those related to falls, 22% in those caused by auto-pedestrian incidents, 8% in those associated with motorcycle accidents, and 50% in those resulting from crush injuries.[11]

Anatomy

A thorough understanding of the anatomy of the pelvis is essential in designing, implementing, and evaluating the success of therapy for pelvic fracture. The fusion of the ilium, ischium, and pubis forms the innominate bone. The bony pelvis is stabilized by the ligamentous union of the innominate bones anteriorly at the pubis symphysis and posteriorly to the sacrum at the sacroiliac (SI) joints. The ring structure formed by this marriage of bones and ligaments represents a fortress designed to provide protection as well as facilitate locomotion. The pelvic ring functions to support the basis of truncal balance and pedal locomotion by providing transference of weight from the vertebral column to the lower extremities and provides a point of attachment and force generation for many muscle groups. It also serves as a protective shield for the bowel, urinary structures, reproductive organs, and other structures that venture below the brim.

Major vascular structures existing under this bony support system include the iliac arteries and veins and their branches. These vessels can be subjected to direct trauma and tremendous shear energy when enough force is generated to fracture the pelvic ring. Peripheral nerves supplying the pelvis and lower extremities lie adjacent to and are tethered by the bones of the pelvis, and are at risk for stretch and transection injury during pelvic trauma.

Classification

Many attempts have been made to classify pelvic fractures. In 1938, Watson-Jones developed a system based on the type and location of the fracture.[12] Thirty years later, Conolly and Hedberg published a classification based on the interruption of the major line of weight transmission.[13] After a review of 173 pelvic fractures treated at San Francisco General Hospital, Trunkey and colleagues in 1974 proposed a classification system designed to include associated soft-tissue injury and treatment considerations.[14] This system categorized pelvic fractures according to stability. Type I fractures were comminuted (crush) injuries that usually involved at least three structural rents. These commonly unstable fractures often were accompanied by severe hemorrhage and other soft-tissue injuries. Type II injuries, also unstable fractures, included the diametric (Malgaigne), open-book, and acetabular fractures. Type III fractures were stable injuries and included both isolated fractures and disruptions of the pubic rami.

Pennal and associates designed a classification system based primarily on the mechanism of injury that incorporated the direction and force of the traumatic event.[15] This system, which has since undergone modification by Tile[16] and by Young and Resnick,[17] stratifies pelvic disruptions into lateral compression (LC), anteroposterior compression (APC), and vertical shear (VS) injuries. The Young modification adds a fourth class, combined mechanical (CM) injury, and incorporates subcategories in an attempt to measure the extent of the applied force. The LC injury involves the transmission of force by a lateral impact directly on the innominate bone or through the axis of the proximal femur and iliac crest. The major ligamentous structures and vasculature actually are shortened during the injury rather than stretched and, therefore, are disrupted less frequently (unless by direct bony fragment involvement). The LC category is subdivided according to the extent of injury into LC-I (Fig 1, A; pubic ramus fracture and sacral compression injury), LC-II (see Fig 1, B; pubic ramus fracture and iliac wing fracture), and LC-III (see Fig 1, C; additional contralateral open-book injury).

APC injuries are caused by the application of force from either the front or the back with sufficient energy to fracture the pelvic ring. Three fracture patterns also are seen with this mechanism of injury. APC-I injuries (Fig 2, A), the least severe variant, demonstrate slight widening of the pubic symphysis and, sometimes, the SI joint. These are stable fractures with few complications. APC-II injuries (see Fig 2, B) manifest as symphyseal distraction with associated SI anterior ligamentous disruption resulting in the typical "open-book" appearance on the anteroposterior (AP) radiograph. APC-III fractures (see Fig 2, C) involve complete separation of the innominate bone from the pelvic ring. The SI joint and pubic symphysis are disrupted completely, but no vertical displacement is present. This variant is caused by extreme force and often is associated with other injuries.

VS fractures are anterior injuries through the pubic symphysis or fractures of the rami associated with posterior disruption through the sacrum, iliac wing, or SI joint allowing vertical displacement of the hemipelvis (Fig 3). The historical fracture of Malgaigne is the classic example of this type of injury. The usual mechanism described involves substantial axial loading of the hemipelvis, as occurs with a fall or sudden deceleration onto an extended leg. The cephalad displacement, combined with the described direction of involved force, differentiates VS injury from the APC-III variant of this classification system.

Periodically, pelvic fractures with characteristics of several of these variants arise, and Young's CM category accommodates these injuries. The combination of force and direction in these fractures results in a multitude of possible presentations.

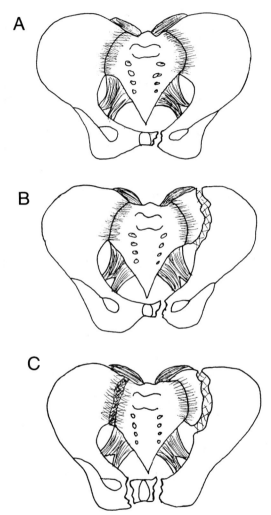

FIG 1.
A, lateral compression type I injury. Sacral compression may occur, but ligamentous support remains intact. **B,** lateral compression type II injury. Note disruption of the iliac wing and ipsilateral ramus. **C,** lateral compression type III injury. Note contralateral injury.

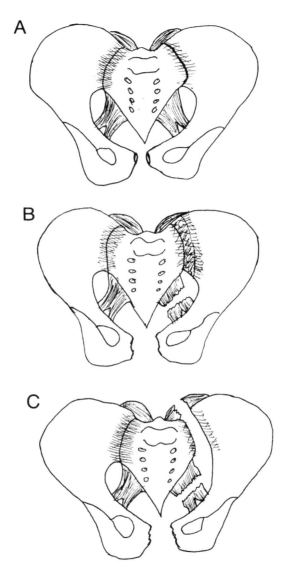

FIG 2.
A, anteroposterior compression (APC) type I injury. Note slight sacroiliac widening, but ligamentous integrity. **B,** APC type II injury. Note injury at the sacroiliac joint and sacrospinous and sacrotuberous ligaments, as well as distraction of the symphysis. **C,** APC type III injury. Note complete dissociation of the left side of the ring structure without vertical displacement.

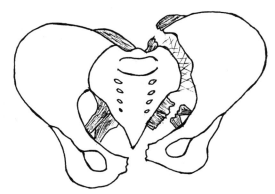

FIG 3.
Vertical shear type of injury. Note cephalad displacement of the left pelvis.

Concomitant Injuries

Substantial force is required to disrupt the bony pelvis, given its shape and construction, and the support that is provided by strong ligamentous structures that can absorb some force. The destruction caused by this energy is not limited to the pelvis; consequently, many patients have involvement of other organ systems. The trauma surgeon must determine how to treat not only the pelvic fracture, but also associated injuries, to guarantee an appropriate systematic focus on diagnosis and therapy that will assure an optimal outcome.

Multisystem involvement in trauma victims with pelvic fracture is common. These associated injuries have been outlined in several reports. Trunkey and coworkers[14] reviewed 173 patients with pelvic fracture and found that 116 (67%) had fractures of the skull, spine, face, or ribs; 93 (54%) suffered lower extremity fractures; 24 (14%) received significant head injuries; and 32 (19%) had liver or spleen injury. In a review of 236 injured patients with pelvic fractures, Poole and colleagues reported similar findings.[5] Because associated injuries vary widely, extreme diligence is necessary to avoid focusing on the pelvic fracture and overlooking other sites of trauma. A systematic, thorough evaluation following Advanced Trauma Life Support course principles is paramount in the identification of associated injuries.[18] After attention has been given to the ABCs of the initial survey, a complete physical examination combined with diagnostic radiographs and laboratory evaluations will reveal organ system involvement and enable further diagnostic and treatment modalities to be prioritized.

The pelvic fracture itself transmits its energy to adjacent tissues and organs, leading to associated injuries that may require immediate lifesaving therapeutic intervention. These injuries are partially responsible for the high morbidity and mortality associated with pelvic trauma, and may take initial priority over actual treatment of the fracture. The most common of these potentially catastrophic injuries are hemorrhage, soft-tissue injury (open pelvic fracture), colon/rectum violation, genitourinary involvement, and compromise of pelvic nerves and surrounding neural tissue. Each of these carries potentially devastating consequences and warrants discussion.

Hemorrhage

Life-threatening hemorrhage occurs in pelvic fractures as a result of bony penetration of the vessel walls as well as a shearing effect on the vast network of arterial and venous structures within the pelvis. The energy required to fracture the resilient construct of the pelvic ring also can cause organ injury remote from the pelvis, producing ongoing blood loss. In 10% to 12% of patients with pelvic fracture, hemodynamic instability is present on arrival at the emergency department or develops shortly thereafter. The general surgeon must determine rapidly whether the pelvis is the source of exsanguinating hemorrhage or associated injury distant from the pelvic fracture is responsible to proceed with lifesaving intervention.

Physical examination and a chest radiograph usually reveal bleeding into the external environment and the chest, but excluding intra-abdominal sources is more difficult. In the absence of absolute indications for celiotomy, the surgeon must use diagnostic methods to determine whether a significant hemoperitoneum is present. The debate in the literature regarding computerized tomography (CT), diagnostic peritoneal lavage (DPL), and ultrasound continues; however, each of these techniques has convincing attributes and defined limitations.

CT not only allows for the identification of intraperitoneal blood but provides additional information as well. The amount of free blood within the peritoneum can be estimated, which may be important in assigning treatment priorities in the trauma patient with multiple sites of blood loss. In addition to allowing examination of the retroperitoneal organs, CT also visualizes the pelvic hematoma. This allows the surgeon to pinpoint the location of the blood collection, assess the extent of its dissection within the retroperitoneal tissues, and measure the amount of blood lost at this site. CT scanning also provides reconstructed images detailing the fracture site, fragments, and involved structures that allow the orthopaedic surgeon to plan better the approach to repair. This diagnostic modality is not suited for injured patients who are hemodynamically unstable. The delay involved in administering enteral contrast media, transporting the patient to the scanner, and performing the abdominal/pelvic scan precludes its use in unstable patients. Physician access to the patient during the test is also limited, placing the hemodynamically unstable patient at increased risk. With the advent of new CT scanners that require significantly less scanning time and their potential for placement within the resuscitation area, these drawbacks may be ameliorated.

Ultrasonography of the peritoneal cavity also can be used to identify solid organ injury and subsequent hemorrhage. This technique can be performed rapidly in the resuscitation room and does not limit patient accessibility for resuscitative efforts. Therefore, ultrasound can be used safely in a hemodynamically unstable trauma patient. The amount of blood within the peritoneal space can be assessed initially and the study can be repeated frequently during the resuscitation. Repeated examinations disclose the volume of ongoing blood loss, which may dictate the urgency of laparotomy. Although it is noninvasive and provides information rapidly, ultrasonography has limitations. Most trauma surgeons have little experience in performing and interpreting ultrasound. Because trauma often occurs at times when radiologists and ultrasound technicians may not be available, timely evaluation may not be possible. Centers that use this technique for trauma evaluation provide their own equipment and provide training for their trauma surgeons.

Many studies have established the value of DPL in patients with pelvic fracture in providing information that directs the sequence of lifesaving intervention. The value of this technique is compromised, however, by an increased rate of false-positive results in patients with pelvic fracture. Thus, the technique used and the interpretation of study results require special consideration. Hubbard[19], Flint,[20] and Zannis[21] reported false-positive rates as high as 50% for DPL performed in patients with pelvic fracture, resulting in numerous nontherapeutic celiotomies. This not only subjects patients to unnecessary risks of operation, but may substantially delay other therapeutic interventions. This high percentage of false-positive results may result from placement of the lavage catheter through the anterior extension of the pelvic hematoma, or from permeation of red cells from the hematoma into the peritoneal space. Recently, several reports have refined the utility and safety of peritoneal lavage in patients with pelvic fracture. Evers and coworkers,[6] and Moreno and associates[11] reported that DPL performed through a supraumbilical approach was associated with lower false-positive rate ($\leq 9\%$). In patients with a positive red cell count on lavage but no gross blood, no intraperitoneal injury was found to account for the ongoing hemorrhage and hemodynamic instability. The supraumbilical approach to open peritoneal lavage permits exposure of the peritoneal cavity at a site distant from the usual extent of a pelvic hematoma. Careful incision and catheter placement reduce the risk that the hematoma will be opened, which may result in loss of tamponade as well as unreliable test results. If more than 10 cc of gross blood is obtained through the lavage catheter, urgent laparotomy is necessary. If the lavage sample yields fewer than 20,000 red blood cells per cubic millimeter, the peritoneal space can safely be excluded as the source of blood loss and hypotension. Lavage effluent with a high red blood cell count indicates the possibility of ongoing bleeding within the abdominal cavity. If the patient remains hemodynamically unstable, however, the pelvic fracture site and a retroperitoneal hematoma should be suspected as bleeding sources, and may require stabilization and angiographic intervention before celiotomy is undertaken.

Once life-threatening hemorrhage from a distant site has been excluded safely, ongoing blood loss within the pelvic fracture must rapidly be addressed to avoid exsanguination. Open surgical intervention, including ligation of the hypogastric arteries, has repeatedly met with negative results.[4, 22, 23] Thus, most authorities recommend that pelvic hematomas not be opened. Spontaneous rupture into the peritoneal cavity is common, however, in patients with large pelvic hematomas extending into the flanks. In this situation, packing into the hematoma and tight closure of the abdomen may be the only method available to arrest the hemorrhage. Simple packing into the pelvis itself usually is not successful because tamponade of the vast vascular network is made difficult by the constraints of the pelvic organs. Furthermore, opening the hematoma to allow tighter packing is likely to increase the volume of blood shed, because the tamponade effect of the pelvic peritoneal cover is violated. In rare cases, and depending on associated injuries, hemipelvectomy or hemicorpectomy may be used as a lifesaving alternative to hemorrhage control.[24] The decision to proceed with this radical therapy is difficult unless obvious tissue loss is present. This delay in decision-making may be partially responsible for the technique's dismal rate of success. Periodically, major vessel involvement (iliac or femoral) is identified on arteriography or suspected based on the discovery of a rapidly expanding or pulsatile hematoma at laparotomy. In these unusual cases, exploration of the hematoma and direct surgical repair of the injury is required.

Other means of achieving hemostasis include early fracture stabilization and arteriographic intervention. Fracture stabilization provides improved hemostasis from small and medium-sized vessels, and from the fractured cancellous bone. Postmortem injection studies performed by Huittenen and Slatis indicate that most bleeding from pelvic fractures occurs in small and medium-caliber vessels near the fracture site and the disrupted ligamentous supports.[25] This substantiates the belief that early stabilization may limit the extent of blood loss. Three models of fracture stabilization have been described in the literature and are in current use. Pneumatic antishock garments have received significant attention recently, and indications for their use are frequently debated. Their ability to create hemodynamic improvement in patients with ongoing abdominal or thoracic hemorrhage is questionable at best; however, their use for pelvic fracture stabilization in both the prehospital arena and the trauma center setting has been well documented. In 1986, Moreno and Moore reported a series in which 47 patients received pneumatic antishock garments for fracture stabilization, resulting in a 71% success rate.[11] Flint echoed the abilities of these garments, using them successfully in 11 of 12 patients.[26] Pneumatic antishock garments carry some risks, however. The compression they provide (40 to 50 mm Hg) reduces capillary flow and poses a risk of compartmental syndrome and neurologic compromise. The trousers also may make the treatment of other injuries difficult, particularly those involving the lower extremity. They have been used without sequelae for periods exceeding 48 hours, but extreme care must be taken to avoid injury.

Various techniques of fracture site fixation have been described to achieve stabilization. The placement of external fixators gained popularity over the past 2 decades, with significant success in a subset of patients with pelvic fracture (Fig 4). Flint,[26] Evers,[6] Burgess,[8] and Moreno[11] describe success rates as high as 95% using these devices. Open-book fractures and those with posterior column disruption require multiple transfusions in most cases,[10] and it is these fractures that appear to respond to stabilization. Several systems for external fixation have emerged in an attempt to provide both initial compression for hemostasis and secure fixation for adequate immobilization during the healing process. External fixators used in the anterior position compress open-book fractures, resulting in hemostasis, but cannot provide adequate immobilization if the posterior column is significantly involved. Those placed more posteriorly may provide both hemostasis and immobilization of VS injuries, but are somewhat less effective in APC fractures. The type of fixator used, therefore, depends on the type of fracture, the experience of the surgeon, and device availability within the institution.

The mechanics of and placement techniques for these fixation devices, as well as those of internal fixators, are beyond the scope of this text. Trauma surgeons should have a basic understanding of the principles, design, and limitations of frequently used systems, however. Ganz developed a relatively simple system for compression and stabilization of the VS injury. This device is secured into the posterior ilium by one pin on each side and the "C" clamp is tightened until the desired amount of compression is achieved. The Ganz system has been shown to be beneficial in the poste-

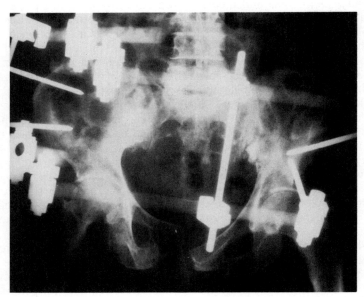

FIG 4.
External pelvic fixator using bilateral two-pin placement for stabilization.

rior injury, but provides less compression anteriorly and may not be as useful for the open-book fracture. The Slatis frame provides anterior compression and support through fixation centered on three pins placed percutaneously into both iliac crests to which a structural support is attached. Anterior compression is sufficient, but posterior support may not be adequate for long-term immobilization. Other systems (e.g., Johnson, Ace-Fischer) also rely on two- or three-pin fixation through the iliac crest and have benefits and limitations similar to those of the Slatis frame.

All systems of external fixation share some inherent limitations and possible complications. Percutaneous pin placement offers a portal of invasion for microbes, which thrive in the hematoma. Aggressive pin wound care with peroxide cleansing and topical antibacterial agents may limit infection, but cannot completely prevent contamination of the subcutaneous tissues and hematoma. Superficial cellulitis and deep-seated infection are clinically significant when optimal treatment of the pelvic fracture requires internal fixation. In addition, the hardware required for external fixation is bulky and may present a spatial barricade to other required procedures and maneuvers, and impose limitations on patient positioning and transportation.

Open reduction and internal fixation of pelvic fractures within the first 48 hours after injury provides permanent fixation and early mobility, and should be considered in patients in whom hemodynamic stability has been achieved.[26] Those injuries that have rendered the pelvic construct unstable for support or gait often are amenable to open reduction and internal fixation, which allows for early rehabilitation. APC injuries with more than 3-cm diastasis of the symphysis may be amenable to an anterior approach and plating of the symphysis to achieve closure and stabilization. Open reduction and internal fixation also has been the mainstay of therapy for posterior element instability after adequate resuscitation has been achieved. Nelson and Duwelius demonstrated an alternative technique using CT-guided percutaneous screw fixation.[27] This method results in less blood loss and rapid fixation, and may allow quicker use of posterior fixation. Modern orthopaedic surgeons possess a vast array of screws, plates, pins, guides, and cabinets of tools that would allow even the successful restoration of Humpty Dumpty. This hardware, combined with the skill of an experienced orthopaedic trauma surgeon, can provide rapid and safe internal fixation of most unstable pelvic fractures using both open and fluoroscopically guided percutaneous techniques.

Estimates of the incidence of pelvic arterial injury in fractures that involve the posterior structural supports range from 6% to 18%.[10] Most of these do not respond to fracture-site stabilization alone, and arterial embolization techniques provide lifesaving hemostasis when branches of the hypogastric artery are bleeding.[8, 10, 11, 25, 28] Arterial embolization was introduced in the 1930s, but has been used widely only within the last 10 to 20 years. Safe access to the vascular tree for this procedure can be achieved through either an axillary or a femoral artery. The right femoral approach is most commonly used, usually by the percutaneous route, although surgical exposure may occasionally be necessary. The catheter is advanced into the distal aorta and initial images are obtained to outline the iliac and femoral systems. Surgical intervention is required if injury to these major vessels in the pelvis is identified; however, temporary balloon occlusion at the time of angiography can be lifesaving. Most bleeding occurs from branches of the hypogastric vessels, and selective catheterization of these branches will localize the site of ongoing blood loss (Fig 5). After the offending vessel has been identified, transcatheter embolization usually provides hemostasis (Fig 6). Original attempts at embolization therapy used muscle as the occlusive agent, but many substances and techniques are part of the armamentarium of today's invasive radiologist. Gelfoam is the most common material used and is administered in small pieces or as a prepared slurry. The vessel is occluded by the Gelfoam and subsequent clot for 2 to 3 weeks, after which recanalization may occur. Steel coils (Gianturco) placed by the transcatheter approach permit permanent occlusion of larger vessels, especially when they are used in conjunction with Gelfoam or similar substances. The technique used varies according to the size of the vessel, the length of time for which occlusion is needed, and the ex-

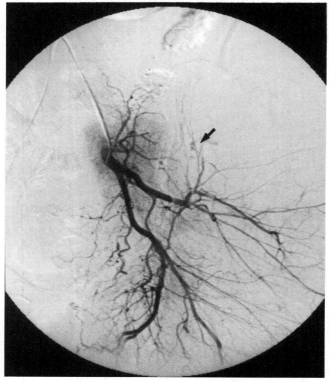

FIG 5.
Selective angiography of the hypogastric system showing extravasation consistent with ongoing hemorrhage *(arrow).*

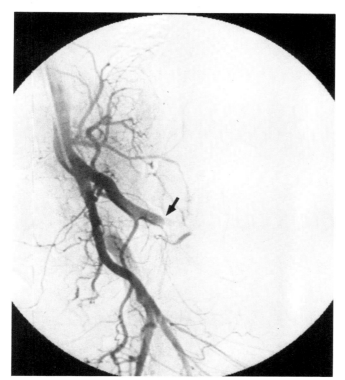

FIG 6.
Selective angiography showing vessel occlusion after placement of coils and Gelfoam *(arrow)*.

perience and preference of the radiologist. Complications of transcatheter embolization can occur and include migration of the embolus, incomplete occlusion, and myonecrosis with myoglobinuria. It is imperative that the trauma surgeon remain involved during the radiologic procedure. Because of ongoing blood loss and other injuries, these patients often are hypotensive and require ongoing resuscitation. They also may require intubation, mechanical ventilation, and, at times, controlled general anesthesia within the angiography suite.

The value of these techniques for arresting hemorrhage are well accepted by experienced trauma surgeons, although their timing and priority vary from center to center. The staff of every institution that treats pelvic injuries should prospectively consider the capabilities of their facility and outline a standard treatment plan for a patient with a severe pelvic fracture that continues to bleed. Facilities that do not have immediately available the personnel and equipment necessary to proceed urgently with either orthopaedic stabilization or arteriographic intervention should develop a procedure for rapid transportation of the patient to another institution. Achieving optimal results in severe pelvic fractures requires a team approach to hemorrhage using all available methods (Fig 7). In our institution, we proceed with arteriographic investigation once the transfusion threshold of 4 units of packed red blood cells is reached, assuming that no other sources of blood loss exist. We also use early arteriographic approaches in patients

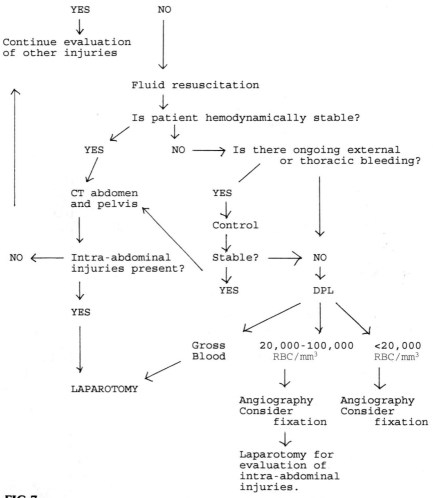

FIG 7.
Evaluation of hemorrhage in patients with pelvic fractures. CT = computed tomography; DPL = diagnostic peritoneal lavage; RBC/mm^3 = red blood cells per mm^3.

who remain hypotensive despite ongoing initial resuscitation after excluding hemorrhage into the chest, abdomen, and external environment. If the fracture involves widening of the pubic symphysis by more than 3 cm or significant posterior disruption with SI widening, orthopaedic surgeons consider optimal methods for rapid fracture stabilization. Fracture stabilization is coordinated with angiographic embolization so that both procedures can be performed as quickly as possible. An established protocol that takes into consideration the capabilities of the institution allows for a smoothly coordinated attempt to save patients with these critical injuries.

Soft-Tissue Injury/Open Pelvic Fracture

Disruption of the protective barrier of the skin and subcutaneous tissues by fracture fragments, exogenous materials, or the shearing forces of transmitted energy potentiates the complications of bleeding and infection (Fig 8). External blood loss is often pronounced and hemorrhage can be massive as the ability of the pelvic structure to provide effective tamponade is lost. Richardson and colleagues reported an average blood loss of 15 units despite aggressive treatment protocols including fracture stabilization, ligation, and arteriography when indicated.[29] If the patient survives resuscitation, invasive infectious complications pose a severe threat to long-term survival. Portals of entry for the offending organisms include invasion from skin disruption and contamination from the rectum and genitourinary structures. In addition, many patients have deep inoculation of the wounds and contamination from dirt, grass, and other foreign material. A protocol must be

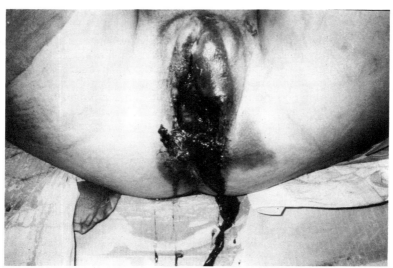

FIG 8.
Open pelvic fracture demonstrating significant soft-tissue injury and blood loss.

followed in which all hemorrhage is addressed first. Bleeding from superficial wounds can usually be managed by surgical exploration of the soft tissue and direct cautery or suture ligation of involved vessels. This should be performed in the operating room under general anesthesia to facilitate adequate exposure and debridement. The patient should be positioned so that the surgeon, wearing a headlight, can visualize the soft-tissue involvement directly. Dissection and removal of all nonviable tissue is essential to allow localization and suture ligation of injured vessels. Some patients with open pelvic fracture have massive bleeding, however, and cannot tolerate prolonged exposure of deep perineal wounds. In such cases, exsanguination must be arrested by tight packing of the wound, often combined with suture closure to achieve tamponade. After the condition of these patients has stabilized and bleeding has stopped, they should be returned to the operating room for repeated exploration and complete debridement of the wound. Fracture stabilization and arteriographic intervention also should be undertaken.

Once life-threatening hemorrhage has been arrested, attention should be turned immediately to treating soft-tissue injury and avoiding infection. Foreign material must be removed from the wound and nonviable tissue debrided. Aggressive wound care with repeated dressing changes and scheduled reoperation for irrigation are vitally important. Antibiotics effective against *Staphylococcus aureus* and enteric pathogens should be initiated immediately. Even wounds that appear to be small or trivial should be treated with respect, because communication with the pelvic injury carries significant morbidity and mortality. The size and depth of the wound and the extent of contamination dictate the need for general anesthesia to allow adequate dressing changes. Daily trips to the operating room often are required to achieve control of these wounds. Perineal and buttock wounds require fecal diversion in addition to aggressive wound care, even in the absence of direct rectal or anal injury. Richardson and associates reported the development of life-threatening infections when colostomy was not used in patients with perineal or buttock wounds and pelvic fracture.[29] The temptation to avoid colostomy in patients with small perineal wounds must be tempered by the realization that, once pelvic sepsis is established, it is difficult to control and may result in the death of the patient.

Rectal Injury

Deep lacerations of the perineum involving the anus and extending into the rectum sometimes occur. Injury to the rectum without a perineal wound can result from direct penetration by bony spicules or from a tearing effect as the pelvic supports shift at the time of fracture. Rectal examination during the initial evaluation in the emergency department is mandatory to identify most of these injuries. In the presence of gross blood, clinical suspicion based on the physical examination, or perineal or buttock laceration, sigmoidoscopy (ideally, performed in the operating room) is indicated to determine the presence and extent of the rectal injury. Disruption of the sphincter, perianal tissues, or rectum requires complete fecal diversion. Distal segment colonic washout using dilute povidone-iodine (Betadine) solutions is warranted if it does not prolong or delay other needed interventions. Closure of the rectal injury or repair of the anal sphincter at the same procedure as colostomy is dependent on the extent of that injury and on the patient's overall condition. If a localized posterior rectal tear is diagnosed in a hemodynamically stable patient, suture repair with presacral drainage allows local hemostasis and definitive care. We prefer to use closed-system drains brought out through the perineum. If the sphincter has been destroyed or the patient is unstable, irrigation and debridement with delayed repair at the time of colostomy closure is recommended. Any attempt at primary repair in a patient who is hemodynamically unstable is dangerous and must be avoided. Injury to the anterior rectum is sufficient to warrant thorough evaluation of the genitourinary structures as well.

The position and type of colostomy must be considered carefully in patients with open pelvic fractures. A loop sigmoid colostomy with a stapled occlusion is one alternative. This technique is quick, permits distal irrigation, is usually easy to accomplish in thin patients, and avoids a formal laparotomy. A sigmoid colostomy can be difficult, however, in patients with pelvic fractures that require incisions for open reduction and internal fixation. Similarly, we have noted that colostomies located adjacent to external fixator pin wounds can create a nidus for pin tract infection and provide a portal of entry for deep hematoma infection. In selected patients, a transverse colon stoma with or without a mucous fistula may be preferable because of its position high in the epigastrium.

Vaginal Injuries

Vaginal perforations, similar to rectal injuries, may result from penetration of the wall by bone, particularly when the pubic rami are fractured. Perineal lacerations also can extend into the vagina. Although most of these patients have documented vaginal bleeding, its absence is not sufficient evidence to exclude vaginal wall penetration. Digital and speculum examination is necessary to identify nonbleeding injuries and evaluate the extent of the violation. Vaginal bleeding in women of childbearing age mandates the performance of a pregnancy test before speculum examination to rule out diagnoses such as abruptio placentae. Speculum examination in the presence of placental disruption can accentuate the hemorrhage and require urgent surgical therapy. In the pregnant patient with a pelvic fracture, regardless of vaginal or obvious uterine injury, early involvement of an obstetrician in the emergency department is required to ensure the well-being of both the mother and the fetus. Immediate evaluation of fetal viability and the status of the placenta, as well as establishment of fetal monitoring is essential.

In patients with simple vaginal perforations, examination in the operating room, irrigation and debridement, and direct suture repair using absorbable suture is appropriate. Perioperative antibiotic coverage should be provided because this is an open fracture and carries a risk of infectious complications. Further evaluation of the urinary tract is warranted in this small group of patients with pelvic fracture.

Urinary Tract Injury

Urethral injuries occur in only a few men with pelvic fracture and even fewer women. Disruption of the urethra can be a source of protracted problems, however, and optimal therapy depends on prompt diagnosis. The classic signs of urethral injury are blood at the meatus, a high-riding prostate on rectal examination, and inability to void spontaneously. These indicators are unfortunately not always present. A high index of suspicion must be maintained to avoid exacerbating urethral disruption by imprudent insertion of a Foley catheter. Such manipulation can easily convert a partial transection into a complete disruption. The urethra is disrupted most often in blunt trauma at the level of the urogenital diaphragm as the puboprostatic ligament is torn, allowing the prostate to be propelled away from the membranous urethra. The diagnosis is confirmed by retrograde urethrography (Fig 9). This test should be performed in patients with the classic signs of disruption as well as those with pelvic fractures that have considerable displacement. Comminuted fractures of the anterior pelvic

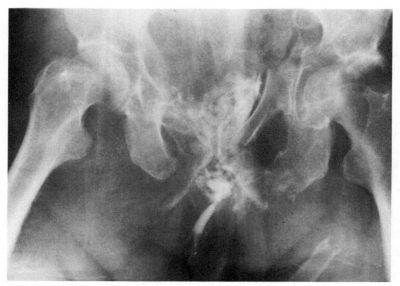

FIG 9.
Retrograde urethrogram demonstrating complete urethral disruption requiring alternate bladder drainage.

ring, such as are frequently seen in crush injuries, also warrant a urethrogram. When a Foley catheter is passed in a patient with a pelvic fracture, it must gently be inserted and the balloon not inflated if resistance is encountered, urine does not flow, or gross blood drains from the catheter. A urethrogram should be obtained in these patients before further attempts are made to pass a urethral catheter. The ideal urethrogram is performed using fluoroscopy; however, a single-view study obtained during resuscitation in the emergency department often is sufficient. Retrograde urethrography is performed with the injection of 20 to 30 cc of water-soluble contrast into the distal urethra through a 12- or 14-French Foley catheter inserted 1 to 2 cm into the meatus or through an irrigating syringe. The presence of extravasation or the inability to propel contrast into the bladder with gentle pressure confirms disruption, complete or incomplete, and mandates alternate bladder drainage and further urologic studies. Suprapubic cystostomy can be used to achieve urinary diversion in most patients. The suprapubic tube can be inserted percutaneously or by direct exploration through the dome of the bladder. One consideration in patients with pelvic fracture who are candidates for open reduction and internal fixation is delivery of the suprapubic tube through the skin off to the side opposite the site of planned incisions. In selected patients with partial disruption, a transurethral catheter can be inserted with the aid of cystoscopy or fluoroscopy by an experienced urologist.

Suprapubic drainage is usually maintained for 2 to 3 months. This allows the hematoma to resolve, with reapproximation of the totally disrupted urethra or healing of the partially torn urethra. Follow-up evaluation with urethral radiography will identify stricture formation that requires surgical correction. Partial transection and anterior injuries frequently heal without significant stricture, whereas complete prostatomembranous disruption usually requires operative correction. Some authors have recommended initial urethral alignment,[30, 31] but multisystem injury may preclude this approach.

Bladder perforation is the most common genitourinary injury associated with pelvic fracture and occurs in 3% to 16%[5, 8, 26] of patients with pelvic trauma. Most of these patients (>90%) have either gross hematuria or microscopic hematuria with more than 40 red blood cells per high-power field on initial urinalysis.[32] Cystography is the diagnostic modality of choice to define both intraperitoneal and extraperitoneal bladder disruption. After urethral injuries are excluded, a Foley catheter is advanced into the bladder and 200 to 300 cc of water-soluble contrast is gravity-infused. An AP radiograph is performed, followed by evacuation of the contrast and a post-drainage radiograph. Patients with intraperitoneal rupture demonstrate extravasation of the contrast medium into the peritoneal cavity, frequently outlining other viscera (Fig 10). Extraperitoneal rupture is characterized by extravasation confined to the immediate retroperitoneal area. Because this extravasation may be limited to the space posterior to the bladder, 15% of these injuries may not be visible on the initial AP view and will be identified only on the post-drainage film (Fig 11).

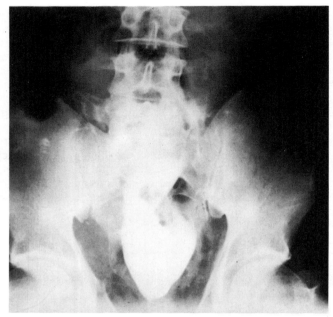

FIG 10.
Cystogram demonstrating intraperitoneal bladder rupture.

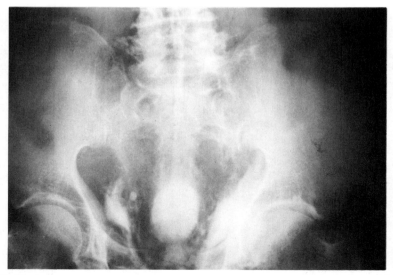

FIG 11.
Cystogram demonstrating extraperitoneal bladder rupture identified on postvoid film only.

Bladder rupture can be managed without operative intervention if it is entirely confined to the extraperitoneal space. Bladder drainage by Foley catheterization for 14 days, followed by gentle repeat cystography will demonstrate healing in most patients. Intraperitoneal rupture occurs most often at the dome as a result of explosive forces during anterior compression injury. The risk of rupture is increased if the bladder is full, and may then occur even without pelvic fracture. Surgical repair is mandated in cases of intraperitoneal extravasation. The surgeon should examine the inside of the bladder through the rent in the dome for additional injuries. Perforation of the bladder by shards of fractured pubic ramus can be identified. Careful examination of the trigone from inside the bladder must begin with identification of the ureteral orifices. If question arises regarding the patency of the ureteral orifices, 5 cc of indigo carmine should be administered intravenously, and dye-stained urine should pass from the orifice within 10 to 15 minutes. Bladder perforations outside the dome are often best treated from inside the bladder using a single-layer closure with the adjacent ureteral orifice cannulated to avoid injury. Lacerations in the dome of the bladder are repaired in multiple layers. Absorbable suture is always used to repair the bladder to avoid leaving a nidus of infection. A standardized protocol ensures that injury to the urinary system will not be overlooked (Fig 12).

Neurologic Injury

Sacral fracture and SI separation may involve destruction or compromise of the neural foramina, leading to nerve root dysfunction and shear injury to the lumbosacral plexus. The true incidence of this injury is not well documented in the literature, but it appears to be relatively uncommon. Upper sacral fractures may lead to S1 and S2 radiculopathy with associated paresthesia of the lateral foot and decreased flexion strength across the ankle. Lower sacral fractures are more likely to produce urinary retention, fecal incontinence, or impotence. Treatment for neural involvement in the initial period after injury consists of fracture stabilization and symptomatic support. Appropriate orthotics and physical therapy aid in minimizing the long-term sequelae of nervous system dysfunction. Richardson reported eight cases of lax sphincter tone after pelvic fracture, all of which resolved completely, with return of fecal continence.[29]

Complications

Respiratory Failure

Respiratory complications continue to plague patients with pelvic fractures. Trunkey and colleagues demonstrated an overall pulmonary complication rate of 34.6%, and many of the patients required mechanical ventilation.[14] There are many causes of respiratory failure, and most cases are probably

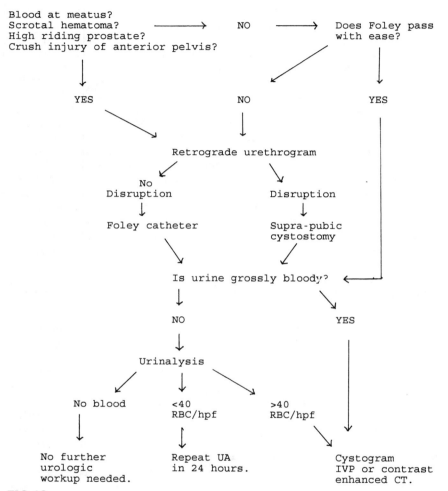

FIG 12.
Evaluation of urinary tract injuries in patients with a pelvic fracture. RBC/hpf = red blood cells per high-power field; UA = urinalysis; IVP = intravenous pyelogram; CT = computed tomogram.

multifactorial. Adult respiratory distress syndrome is responsible for a significant amount of respiratory failure in these patients. Although it is not a direct result of the fracture itself, the lung is injured as a consequence of the inflammatory response to injury. Untimely or inappropriate treatment of the adult respiratory distress syndrome may rapidly lead to the demise of the patient. The mainstay of therapy consists of mechanical ventilation and concurrent treatment of the underlying pathology. Positive-pressure ventilation, adequate resuscitation and hydration, and nutritional support increase the chances of recovery in these critically ill patients. Advanced modes of ventilation, positive end-expiratory pressure, including pressure-controlled ventilation with reversed I:E ratio, and high-frequency jet ventilation, may be required to provide adequate oxygenation.

Nosocomial pneumonia occurs in a large percentage of severely injured patients, especially those who require mechanical ventilation. Pneumonia may further exacerbate a significant pulmonary shunt, causing catastrophic hypoxia. Pneumonia must be diagnosed early and treated aggressively with pulmonary toilet and appropriate antibiotics. Both gram-negative and gram-positive bacteria, as well as opportunistic organisms, may be responsible for this infectious complication. Identification of the offending microbe first by Gram stain and then by culture and sensitivity is essential to guide antibacterial therapy. While this evaluation is under way, the patient should be treated empirically with broad-spectrum antibiotics. These can be tailored to the specific organisms once it is isolated.

Other causes of progressive respiratory failure in patients with pelvic fracture include pulmonary embolism from venous thrombosis, fat emboli (although these are less common in pelvic fractures than in long-bone fractures), and concurrent pulmonary injury. The trauma surgeon treating a patient with a complicated pelvic fracture must maintain a careful watch for the onset of pulmonary complications and be prepared to respond promptly. Both the surgeon and the staff must have a thorough understanding of various modes of mechanical ventilation, antibiotic regimens, and critical care support.

Thrombosis

Stagnation of flow resulting from prolonged immobilization, combined with direct vessel injury, place patients with pelvic fracture at substantial risk for deep venous thrombosis and pulmonary embolism. Various prevention strategies have been shown to decrease the risk of deep venous thrombosis, including early mobilization, pneumatic compression sleeves, low-dose heparin, low-molecular-weight heparin, and warfarin therapy. Depending on the presence of concurrent injuries and hemostasis, however, patients with pelvic fracture may not tolerate these forms of prophylaxis. Experience with the use of prophylactic vena caval filter placement in high-risk patients is growing, although it is not universally accepted. Our protocol for deep venous thrombosis prophylaxis begins with pneumatic compression sleeves if the lower extremities are available. After 48 hours, if hemorrhage has stopped, patients without serious head injury receive further prophylaxis with a low-dose continuous intravenous heparin infusion, or subcutaneous administration of low-dose heparin three times a day or low-molecular-weight heparin daily. In patients who have contraindications to heparin and require prolonged bed rest, percutaneous insertion of caval filtration may be warranted.

Sepsis

Patients with multiple trauma have many possible sources of sepsis, and surveillance and early treatment are important. Line sepsis from central venous catheters remains a potential source of bacteremia that can cause secondary infection of the hematoma associated with the pelvic fracture. Venous access should be removed as soon as possible. Some patients may require prolonged central venous access, these lines must be monitored carefully for early signs of infection. Signs of line sepsis include redness or purulence at the puncture site, unexplained fever, and positive blood culture results. Infected or contaminated catheters should be removed immediately. Other sources of infection, such as abscess, cellulitis, urinary tract infection, and pneumonia, must be monitored and treated aggressively to decrease the mortality and morbidity of pelvic fractures.

Acetabular Fractures

Acetabular fractures comprise a subset of pelvic ring injuries. Because the weight-bearing function of the pelvis is provided through the acetabulum, these fractures often require fixation for optimal functional outcome. Isolated acetabular fractures usually are not associated with the risks of hemorrhage and the complications of other pelvic fractures and, thus, are addressed separately.

The acetabulum is composed of the confluence of the ischium, the ilium, and the pubis. It provides the "home" for the femoral head, allowing motion that facilitates flexion, extension, and rotation of the hip and leg. From the lateral view, it appears as an inverted "Y" and can be divided into anterior and posterior columns. The anterior column includes the anterior wall of the acetabulum and extends downward from the iliac crest to the pubic symphysis. The posterior column includes the posterior wall and extends from the superior gluteal notch down through the obturator foramen and inferior pubic ramus.

An acetabular fracture is usually caused by the hammerlike action of the femoral head as it is driven into the acetabulum. Therefore, the anatomy of the fracture depends on the magnitude of the force and the position of the femoral head at the time of impact. Internal rotation of the femur results in a fracture of the posterior column and external rotation leads to anterior column disruption. Significant fracture and ligamentous disruption are frequently associated with dislocation of the femoral head. This dislocation must be corrected urgently to prevent significant long-term effects. Reduction often can be performed in the emergency department with the aid of significant intravenous sedation, but may require general anesthesia.

As with other pelvic fractures, more than one classification system exists. Judet and coworkers described a system that has changed minimally since its inception.[33] This scheme divides acetabular fractures into those of the posterior wall, posterior column, anterior wall, anterior column, and transverse direction. The AO group standardized this group of fractures by severity, and Tile proposed a classification scheme based on the direction of force.

In the past, the acetabular fracture was treated nonoperatively, often with prolonged bed rest and traction. Good results were obtained if anatomic alignment was achieved. The current orthopaedic literature supports early internal fixation as a means of obtaining superior functional results and early patient mobilization.[34]

Orthopaedic Considerations

The involvement of orthopaedic surgeons with an interest in trauma is essential to the optimal functional outcome of patients with pelvic fracture. The method used for fracture fixation must be chosen by the orthopaedic surgeon, but the timing of the procedure is often a joint decision involving the trauma surgeon. Orthopaedic consultation also may be necessary when general surgical procedures are performed. For example, a misplaced ostomy or drainage tube may interfere with internal fixation approaches and alter the patient's recovery. To minimize such problems, the trauma surgeon must communicate with the orthopaedic surgeon before intervention is undertaken, if possible.

Summary

Pelvic fractures remain a challenge for the trauma surgeon, even in the most sophisticated trauma centers. The potential for loss of life as well as long-term disability must not be underestimated. A multidisciplinary approach to this complex injury provides optimal care and the best chance for the patient to regain functional capacity. The trauma surgeon must coordinate a team that provides resuscitation and treatment of all injuries, and addresses such complex postoperative issues as nutrition and infection. The expertise of professionals such as the orthopaedic surgeon, radiologist, and blood bank staff must be called on from the outset.

The formulation of a prioritized protocol that uses the capabilities of the personnel and equipment available in each institution is vital to decrease the morbidity and mortality of pelvic injuries. Initial attention to the ABCs of resuscitation, followed by systematic evaluation of the patient to identify all injuries must precede attempts at fracture treatment. After other life-threatening injuries have been controlled, attention can be turned to the pelvic fracture and its potential complications. Early intervention facilitates rapid stabilization and return of function. The trauma surgeon must maintain vigilant surveillance for the onset of complications and initiate therapy early. Finally, those centers that do not have the capability to meet needs of the trauma patient with a pelvic fracture should stabilize the patient and arrange for transportation to an appropriate trauma center.

References

1. Kane WJ: Fractures of the pelvis, in Rockwood, Calif, Green DP (eds): *Fractures*. Philadelphia, JB Lippincott, 1984, p 1093.
2. Rothenberger DA, Velaseo R, Strate R, et al: Open pelvic fractures: A lethal injury. *J Trauma* 1978; 18:184.
3. Perry JF Jr, McClellan RJ: Autopsy findings in 127 patients following fatal accidents. *Surg Gynecol Obstet* 1964; 47:581.
4. Gilliland MD, Ward RE, Barton RM, et al: Factors affecting mortality in pelvic fractures. *J Trauma* 1982; 22:691.
5. Poole GV, Ward EF, Griswold JA, et al: Complications of pelvic fractures from blunt trauma. *Am Surg* 1992; 58:225.
6. Evers BM, Cryer HM, Miller FB, et al: Pelvic fracture hemorrhage. *Arch Surg* 1989; 124:422.
7. Dalal SA, Burgess AR, Siegel JH, et al: Pelvic fracture in multiple trauma: Classification by mechanism is key to pattern of organ injury, resuscitative requirements, and outcome. *J Trauma* 1989; 29:981.
8. Burgess AR, Eastridge BJ, Young JW, et al: Pelvic ring disruptions: Effective classification system and treatment protocols. *J Trauma* 1990; 30:848.
9. Naam NH, Brown WH, Hurd R, et al: Major pelvic fractures. *Arch Surg* 1983; 118:610.
10. Cryer HM, Miller FB, Evers BM, et al: Pelvic fracture classification: Correlation with hemorrhage. *J Trauma* 1988; 28:973.
11. Moreno C, Moore EE, Rosenberger A, et al: Hemorrhage associated with major pelvic fracture: A multispecialty challenge. *J Trauma* 1986; 26:987.
12. Watson-Jones R: Dislocations and fracture-dislocations of the pelvis. *Br J Surg* 1938; 25:773.
13. Conolly WB, Hedberg EA: Observations on fractures of the pelvis. *J Trauma* 1969; 9:104.
14. Trunkey DD, Chapman MW, Lim RC, et al: Management of pelvic fractures in blunt trauma injury. *J Trauma* 1974; 14:912.
15. Pennal GF, Tile M, Waddell JP, et al: Pelvic disruption: Assessment and classification. *Clin Orthop* 1980; 151:12.
16. Tile M: *Fractures of the Pelvis and Acetabulum*. Baltimore, Williams & Wilkins, 1984.
17. Young JW, Resnick CS: Fracture of the pelvis: Current concepts of classification. *Am J Radiology* 1990; 155:1169.
18. Alexander RH, Proctor HJ: *Advanced Trauma Life Support Course for Physicians*. Chicago, American College of Surgeons, 1993.
19. Hubbard SG, Bivins BA, Sachatello CR, et al: Diagnostic errors with peritoneal lavage in patients with pelvic fracture. *Arch Surg* 1979; 114:;844–846.
20. Flint LM, Brown A, Richardson JD, et al: Definitive control of bleeding from severe pelvic fractures. *Ann Surg* 1979; 189:709–716.
21. Zannis VJ, Wood M: Laparotomy for pelvic fractures. *Am J Surg* 1980; 140:841–846.
22. Hawkins L, Pomerantz M, Wiscoan B: Laparotomy at the time of pelvic fracture. *J Trauma* 1970; 10:619–623.
23. Patterson FP, Morton KS: The cause of death in fractures of the pelvis: With a note on treatment by ligation of the hypogastric (internal iliac) artery. *J Trauma* 1973; 13:849.

24. Morales GR, Phillips R, Conn AK, et al: Traumatic hemipelvectomy: Report of 2 survivors and review. *J Trauma* 1983; 23:615–620.
25. Huittenen V, Slatis P: Postmortem angiography and dissection of the hypogastric artery in pelvic fractures. *Surgery* 1973; 73:454–462.
26. Flint L, Babikian G, Anders M, et al: Definitive control of mortality from severe pelvic fracture. *Ann Surg* 1990; 211:703–707.
27. Nelson DW, Duwelius PJ: CT guided fixation of sacral fractures and sacro-iliac joint disruptions. *Radiology* 1991; 180:527–532.
28. Yellin AE, Lundell CJ, Finck EJ: Diagnosis and control of posttraumatic pelvic hemorrhage. *Arch Surg* 1983; 118:1378.
29. Richardson JD, Harty J, Amin M, et al: Open pelvic fractures. *J Trauma* 1982; 22:533.
30. Morehouse DD, MacKinnon KJ: Management of prostatomembranous urethral disruption: 13-Year experience. *J Urol* 1980; 123:173.
31. Gibson GR: Impotence following fractured pelvis and ruptured urethra. *Br J Urol* 1970; 42:86.
32. Carroll PR, McAninch JW: Bladder trauma: Mechanisms of injury and a unified method of diagnosis and repair. *J Urol* 1984; 132:254.
33. Judet R Judet J, Letournal E: Fractures of the acetabulum: Classification and surgical approaches for open reduction. *J Bone Joint Surg* [Am] 1964; 46A:1615–1638.
34. Ylinen P, Santavirta S, Slatis P: Outcome of acetabular fractures: A 7-year follow-up. *J Trauma* 1989; 29:19.

Opportunistic *Candida* Infection Complicating Major Injury: A Consequence of Immune Suppression

Alexander S. Rosemurgy, II, M.D.

Associate Professor of Surgery, Department of Surgery, University of South Florida, Tampa, Florida

John F. Sweeney, M.D.

Surgery-Immunology Research Fellow, Department of Surgery, University of South Florida, Tampa, Florida

---

Trauma is the leading cause of death for individuals aged 1 to 39 years, and more money is spent on the care of trauma patients than on the care of patients with heart disease, cancer, and neurologic disorders combined.[1, 2] In our society, the effect of accidental death and trauma care as a whole is tremendous.

Injured patients can be divided into three groups. The first and largest group are those patients who sustain minor injuries. Most trauma victims are in this group, and virtually none die. The second group of patients consists of those who die within 10 minutes of injury. Although only 5% of all injured patients fall into this group, it accounts for about half of all patients who die. In general, these patients die of massive head injuries, airway problems, or exsanguination. To decrease the size of this group, national efforts must be made to eliminate drinking and driving, improve motor vehicle safety, and decrease urban crime. The third group of trauma patients, and those who are the focus of this chapter, consists of patients who sustain urgent, life-threatening injuries. This category includes only about 15% of all trauma patients, but accounts for the other 50% of patients who die after injury. These patients experience major intracranial injuries, airway problems, hemorrhage, multiple organ trauma, or major burns. They are injured seriously, yet live long enough to be resuscitated in the hospital.

One of the consequences of resuscitation, including blood transfusions, may be significant immune defects that exacerbate the underlying immune alterations related to major trauma.[3, 4] Although early survival depends on vigorous resuscitation, sepsis often develops as a cause of late death after injury in seriously injured patients who receive invasive intervention.[5, 6]

Included in the spectrum of late sepsis after injury is the development of opportunistic fungal infections. Many reports of seriously injured patients document an increasing frequency of *Candida* infections.[7-9] Surprisingly, despite increased interest in opportunistic infections after injury, controversy continues regarding fundamental aspects of *Candida* "infections." For example, *Candida* "infections" may not be infections at all, but instead may represent either colonization by *Candida* or only localized *Candida* invasion. There is, however, little disagreement that true *Candida* infection is associated with a high mortality rate in ill patients after injury and that systemic antifungal therapy is warranted.[10, 11] Great debate continues regarding what constitutes early, yet significant, *Candida* invasion. Whereas some feel that the growth of *Candida* from superficial sources is significant,[12, 13] others believe that candidemia or tissue invasion by *Candida* is required to constitute true infection.[14, 15] It seems that detection of early or occult *Candida* infection would allow for the best chance of cure, but in the absence of a consensus regarding what constitutes occult *Candida* invasion, there is no agreement as to when antifungal therapy should be initiated. Therefore, clinical impressions and practical experience continue to guide antifungal therapy in ill patients who have sustained accidental or surgical trauma. With the recent advent of nontoxic, efficacious agents, antifungal therapy has improved, but not the logic with which such therapy is applied.[16]

In an attempt to initiate early antifungal therapy, many investigators have sought better ways to detect occult *Candida* infection reliably and accurately. Antibody titers have been investigated as one option, but have been found to correlate poorly with known *Candida* infections.[17] The delayed antibody response to *Candida* invasion presumably is a result of the depressed immune status of seriously ill or injured patients. *Candida* cell wall metabolites also have been sought in serum and urine to document host response to a systemic *Candida* challenge.[18] Unfortunately, the assays for such cell wall metabolites are not commonly or commercially available, and testing for them has not gained widespread acceptance. Others have sought the presence of fungal cytoplasmic antigens in the serum of ill or injured patients as evidence of host response to *Candida*.[19] As with the assays for cell wall metabolites, the assays for cytoplasmic antigens are not widely available and have been reviewed with mixed, though mostly poor, reviews. In contrast, tests for *Candida* antigen have been used widely by numerous investigators to determine occult *Candida* invasion. Most experience has been with a commercially available latex agglutination test that detects an uncharacterized cell wall antigen of *Candida*.[20-25] This substance actually may be a *Candida* cell wall antigen that has been modified by host response. Studies using the antigen have focused on the sensitivity and specificity of the test in patients with hematologic malignancies with and without chemotherapy, and often with neutropenia. In these patients, the test was found to have a mixed sensitivity and specificity in detecting

Candida invasion. This is unfortunate, because it is doubtful that this is the correct methodology to assess the value of such a test. If the test for *Candida* antigen is to detect occult invasion, a comparison of test results with known culture results seems shortsighted because an elevated antigen titer in a patient with a negative culture would be considered a false-positive result. The focus should be on the implications of elevated *Candida* antigen titers, rather than on the correlation of the titers with culture results.

We have studied the implications of elevated *Candida* antigen titers in injured patients, especially those with Injury Severity Scores of 18 or more in the intensive care unit.[26] When these patients were noted to have clinically apparent sources of *Candida* (e.g., skin, oropharynx), culture evidence of *Candida,* or unexplained clinical deterioration despite aggressive support, *Candida* antigen titers were determined. The titer results were not known to the treating physicians so that therapeutic decisions, including antifungal therapy, were based on the clinical impression and practical experience of the attending physician. After clinical outcomes were correlated with titer status, we were able to separate seriously injured patients into those with and without elevated *Candida* antigen titers, and to determine the implications of elevated titers.

Sixty-six patients were entered into this protocol, and all were receiving intravenous antibiotics to treat documented or suspected bacterial infections. Bacterial infections were documented in 65 of the patients. Most patients had polymicrobial infections (Table 1).

When patients were grouped by titer status, an elevated titer was noted to have developed during hospitalization in 42 patients. Patients with elevated titers were marginally older (44 years $\pm$ 3 (SEM) vs. 37 years $\pm$ 4) and had a longer duration of antibiotic therapy (53 $\pm$ 5.2 vs. 38 $\pm$ 6.1) than did patients with negative titers, although their Injury Severity Scores were somewhat lower (27 $\pm$ 1.5 vs. 30 $\pm$ 3.0). Sources of *Candida* were equally common in both groups (50% vs. 46%), but patients with elevated

TABLE 1.
A Comparison of Ill and Injured Patients With vs. Without Elevated *Candida* Antigen Titers (Cand-Tec)

Parameter	All Patients	Elevated Titer	Negative Titer
Number	66	42	24
Age	42 yr $\pm$ $\geq$(SEM)	41 $\pm$ 3	43 $\pm$ 2
Antibiotics (%)	100	100	100
Antibiotic days	48 $\pm$ 3.0	53 $\pm$ 5.2	38 $\pm$ 6.1
Bacterial infections (%)	98	100	96
Multiple bacterial infections (%)	79	83	71

titers more frequently had a deep or invasive source of Candida (38% vs. 18%) such as a subdural hematoma or a blood culture.

Reflecting their lower injury severity score (ISS), patients with elevated titers had a higher predicted survival 0.82 ± 0.04 vs. 0.76 ± 0.06) using TRISS methodology. Unexpectedly, mortality was twice as high in patients with elevated titers (24% vs. 12%; Table 2). Interestingly, the presence or absence of a source of Candida had no bearing on clinical outcome. Patients with documented Candida by culture had a 22% mortality rate, whereas those with Candida from a superficial source or an invasive or deep source had mortality rates of 23% and 20%, respectively. Patients without a source of Candida had a mortality rate of 18%. Because culture results do not correlate with mortality, it seems questionable that they should be used to guide antifungal therapy. This disagrees with the findings of others, but has been a consistent finding in our subsequent studies. In addition, the poor correlation between mortality and cultures of Candida in recent studies may reflect our use of titers with early detection and initiation of antifungal therapy for occult Candida infection.

In this study, three patients with negative titers died, all because of bacterial sepsis. Ten patients with elevated titers died, seven because of bacterial sepsis and three because of trauma-related injuries. No deaths apparently were caused by Candida infections or systemic candidiasis. When mortality was analyzed in light of antifungal therapy, however, there was a decrease in mortality among treated patients with elevated titers from 35% to 16%. Systemic antifungal therapy in patients with negative titers brought about no such reduction in mortality (11% without therapy vs. 20% with therapy). Patients with elevated titers are more likely to die, and when they do, the usual cause of death is bacterial sepsis. Antifungal therapy seems to decrease the mortality associated with elevated titers, suggesting that it protects against bacterial septic demise in patients with elevated titers.

This study supports the contention that severely injured adults who are receiving prolonged antibiotic therapy for bacterial infections have a mortality rate that is associated more with Candida antigen titer status than with ISS or predicted survival using TRISS methodology. It tentatively sup-

TABLE 2.
A Comparison of Ill Injured Patients With vs. Without Elevated Candida Antigen Titers (Cand-Tec)

Parameter	Elevated Titer	Negative Titer
Injury Severity Score	27 ± 1.5 (SEM)	30 ± 3.0
Predicted mortality (%)	18	24
Actual mortality (%)	24	12
Number of septic deaths	7	3

ports the use of systemic antifungal therapy in patients with elevated titers, but is being repeated in a prospective, placebo-controlled, randomized trial.

The dimorphic fungus Candida albicans is an opportunistic organism that colonizes mucosal surfaces in man shortly after birth.[27] Depending on growth conditions, Candida can be found in a yeast or a hyphal form, although the hyphal form is believed to be responsible for tissue invasion.

Despite daily exposure to this organism, invasive Candida infections are uncommon and are seen only in the setting of immune suppression. Recipients of solid organ transplants undergoing active immune suppression and patients with cancer who are receiving chemotherapy or radiation therapy for reduction of tumor load both are at increased risk for the development of invasive Candida infections.[28, 29] In addition, patients with the acquired immunodeficiency syndrome often succumb to opportunistic Candida infections.[30] These observations underscore the importance of an intact immune system to combat life-threatening infections by this organism.

Candida invasion generates humoral and cell-mediated immune responses, although the relative importance of each is a source of debate. Phagocytes, particularly polymorphonuclear leukocytes (PMNs), are generally believed to be the key effector cells responsible for controlling Candida growth.[31, 32] This is achieved through a combination of intracellular and extracellular PMN pathways. PMNs coming into contact with a pathogen respond with a burst of metabolic and respiratory activity.[33, 34] Increased oxygen consumption leads to the production of superoxide radicals, which are transformed enzymatically to hydrogen peroxide, and then are transformed further into more toxic substances by the myeloperoxidase/halide system. PMNs also control C. albicans growth through nonoxidative pathways by the degranulation of cationic proteins and lytic enzymes from primary and secondary granules. Both the highly reactive superoxide radicals and the lytic enzymes then are released into the phagosome-containing ingested pathogens and are most likely responsible for the intracellular killing of Candida yeast cells.[31, 32] Although superoxide radicals and lytic enzymes also can be released into the extracellular environment to act on larger hyphae that cannot be ingested, these factors are rapidly broken down by proteases and other endogenous substances. Extracellular Candida growth is more likely to be controlled by lactoferrin, which is released from the secondary or specific granules of PMNs.[32] This iron-binding glycoprotein has been shown to possess potent anticandidal function.[35, 36]

Although PMNs are the primary effector cells responsible for controlling Candida growth and proliferation, they do not act alone. PMNs require the presence of cytokines to induce maturation,[37, 38] stimulate migration,[39–41] and activate antimicrobial functions.[42, 43] These cytokines are released to a large degree by T lymphocytes, macrophages, and large granular lymphocytes after exposure to Candida. Despite possessing minimal anticandidal activity themselves, these cells indirectly play a significant role in cell-mediated immunity to *Candida* through the production of these PMN-activating factors.

Recent advances in gene cloning and protein purification techniques have enabled the creation and availability of recombinant human cytokines. Using several of these newly synthesized products, investigators have evaluated the effects of specific cytokines on PMN function against *C. albicans*. Granulocyte-macrophage colony-stimulating factor (GM-CSF) is known to be a potent stimulator of the differentiation of hematopoietic stem cells in the marrow and improves leukocyte counts rapidly in recipients of bone marrow transplants and in patients with cancer who have neutropenia as a result of chemotherapy.[44–46] In addition to its hematopoietic properties, GM-CSF has been shown to exert potent effects on the anticandidal function of mature PMNs.[47] This cytokine is produced by lymphocytes after exposure to *Candida* and stimulates the intracellular and extracellular anticandidal pathways previously discussed. Interleukin-8 (IL-8) is produced by activated monocytes, alveolar macrophages, and endothelial cells.[48] This novel cytokine induces chemotaxis, degranulation, respiratory burst, leukotriene formation, and Ca^{2+} mobilization in human PMNs.[39, 49–51] In addition to its proinflammatory effects, IL-8 also is known to activate PMN anticandidal function, most likely through the upregulation of intracellular anticandidal mechanisms (superoxide production and degranulation of lytic enzymes).[52] Interferon-γ (IFN-γ) is produced primarily by activated T lymphocytes. This cytokine induces major histocompatibility class I and II antigen expression on antigen-presenting cells, promotes the differentiation of B and T lymphocytes, activates mononuclear phagocytes, and has potent antiviral properties.[53–56] IFN-γ also has been shown to activate PMNs, augmenting anticandidal function through the stimulation of intracellular anticandidal mechanisms.[57]

Although they once were felt to be terminally differentiated effector cells, there is increasing evidence that PMNs play a larger role in the immune response than previously recognized. For example, tumor necrosis factor (TNF) is known to be an activator of the anticandidal function of PMNs, and it has recently been documented that PMNs cultured with *C. albicans* release TNF.[57, 58] The ability of PMNs to produce TNF suggests an autocrine system of self-activation of PMNs against pathogenic organisms. Several investigators have reported the production of interleukin-1α, interleukin-1β, granulocyte colony-stimulating factor, macrophage colony-stimulating factor, interferon-α, and IL-8 by activated PMNs.[59–62] By releasing these cytokines, PMNs are able to activate and recruit neighboring PMNs, macrophages/monocytes, and T cells to the site of inflammation. Therefore, in addition to being the primary effector cells in the host response to injury and infection, PMNs actively participate in the amplification of the immune cascade by releasing cytokines.

Our early clinical investigations focused on the implications of an elevated *Candida* antigen titer after injury. We have demonstrated that injured patients with an elevated *Candida* antigen titer have an increased mortality rate compared with matched patients with negative *Candida* antigen titers.[26] In addition, death in patients with elevated titers usually results from sepsis and multisystem organ failure.

Considerations of host immunity led us to investigate the anticandidal function of PMNs isolated from injured adults with elevated Candida antigen titers. Initial studies in our laboratory demonstrated that PMNs from these patients have impaired function against C. albicans compared with PMNs obtained from healthy volunteers.[63] The possibility exists, however, that the defect in PMN anticandidal function is a generalized finding after major trauma and not one that is specific to injured adults with elevated Candida antigen titers. To address this issue, the anticandidal function of PMNs from injured adults with elevated Candida antigen titers, from matched injured patients with negative Candida antigen titers, and from healthy volunteers was evaluated using an ^{3}H-glucose incorporation assay. Our hypothesis in undertaking this study was that PMNs from severely injured adults with elevated Candida antigen titers have defective anticandidal function that is not seen in matched patients with negative Candida antigen titers. If a defect in PMN anticandidal activity was present, we hypothesized that stimulation of these PMNs with exogenous GM-CSF, IFN-γ, or IL-8 could reconstitute their function against C. albicans.

To undertake this study of PMN anticandidal function, all patients admitted to the hospital with an ISS of 18 or more had Candida antigen titers drawn at the time of admission and then weekly during hospitalization. Patients in whom a titer of 1:4 or greater developed were considered to have an elevated titer. With the development of an elevated titer and before the initiation of antifungal treatment, patients had 20 cc of whole blood drawn into heparinized Vacutainer tubes. Simultaneously, whole blood was drawn from patients matched in age (± 5 years), gender, mechanism of injury, and severity of injury who had negative Candida antigen titers, and from healthy volunteers for concurrent study. PMNs from each blood sample were studied using the same reagents, growth medium, cytokines, and C. albicans preparations. Data describing the injured patients were collected and included age, gender, race, mechanism of injury, organs injured, use of antibiotic therapy, presence of bacterial or fungal infections, and ISS calculated at hospital discharge or autopsy.

Twenty injured adults had elevated Candida antigen titers during their hospital course. Seven patients had titer dilutions of 1:4, 7 had titers of 1:8, 4 had titers of 1:16, and 2 had titers of 1:32. The severely injured adults with elevated Candida antigen titers were not different from injury-matched patients with negative Candida antigen titers in terms of age, severity of injury, mechanism of injury, gender, incidence of concomitant bacterial infections, and units of blood transfused (Table 3). All patients in both groups received aggressive broad-spectrum antibiotic therapy at some point during their admission and had a similar duration of antibiotic therapy. Only 2 of the 20 patients with elevated Candida antigen titers had culture evidence of Candida (sputum and urine, respectively), whereas 1 of the 20 patients with negative titers had Candida in culture (urine). None

TABLE 3.
Patient Demographics for Polymorphonuclear Leukocyte Anticandidal Function Study

Parameter	Titer-Negative	Titer-Positive
Number	20	20
Age (yrs)	43 ± 4(SEM)	35 ± 2
Percent male sex	80	90
Percent with blunt injury	85	90
Injury Severity Score	26 ± 2	28 ± 2
Blood transfused (units)	3 ± 1	6 ± 2
Percent bacterial infections	45	75
Percent with Candida in culture	5	10

of the patients in either group had visceral biopsies or blood cultures that were positive for Candida.

PMNs from all three groups of patients inhibited Candida growth in vitro (Fig 1). This was manifested in a dose-dependent manner, with higher growth inhibition present at the larger PMN:Candida ratios. Compared with the anticandidal function of PMNs from the healthy volunteers and the injured adults with negative Candida antigen titers, the anticandidal function of PMNs from the patients with elevated Candida antigen titers was impaired significantly. GM-CSF, IFN-γ, and IL-8 each significantly in-

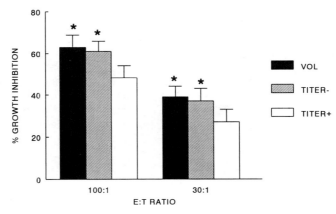

FIG 1.
The mean anticandidal function of PMNs from 20 injured adults with elevated Candida antigen titers, 20 matched injured patients with negative Candida antigen titers, and 20 healthy volunteers. Error bars represent SEM. The asterisks indicate greater growth inhibition than in injured adults with elevated Candida antigen titers; $P < .05$, paired Student's t-test.

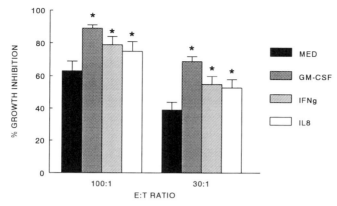

FIG 2.
Cytokine stimulation improves the anticandidal function of PMNs from healthy volunteers. IL-8 = interleukin-8; $IFNg$ = interferon-γ; GM-CSF = granulocyte-macrophage colony-stimulating factor; MED = medium. Error bars represent SEM. The asterisks indicate greater anticandidal function than in respective PMNs incubated in medium alone; $P < .0001$, paired Student's t-test.

creased PMN anticandidal function of PMNs obtained from these patients (Figs 2 to 4), with GM-CSF being the most potent activator of the three. Interestingly, the percent increase in anticandidal function above baseline manifested by cytokine-stimulated PMNs from the injured adults with elevated Candida antigen titers was comparable to or greater than that

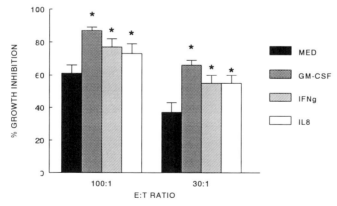

FIG 3.
Cytokine stimulation improves the anticandidal function of PMNs from injured adults with negative Candida antigen titers. IL-8 = interleukin-8; $IFNg$ = interferon-γ; GM-CSF = granulocyte-macrophage colony-stimulating factor; MED = medium. Error bars represent SEM. The asterisks indicate greater anticandidal function than in respective PMNs incubated in medium alone; $P < .0001$, paired Student's t-test.

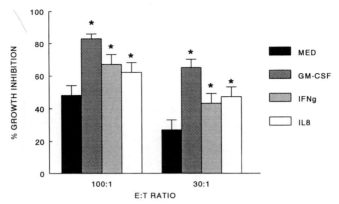

FIG 4.
Cytokine stimulation reconstitutes the anticandidal function of PMNs from injured adults with elevated *Candida* antigen titers. IL-8 = interleukin-8; IFNg = interferon-γ; GM-CSF = granulocyte-macrophage colony-stimulating factor; MED = medium. Error bars represent SEM. The *asterisks* indicate greater anticandidal function than in respective PMNs incubated in medium alone; $P < .0001$, paired Student's *t*-test.

manifested by PMNs from the matched patients with negative *Candida* antigen titers. Although PMNs from injured patients with elevated titers have impaired function against *C. albicans,* these results suggest that the mechanisms and pathways required for cytokine stimulation of PMN anticandidal function remain generally intact. Work is under way in our laboratory to determine which anticandidal pathway(s) is defective within these PMNs. In addition to anticandidal function, investigations concerning antimicrobial function against gram-positive and gram-negative organisms are planned. We have also recently begun evaluating cytokine production by PMNs from injured adults with elevated *Candida* antigen titers. Preliminary results suggest that PMNs from these patients produce ample amounts of TNF and IL-8 in response to *C. albicans,* implying that mechanisms for cytokine production and PMN autocrine activation also remain intact, although killing is defective.

In vivo, the endogenous cytokines that reconstitute anticandidal function in injured adults with elevated *Candida* antigen titers are produced primarily by monocytes and lymphocytes in response to *C. albicans* stimulation. Because lymphocytes play an important role in the activation of PMN function against *C. albicans,* it was believed to be important to evaluate the ability of lymphocytes from severely injured adults with elevated *Candida* antigen titers to stimulate the anticandidal function of normal PMNs. Lymphocytes from 13 injured adults with elevated *Candida* antigen titers were isolated and incubated with or without heat-killed *C. albicans*. After 48 hours, cell culture supernatants were harvested, diluted serially tenfold from 1:10 to 1:1,000, and tested for the ability to activate the anticandidal

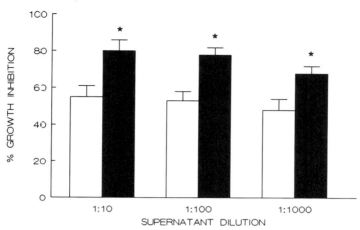

FIG 5.
Dose response of supernatants (sup) from volunteer lymphocytes. Lymphocytes were incubated with heat-killed Candida albicans (solid bars) or in medium alone (open bars) for 48 hours. Supernatants were collected, serially diluted, and tested for the ability to augment PMN function against C. albicans. The asterisks indicate a significant increase in PMN function against C. albicans; $P < .05$, paired Student's t-test. Error bars represent SEM.

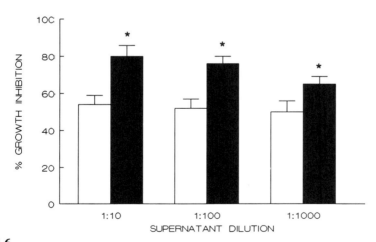

FIG 6.
Dose response of supernatants (sup) from lymphocytes of injured adults with negative Candida antigen titers. Lymphocytes were incubated with heat-killed Candida albicans (solid bars) or in medium alone (open bars) for 48 hours. Supernatants were collected, serially diluted, and tested for the ability to augment PMN function against C. albicans. The asterisks indicate a significant increase in PMN function against C. albicans; $P < .05$, paired Student's t-test. Error bars represent SEM.

function of normal PMNs. Lymphocytes from 13 volunteers and 13 patients with negative *Candida* antigen titers were studied for comparison. The patients with or without elevated titers were well-matched in age, gender, Injury Severity Score, units of blood transfused, and length/breadth of antibiotic therapy (Table 4). Patients with elevated titers had a higher incidence of bacterial infections than did patients with negative titers. Two of the 13 patients with elevated titers and 1 of the 13 patients with negative titers had *Candida* grown in culture. Lymphocytes from the volunteers and from the patients with negative titers released large amounts of a PMN-activating factor(s) when they were exposed to *C. albicans* (Figs 5 and 6). Supernatants from these lymphocytes that had been incubated with heat-killed *C. albicans* significantly augmented the anticandidal function of normal PMNs compared to supernatants from respective lymphocytes that had been incubated in medium alone. This was manifested in a dose-dependent fashion, with greater augmentation of PMN function seen at the more concentrated supernatant dilutions. Lymphocytes from patients with elevated titers were defective in their ability to release this activating factor(s) after exposure to *C. albicans* (Fig 7). Supernatants from these cells did not augment anticandidal function at any dilution tested.

The results of these studies provide further insight into our understanding of the association between increased mortality and impaired immune function in injured adults with elevated *Candida* antigen titers. Lymphocytes play a vital role in cell-mediated immunity to *C. albicans* through the release of cytokines, which induce maturation and functional activation of phagocytes. Impaired production of PMN-activating factors by lympho-

TABLE 4.
Patient Demographics for Lymphocyte Dysfunction Study

Parameter	Titer-Negative	Titer-Positive
Number	13	13
Age (yrs)	39 ± 5(SEM)	34 ± 4
Percent male sex	77	77
Percent with blunt injury	85	92
Injury Severity Score	26 ± 2	26 ± 2
Blood transfused (units)	3 ± 1.3	3 ± 0.7
Percent bacterial infections	39	85
Percent with *Candida* in culture	8	15
Antibiotic days	24 ± 7.3	28 ± 3.4

*Greater than titer-negative, $P < .05$, Fisher exact test.

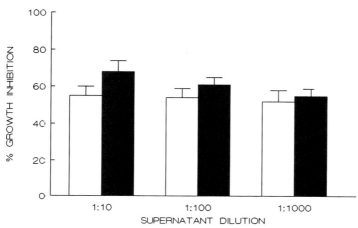

FIG 7.
Dose response of supernatants *(sup)* from lymphocytes of injured adults with elevated *Candida* antigen titers. Lymphocytes were incubated with heat-killed *Candida albicans (solid bars)* or in medium alone *(open bars)* for 48 hours. Supernatants were collected, serially diluted, and tested for the ability to augment PMN function against *C. albicans*. No significant increase in PMN function against *C. albicans* was seen; $P < .05$, paired Student's *t*-test. Error bars represent SEM.

cytes from injured adults with elevated *Candida* antigen titers, could therefore, lead to improper maturation and activation of effector cells, partially explaining the defect in anticandidal function that is found in PMNs from these patients. This is further supported by our observation that exogenous cytokines can reconstitute the anticandidal function of PMNs from injured adults with elevated *Candida* antigen titers. Interestingly, seriously injured adults with negative titers have PMN and lymphocyte function similar to that of healthy volunteers.

Investigators have previously reported the immunoinhibitory effects of various *Candida* cell wall metabolites on lymphocyte responses in vitro.[64, 65] In vivo evidence of depressed immune function also has been found in patients with chronic mucocutaneous *Candida* infections.[66] In our clinical experience, microbiologic evidence for *Candida* invasion in injured adults with elevated *Candida* antigen titers is uncommon. More likely, the *Candida* antigen titer is a marker of occult *Candida* invasion. It is believed that the antigen measured by the Cand-Tec latex agglutination assay is a *Candida* cell wall antigen that has been modified by interaction with the host effector cell.[67] The possibility exists, therefore, that during host response to occult *Candida* invasion, catabolites causing immune suppression are released. These catabolites may lead to the host immune dysfunction that is found in injured adults with elevated Candida antigen titers.

In summary, when discussing the utility of measurements of the Candida antigen titer in severely injured adults, it is important to focus on the implications of an elevated titer rather than on the sensitivity or specificity of the assay. Severely injured adults with an elevated Candida antigen titer have an increased mortality rate compared to injury-matched patients with a negative Candida antigen titer. Mortality results from sepsis and multisystem organ failure, and not from apparent Candida infection. Finally, the Candida antigen titer is a marker of broad-based immune dysfunction against C. albicans after major injury, which in part begins to explain the increased mortality rate that is seen in injured adults with elevated Candida antigen titers.

The concept of early therapy in patients with elevated Candida antigen titers is gaining popularity, and for good reason, we believe. Further studies should continue to focus on the diagnosis of early, yet significant, Candida invasion and the timely initiation of antifungal therapy.

References

1. Trunkey DD: Trauma. *Sci Am* 1983; 249:28.
2. Committee on Trauma Research: *Injury in America: A Continuing Public Health Problem.* Washington, DC, National Academy Press, 1985.
3. Wey SB, Mori M, Pfaller MA, et al: Hospital acquired candidemia: The attributable mortality and excess length of stay. *Arch Intern Med* 1988; 148: 2642–2645.
4. Rosemurgy AS, Hart MB, Murphy CG, et al: Infection after injury: Association with blood transfusion. *Am Surg* 1992; 58:104–107.
5. Baker CC, Oppenheimer L, Stephens B, et al: Epidemiology of trauma deaths. *Am J Surg* 1980; 140:144–150.
6. Shackford SR, Hollingworth-Fridlund P, Cooper CF, et al: The effect of regionalization upon the quality of trauma care as assessed by concurrent audit before and after institution of a trauma system. *J Trauma* 1986; 26:810–820.
7. Pfaller MA: Infection control: Opportunistic fungal infections—the increasing importance of Candida species. *Infect Control Hosp Epidemiol* 1989; 10:270–273.
8. Schaberg DR, Culver DH, Gaynes RP: Major trends in the microbial etiology of nosocomial infection. *Am J Med* 1991; 91:72S–75S.
9. Perfect JR, Pickard WW, Hunt DL, et al: The use of amphotericin B in nosocomial fungal infection. *Rev Infect Dis* 1991; 13:474–479.
10. Marsh PK, Tally FP, Kellum J, et al: Candida infections in surgical patients. *Ann Surg* 1983; 198:42–47.
11. Solomkin JS: Pathogenesis and management of Candida infection syndromes in non-neutropenic patients, *New Horizons* 1993; 1:202–213.
12. DeLozier JB, Stratton CW, Potts JR: Rapid diagnosis of Candida sepsis in surgical patients. *Am Surg* 1987; 53:600–602.
13. Solomkin JS, Flohr AB, Quie PG, et al: The role of Candida in intraperitoneal infections. *Surgery* 1980; 88:524–530.

14. Bodey GP, Anaissie EJ, Edwards JE: Definitions of Candida infections, in Bodey GP (ed): *Candidiasis: Pathogenesis, Diagnosis, and Treatment.* New York, Raven Press, 1993, pp 407–408.
15. Rutledge R, Mandel SR, Wild WE: Candida species. Insignificant contaminant or pathogenic species. *Am Surg* 1986; 52:299–302.
16. Robinson PA, Knirsch AK, Joseph JA: Fluconazole for life threatening fungal infections in patients who cannot be treated with conventional antifungal agents. *Rev Infect Dis* 1990; 12(suppl 3):S349–363.
17. Bougnoux ME, Hill C, Moissenet D, et al: Comparison of antibody, antigen, and metabolic assays for hospitalized patients with disseminated or peripheral candidiasis. *J Clin Microbiol* 1990; 28:905–909.
18. Gold JWM, Wong B, Bernard EM, et al: Serum arabinatol concentrations and arabinatol/creatinine ratios in invasive candidiasis. *J Infect Dis* 1983; 147:504–513.
19. Walsh TJ, Hathorn JW, Sobel JD: Detection of circulating Candida enolase by immunoassay in patient with cancer and invasive candidiasis. *N Engl J Med* 1991; 324:1026–1031.
20. Kahn FW, Jones JM: Latex agglutination tests for the detection of Candida antigen in sera of patients with invasive candidiasis. *J Infect Dis* 1986; 3:579–585.
21. Fung JC, Donta ST, Tilton RC: Candida detection systems (Cand-Tec) to differentiate between Candida albicans colonization and disease. *J Clin Microbiol* 1986; 24:542–547.
22. Piens MA, Guyotat D, Archimbaud E, et al: Evaluation of a Candida antigen detection test (Cand-Tec) in the diagnosis of deep candidiasis in neutropenic patients. *Eur J Cancer Clin Oncol* 1988; 24:1655–1659.
23. Cabeyudo I, Pfaller M, Gerarden T, et al: Value of the Cand-Tec Candida antigen assay in the diagnosis or therapy of systemic candidiasis in high risk patients. *Eur J Clin Microbiol* 1989; 8:770–777.
24. Phillips P, Dowd A, Jewesson P, et al: Nonvalue of antigen detection immunoassays for diagnosis of candidemia. *J Clin Microbiol* 1990; 18:2320–2326.
25. Kealey GP, Heimley JA, Lewis RW, et al: Value of the Candida antigen assay in the diagnosis of systemic candidiasis in burn patients. *J Trauma* 1991; 32:285–288.
26. Rosemurgy AS, Sweeney JF, Albrink MH, et al: Implications of Candida antigen titers in injured adults. *Contemp Surg* 1993; 42:327–332.
27. Odds FC: *Candida and Candidiasis. A Review and Bibliography*, 2nd ed. Philadelphia, WB Saunders, 1988.
28. Bach MC, Sahyoun A, Adler JL, et al: High incidence of fungus infections in renal transplantation patients treated with antilymphocyte and conventional immunosuppression. *Transplant Proc* 1973; 5:549–553.
29. Cho YS, Choi HY: Opportunistic fungal infection among cancer patients. A ten year autopsy study. *Am J Clin Pathol* 1979; 72:617–621.
30. Mildvan D, Mathur U, Enlow RW, et al: Opportunistic infections and immune deficiency in homosexual men. *Ann Intern Med* 1982; 96:700–704.
31. Diamond RD, Clark RA, Haudenschild CC: Damage to *Candida albicans* hyphae and pseudohyphae by the myeloperoxidase system and oxidative products of neutrophil metabolism in vivo. *J Clin Invest* 1980; 66:908–917.
32. Schuit KE: Phagocytosis and intracellular killing of pathogenic yeasts by human monocytes and neutrophils. *Infect Immun* 1979; 24:932–938.
33. Babior BM: Oxygen-dependent microbial killing by phagocytes. *N Engl J Med* 1978; 298:659–668.

34. Clark RA: The human neutrophil respiratory burst oxidase. *J Infect Dis* 1990; 161:1140–1147.
35. Palma C, Cassone A, Serbousek D, et al: Lactoferrin release and interleukin-1, interleukin-6, and tumor necrosis factor production by human polymorphonuclear cells stimulated by various lipopolysaccharides: Relationship to growth inhibition of *Candida albicans*. *Infect Immun* 1992; 60:4604–4611.
36. Palma C, Serbousek D, Torosantucci A, et al: Identification of a mannoprotein fraction from *Candida albicans* that enhances human polymorphonuclear leukocyte (PMNL) functions and stimulates lactoferrin in PMNL inhibition of candidal growth. *J Infect Dis* 1992; 166:1103–1112.
37. Gasson JC, Weisbart RH, Kaufman SE, et al: Purified human granulocyte macrophage-colony stimulating factor: Direct action on neutrophils. *Science* 1984; 226:1339–1342.
38. Groopman JE, Molina JM, Scadden DT: Hematopoietic growth factors. Biology and clinical applications. *N Engl J Med* 1989; 321:1449–1459.
39. Yoshimura T, Matsushima K, Tanaka S, et al: Purification of a human monocyte-derived neutrophil chemotactic factor that has peptide sequence similarity to other host defense cytokines. *Proc Natl Acad Sci U S A* 1987; 84:9233–9237.
40. Wang JM, Colella S, Allavena P, et al: Chemotactic activity of human recombinant granulocyte macrophage colony stimulating factor. *Immunology* 1987; 60:439–444.
41. Ming WJ, Bersani L, Mantovani A: Tumor necrosis factor is chemotactic for monocytes and polymorphonuclear leukocytes. *J Immunol* 1987; 138:1469–1474.
42. Perussia B, Kobayashi M, Rossi ME, et al: Immune interferon enhances functional properties of human granulocytes: Role of Fc receptors and effect of lymphotoxin, tumor necrosis factor, and granulocyte-macrophage colony stimulating factor. *J Immunol* 1987; 138:765–774.
43. Weisbart RH, Golde DW, Clark SC, et al: Human granulocyte-macrophage colony-stimulating factor is a neutrophil activator. *Nature* 1985; 314:361–363.
44. Link H, Boogaerts MA, Carella AM, et al: A controlled trial of recombinant human granulocyte-macrophage colony-stimulating factor after total body irradiation, high-dose chemotherapy, and autologous bone marrow transplantation for acute lymphoblastic leukemia or malignant lymphoma. *Blood* 1992; 80:2188–2195.
45. Lazarus HM, Andersen J, Chen MG, et al: Recombinant granulocyte-macrophage colony-stimulating factor after autologous bone marrow transplantation for relapsed non-Hodgkin's lymphoma: Blood and bone marrow progenitor growth studies. A phase II Eastern Cooperative Oncology Group trial. *Blood* 1991; 78:830–837.
46. Neumanaitis J, Rabinowe SN, Singer JW, et al: Recombinant granulocyte macrophage colony-stimulating factor after autologous bone marrow transplantation for lymphoid cancer. *N Engl J Med* 1991; 324:1773–1778.
47. Blanchard DK, Michelini-Norris MB, Djeu JY: Production of granulocyte-macrophage colony stimulating factor by large granular lymphocytes: Role in activation of human neutrophil function. *Blood* 1991; 77:2259–2265.
48. Baggiolini M, Walz A, Kunkel SL: Neutrophil activating peptide-1/interleukin 8, a novel cytokine that activates neutrophils. *J Clin Invest* 1989; 84:1045–1049.
49. Peveri P, Walz A, DeWald B, et al: A novel neutrophil activating factor

produced by human mononuclear phagocytes. *J Exp Med* 1988; 167: 1547–1559.
50. Brom J, Konig W: Cytokine induced (interleukins-3, -6, and -8, and tumor necrosis factor-beta) activation and deactivation of human neutrophils. *Immunology* 1992; 75:281–285.
51. Liu JH, Blanchard DK, Wei S, et al: Recombinant interleukin-8 induces changes in cytosolic Ca^{2+} in human neutrophils. *J Infect Dis* 1992; 166: 1089–1096.
52. Djeu JY, Matsushima K, Oppenheim JJ, et al: Functional activation of human neutrophils by recombinant monocyte-derived neutrophil chemotactic factor/IL-8. *J Immunol* 1990; 144:2205–2210.
53. Abbas AK, Lichtman AH, Pober JS: Cytokines, in *Cellular and molecular immunology*. Philadelphia, WB Saunders, 1991.
54. Nathan CF, Murray HW, Wiebe ME, et al: Identification of interferon-gamma as the lymphokine that activates human macrophage oxidative metabolism and antimicrobial activity. *J Exp Med* 1983; 158:670–689.
55. Nathan CF, Prendergast TJ, Wiebe ME: Activation of human macrophages. Comparison of other cytokines with interferon-gamma. *J Exp Med* 1984; 160:600–605.
56. Murray HW, Byrne GI, Rothermel CD, et al: Lymphokine enhances oxygen-independent activity against intracellular pathogens. *J Exp Med* 1983; 158:234–239.
57. Djeu JY, Blanchard DK, Halkias D, et al: Growth inhibition of *Candida albicans* by human polymorphonuclear neutrophils: Activation by interferon-γ and tumor necrosis factor. *J Immunol* 1986; 137:2980–2984.
58. Djeu JY, Serbousek D, Blanchard DK: Release of tumor necrosis factor by human polymorphonuclear leukocytes. *Blood* 1990; 76:140–146.
59. Lindemann A, Reidel D, Oster W, et al: Granulocyte-macrophage colony stimulating factor induces cytokine secretion by human polymorphonuclear leukocytes. *J Clin Invest* 1988; 83:1308–1316.
60. Lindemann A, Reidel D, Oster W, et al: Granulocyte/macrophage colony stimulating factor induces interleukin 1 production by human polymorphonuclear neutrophils. *J Immunol* 1988; 140:837–845.
61. Shirafuji N, Matsuda S, Ogura H, et al: Granulocyte macrophage-colony stimulating factor stimulates mature neutrophilic granulocytes to produce interferon-α. *Blood* 1990; 75:17–25.
62. Strieter RM, Kasahara K, Allen R, et al: Human neutrophils exhibit disparate chemotactic factor gene expression. *Biochem Biophys Res Commun* 1990; 173:725–730.
63. Sweeney JF, Rosemurgy AS, Wei S, et al: Impaired polymorphonuclear leukocyte anticandidal function in injured adults with elevated Candida antigen titers. *Arch Surg* 1993; 128:40–46.
64. Podzorski RP, Gray GR, Nelson RD: Different effects of native *Candida albicans* mannan and mannan-derived oligosaccharides on antigen stimulated lymphoproliferation in vitro. *J Immunol* 1990; 144:707–716.
65. Podzorski RP, Herron MJ, Fast DJ, et al: Pathogenesis of candidiasis: Immunosuppression by cell wall mannan catabolites. *Arch Surg* 1990; 124: 1290–1294.
66. Dwyer JM: Chronic mucocutaneous candidiasis. *Annu Rev Med* 1981; 32:491–493.
67. de Repentigny L: Serodiagnosis of candidiasis, aspergillosis, and cryptococcosis. *Clin Infect Dis* 1992; 14(suppl 1):S11–22.

Esophageal Injury

Rao R. Ivatury, M.D.
Professor of Surgery, New York Medical College; Director, Trauma, Co-Director, Surgical Intensive Care Unit, Lincoln Medical & Mental Health Center, Bronx, New York

Michael Rohman, M.D.
Professor of Surgery, New York Medical College; Chief, Cardio-thoracic Surgery, Lincoln Medical & Mental Health Center, Bronx, New York

Ronald J. Simon, M.D.
Assistant Professor of Surgery, New York Medical College; Attending Surgeon, Lincoln Medical & Mental Health Center, Bronx, New York

The *Edwin Smith Papyrus* written about 4,000 to 5,000 years ago recorded the first "penetrating wound of the Gullet."[1] Frink, in 1941, reported the first successful drainage of a perforated esophagus.[2] In 1947, Barrett[3] and Clagett[4] independently described the first effective surgical repair of an esophageal perforation. In recent years, treatment of the injured esophagus has ranged from nonoperative therapy to surgical replacement of the organ. Regardless of the approach chosen, early diagnosis and prompt treatment are essential to success. A high index of suspicion and aggressive pursuit with appropriate studies is crucial to early diagnosis. This chapter reviews the varied etiology of esophageal injury and accepted principles of and methods for its treatment, and introduces recent innovations in this field.

Surgical Anatomy

The esophagus is a long, muscular organ that begins at the pharyngoesophageal junction at the level of the sixth cervical vertebra. The organ originates at the cricopharyngeus muscle, which is continuous with the oblique fibers of the inferior pharyngeal constrictor muscle that continues inferiorly as the circular and longitudinal muscle of the esophagus. This area of narrowing was called by Jackson the "pass of Bal-el Mandeb" or the "gate of tears."[5] This is one of the areas that is at risk for injury by an endoscopist or neophyte anesthesiologist, because the esophagus occupies the midline immediately behind the trachea and is vulnerable to injury during intubation. Passing into the thorax, the esophagus and the trachea traverse the superior mediastinum behind the great vessels and, curving slightly, pass behind the left main stem bronchus. From this point, the esophagus curves to the right in the posterior mediastinum, curves back to the left behind the pericardium, and crosses the thoracic aorta. Lying anterior to the thoracic aorta, it reaches the abdomen through the esophageal hiatus of the diaphragm. It ends within the abdomen at the gastroesophageal junction, which is marked by the oblique sling fibers of the stomach known as the loop of Willis or the collar of Helvetius. The surgical anatomy of the esophagus is illustrated in Figures 1 and 2.

The reputation of the esophagus as a surgeon's nightmare stems from the fact that the structure has no serosal covering. The outer layers are

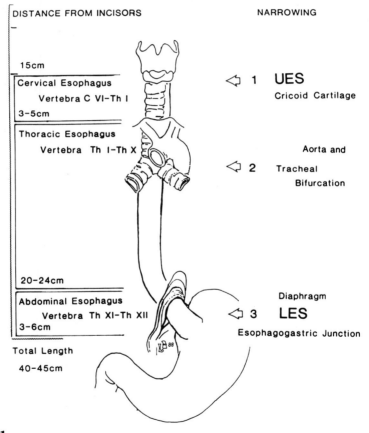

FIG 1.
Classic divisions of the esophagus and its relationship to vertebral levels. LES = lower esophageal sphincter; UES = upper esophageal sphincter. (From Duranceau A, Liebermann-Meffert D: Embryology, anatomy and physiology of the esophagus, in Zuidema GD (ed): *Shackelford's Surgery of the Alimentary Tract,* 3rd ed. Philadelphia, WB Saunders, 1991, p 21. Used by permission.)

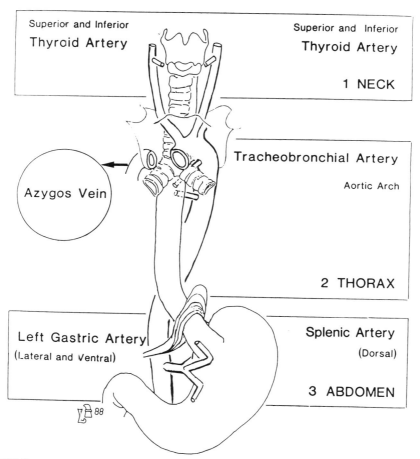

FIG 2.
Arterial supply of the esophagus and its relationship to the azygos vein. (From Duranceau A, Liebermann-Meffert D: Embryology, anatomy and physiology of the esophagus, in Zuidema GD (ed): *Shackelford's Surgery of the Alimentary Tract*, 3rd ed. Philadelphia, WB Saunders, 1991, p 25. Used by permission.)

composed entirely of longitudinal and circular muscle fibers, with squamous epithelium as the mucosal lining. This not only makes the organ more susceptible to rupture, but also creates an unfavorable situation for surgical suturing. The blood supply is derived from branches of the inferior thyroid, bronchial, and intercostal arteries, and from the aorta. The blood supply is segmental, with relatively poor collateralization, and extensive mobilization of the esophagus incurs the risk of devascularization. Venous drainage is through submucosal channels into a periesophageal plexus that eventually enters into the inferior thyroid and vertebral veins in the neck, the azygos and hemiazygos veins in the thorax, and the left gastric vein in the abdomen.

The protected environment of the esophagus makes it less susceptible to external trauma, but increases its vulnerability to intraluminal, iatrogenic injury. Spasm or hypertrophy of the cricopharyngeus, arthritis of the cervical spine and "spurs" in elderly patients, and inadequate anesthesia and relaxation during invasive procedures contribute to an increased risk of perforation of the cervical esophagus. The point at which the thoracic esophagus turns forward and to the left at the level of the diaphragm is another common site of iatrogenic injury.

Etiology of Esophageal Injury

Esophageal injury has a variety of causes that can be classified as either intraluminal or extraluminal forces (Table 1).[6] The relative incidence of each cause is listed in Table 2.

TABLE 1.
Classification of Etiology of Esophageal Injury

I. Intraluminal force
  A. Instrumentation
    1. Endoscopy, dilatation, biopsy
    2. Esophageal intubation
    3. Endotracheal intubation
  B. Foreign bodies, caustic lye ingestion
  C. Blast injury
  D. Spontaneous perforation
II. Extraluminal force
  A. Blunt trauma
  B. Penetrating trauma
  C. Iatrogenic operative injury
III. Perforations in the diseased esophagus
  A. Carcinoma
  B. Esophagitis

TABLE 2.
Etiology of Esophageal Perforation in Recent Large Series

Etiology	Goldstein 1982 (n=44)	Richardson 1985 (n=56)	Nesbitt 1987 (n=115)	Flynn 1989 (n=69)
Iatrogenic				
Total	27	32	65	33
Dilatation	15	8	14	20
Endoscopy	5	6	29	7
Celestin/Souttar tube	—	5	1	—
Sengstaken tube	1	3	3	1
Cantor/feeding tube	—	—	2	1
Intubation	1	2	1	—
Operative injury	5	2	13	1
Sclerotherapy	—	—	1	3
Foreign body extraction	—	6	—	—
Intraoperative temperature probe	—	—	1	—
Spontaneous	7	5	22	8
External trauma	5	19	23	23
Foreign body	1	—	5	3
Others	4	—	—	2

Injury From an Intraluminal Force

Endoscopy and Dilatation

Iatrogenic perforation is the most common cause of esophageal injury. Its overall incidence is small (<0.5%), however, when all procedures on the esophagus are considered. The American Society of Gastrointestinal Endoscopy, in a survey of 211,410 endoscopic procedures, recorded perforations in 0.03% of esophagogastroscopies and 0.25% of dilatation procedures.[7] The incidence of perforation was similar between rigid and flexible esophagoscopy (0.074% and 0.093%, respectively).[8] The areas of the cricopharyngeus, the gastroesophageal junction, and the curve of the esophagus at the diaphragmatic hiatus are the most common sites of perforation. Dilatation and biopsy increase the risk of instrumental perforation, undoubtedly related to the underlying disease. Sclerotherapy of esophageal varices rarely causes perforation. When large amounts of sclerosing solution are injected, extravasation outside the varix can cause a delayed sloughing of the mucosa. Postlethwait reported a 3.8% incidence of this complication in 977 cases of sclerotherapy.[9]

Intraluminal Tubes

Nasogastric tubes have been known to produce esophageal perforation if excessive force is used during their insertion. The incidence probably is much higher than reported in the literature. The Sengstaken-Blakemore tube is associated with a significant potential for esophageal rupture from excessive inflation of the esophageal balloon or pressure necrosis of the esophageal wall, or from a restless patient who pulls on the tube when the balloon is inflated.[5] Commonly, the perforation is related to inflation of the gastric balloon in the esophagus. We have seen several instances of this complication in which the physician either assumed that the tube had been advanced into the stomach or misinterpreted the chest radiograph and inflated the gastric balloon in the esophagus. This complication has uniformly been fatal in our experience because of the inevitable delay in recognition and the poor general condition of the patient. Tube perforation of the esophagus may be prevented by obtaining a chest radiograph after the instillation of a small amount of meglumine diatrizoate (Gastrografin) solution in the gastric balloon to confirm proper positioning of the tube. Esophageal "stents" used to bypass unresectable neoplasms are rare causes of perforation (see Table 2).[10–13]

Repeated attempts at endotracheal intubation by inexperienced personnel have led to pharyngoesophageal perforation, and this complication is reported in almost all series of esophageal trauma. Esophageal temperature probes, stethoscopes, and the esophageal obturator airway, which once was used as an alternative to endotracheal intubation, are rare causes of esophageal perforation.

Foreign Bodies

Impacted foreign bodies, both sharp and blunt, may cause esophageal injury by either direct penetration or erosion. The usual sites of perforation are the areas of anatomic narrowing at which foreign bodies may become impacted: at the level of the cricopharyngeus, at the aortic arch, and just above the cardia. Sharp objects also can cause injury during endoscopic removal. Richardson and associates reported six cases of perforation during foreign body extraction.[11] Injury also may result from the ingestion of caustic or corrosive agents, which may produce a full-thickness burn of the esophagus and secondary perforation.

Michel and coworkers cited two reports of perforation from "esoteric causes": sword swallowing and self-dilatation by the passage of a heavy electric wire into the esophagus![5]

Blast Injury

Blast injury is an interesting, albeit rare, mechanism of esophageal rupture resulting from a sudden rise in intraluminal pressure. The pressure necessary to rupture the organ by distention has been studied experimentally and found to be about 5 psi.[14, 15] Because the lower end of the esophagus is the weakest, this is the most common site of rupture. Guth and colleagues reported a case of rupture of the distal esophagus caused by the explosion of a compressed air tank in front of a construction worker, and summarized 18 other cases from the literature: the initial blast came from compressed air in all but 3 cases.[16] The explosion of a fire extinguisher (1 case) and of a soda bottle (2 cases) accounted for the remainder. A history of external barotrauma in a symptomatic patient should raise suspicion for an esophageal injury.

Spontaneous Rupture of the Esophagus

Spontaneous rupture of the esophagus is related to barotrauma and is strain-induced. Described in 1724 by Boerhaave as a postemetic event, it also may occur after severe straining, such as that associated with defecation, seizures, or weight lifting.[5] The sudden rise in intraluminal pressure against a closed glottis causes the esophagus to rupture, almost always at the lower end, just above the diaphragm on the left lateral aspect. Weakness at this level in the muscular coats of the esophagus, caused by vessel and nerve entry, lack of support, and the acute angulation of the esophagus, are the predisposing factors for rupture at this level.[12] This is a relatively rare cause of esophageal perforation and accounted for 20 of the 115 patients described by Nesbitt and Sawyers.[12]

Abbott and associates presented a large series of 47 cases of strain-induced perforation of the esophagus and postulated three etiologic factors: (1) increased intraluminal pressure, (2) esophageal disease, and (3) neurogenic causes.[17] Preexisting esophageal disease (esophagitis, hiatal hernia, esophageal webs, strictures, achalasia, and neoplasm) may contribute to spontaneous perforation by weakening the esophageal wall. Occasionally, intracranial diseases or operations have been associated with esophageal perforation, presumably related to neurogenic vasospasm, ischemia, and subsequent perforation.[5, 12]

Perforation in Preexisting Esophageal Disease

A relatively rare cause of esophageal perforation is a preexisting carcinoma or esophagitis that leads to full-thickness penetration and perforation. In the series reported by Skinner and colleagues, 13 of 47 patients had perforation from a carcinoma and 2 from esophagitis.[18]

Injury From External Trauma

Iatrogenic Operative Trauma

Esophageal trauma has been reported as a complication of antireflux procedures, pneumonectomy, truncal vagotomy (0.5%), and, rarely, anterior cervical spinal fusion. During esophagomyotomy, a small mucosal perforation may be overlooked.[5]

Blunt External Trauma

Esophageal trauma resulting from blunt external injury is exceedingly rare and often overlooked. Beal and associates reported five cases (an incidence of 0.001% in their institution) and reviewed extensively the literature since 1900.[19] They found a total of 96 reported cases and analyzed 63 patients in detail.

Most cases of blunt esophageal rupture involved motor vehicle crashes (62%). Other causes included falls (11%), motorcycle crashes (5%), assault (3%), blast injuries (3%), Heimlich maneuvers (3%), driving into a suspended wire (3%), diving (2%), being hit by an elevator (2%), and unspecified mechanisms (2%). Extensive steering wheel damage was found in 34% of the motor vehicle collisions. The predominant site of rupture was in the cervical and upper esophageal regions (82.3%), and associated tracheoesophageal fistulas were noted in 28 patients. Middle thoracic (5 cases) and lower thoracic (6 cases) perforations were less frequent.

The exact mechanism of esophageal rupture from blunt external force is not clear. As postulated by Hagan, the lesion may be similar to a blast injury, whereby a sudden increase in intraluminal pressure, by compression of the chest and expulsion of air from the lungs against a closed glottis, produces a rupture at the site of the anatomically weak cervicothoracic esophagus.[20] Beal proposed a deceleration-traction injury that resulted in a compromised blood supply of the organ with a "delayed ischemic" perforation.[19] Another possible mechanism for cervical esophageal rupture is hyperextension of the neck with a shearing injury to the hypopharynx against the cervical vertebral bodies.

Penetrating Injury

Penetrating injury of the esophagus is uncommon. Nesbitt and Sawyers recorded this mechanism in only 14 patients in a series of 115 patients (see Table 2).[12] In a group of 600 patients with penetrating chest trauma, Oparah and Mandal found only 3 patients with esophageal injury.[21] From a busy trauma center, Symbas and associates described 48 patients with bullet wounds who were treated over a 15-year period.[22] Pass and associates, from Parkland Memorial Hospital, reported only 20 cases of esophageal gunshot wounds over a 13-year period.[23] In a 15-year experience, we noted only 21 patients with penetrating esophageal trauma. In most series, the cervical esophagus was involved much more often than was the thoracic esophagus.

Diagnosis of Esophageal Injury

The clinical symptoms early after perforation are nonspecific. Radiologic clues are subtle and easily overlooked. Consequently, delayed diagnosis of esophageal perforation is extremely common. This is especially true in iatrogenic trauma unrelated to endoscopy and after spontaneous perforation. Flynn and associates recorded a delay in diagnosis of more than 24 hours in half their cases.[13] Nesbitt and Sawyers noted a 58% incidence of delayed diagnosis.[12] In the collective series of Beal and colleagues, 68% of the cases had a delay in diagnosis of more than 24 hours.[19] In contrast, delayed diagnosis after penetrating trauma is uncommon, because established protocols usually require investigation of the esophagus for proximity or transmediastinal injuries. Unusual, and curious, delays do occur after penetrating trauma, however: Symbas and colleagues recorded one patient with a gunshot wound of the chest.[22] The bullet was thought to be in the hilum of the left lung on chest radiography. A correct diagnosis of esophageal injury was made when the patient passed the bullet through the rectum.

Because of the increased morbidity and mortality associated with delayed diagnosis, esophageal injury must be considered in every instance of esophageal instrumentation, penetrating injury in the vicinity of the organ, or appropriate clinical circumstances of increased pressure transmission to the structure (i.e., blast injury, forceful vomiting, upper abdominal trauma). Perforation after esophageal instrumentation in the presence of a diverticulum, stenosis, or foreign body is sufficiently common that routine chest radiography is recommended after these procedures.[13] Similarly, pneumatic dilatation of the esophagus should be followed by a routine chest radiograph and esophageal contrast study if the patient complains of pain.[13]

Clinical Symptoms and Signs

Pain is a frequent complaint of patients with esophageal perforation, occurring in 70% to 90% of cases. The pain usually is located in the chest with cervical perforation and may be referred to the abdomen with thoracic perforation.[5] Neck, chest, and abdominal pain were noted in 20 of the 63 patients reviewed by Beal and colleagues (Table 3).[19] Nesbitt and Sawyers recorded abdominal pain in 45% of their patients with spontaneous rupture and noted that the diagnosis was confused with perforated peptic ulcer, pancreatitis, and other conditions.[12] Pain preceded by repeated episodes of vomiting is a particularly important history that must be sought.

Dyspnea is the second most common symptom, especially with thoracic perforation, but is infrequently seen with cervical or abdominal perforation. It is more common in patients with a late diagnosis, and may be accompanied by cyanosis. Fever also may be a late manifestation.[12]

Subcutaneous emphysema and crepitation are seen often with cervical perforation, but may be difficult to elicit in patients with a thoracic or abdominal site of injury. In the series reported by Nesbitt and Sawyers, crepitation was noted in only 18% of patients, 3 of whom had a delayed diagnosis.[12] This study had a predominance of thoracic perforations, however. Pass and coworkers observed the following symptoms in 9 patients with cervical esophageal gunshot wounds: 5 with subcutaneous emphysema, 4 with respiratory distress, 3 with cervical hematoma, and 2 with hoarseness.[23] Subcutaneous emphysema was seen in only 4 of the 10 patients with thoracic perforation. Beal and associates observed crepitation in 36 (neck, 23; chest, 8; face, 5) of 63 patients with blunt esophageal rupture (cervicothoracic, 52; middle thoracic, 5; lower thoracic, 6; see Table 3).[19]

TABLE 3.
Clinical Features in External Esophageal Trauma

Clinical Feature	Symbas, 1980 (Gunshot wound, n=48)	Beal, 1988 (Blunt trauma, n=63)
Symptoms (%)		
Neck and chest pain	—	16(25)
Dyspnea	5(10)	15(24)
Cough	—	14(22)
Dysphagia	2 (4)	8(13)
Hoarseness	2 (4)	7(11)
Hemoptysis	3 (6)	6(10)
Others	9*(19)	10(16)
Physical findings (%)		
Cervical crepitation	10(20)	23(37)
Thoracic crepitation	2 ("crunch"; 4)	8(13)
Facial crepitation		5 (8)
Shock	13(27)	6(10)
Radiographic findings (%)		
Subcutaneous air	11(23)	
Cervical		12(19)
Mediastinal	4 (widening; 8)	10(16)
Thoracic		2 (3)
Hydrothorax or pneumothorax	17(35)	15(24)

*Bleeding from the mouth (8 patients), stridor (1 patient).

Careful examination for crepitation, therefore, is warranted in patients with suspected esophageal injury.

Radiography

Plain Radiographs

Radiographs of the neck and chest should routinely be obtained in patients with a potential for esophageal injury. Findings suggestive of the diagnosis are free air in the soft tissues of the neck and swelling behind the pharynx or trachea. Chest radiographs may reveal free mediastinal or cervical air (Fig 3), mediastinal widening, pneumothorax, or, in delayed cases, pulmonary infiltrates. The findings depend on the time elapsed since the perforation, the site of the perforation, and the integrity of the mediastinal pleura.[24] Mediastinal widening from edema and easily detectable pneumomediastinum are late findings. With an intact mediastinal pleura, hydrothorax or pneumothorax may not occur. Pneumothorax and

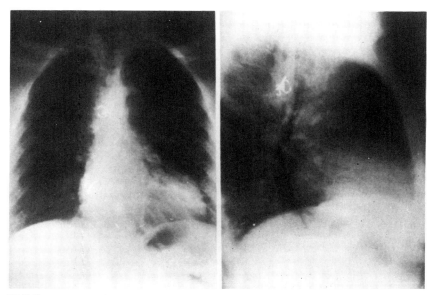

FIG 3.
Esophageal perforation during endoscopic removal of an inadvertently swallowed bridge work. Note the mediastinal air. (From Stirling MC, Orringer MB: Esophageal trauma, in Zuidema GD (ed): *Shackelford's Surgery of the Alimentary Tract,* 3rd ed. Philadelphia, WB Saunders, 1991, p 361. Used by permission.)

hydrothorax were uncommon (10 and 5 cases, respectively) among the 63 patients reviewed by Beal and colleagues.[19] Flynn and associates observed pneumomediastinum, pneumothorax, or effusion in only 20% to 36% of their patients with esophageal perforation.[13] The inconsistency and often subtle appearance of these findings demand careful scrutiny of plain radiographs.

Contrast Studies

Contrast esophagography is indicated to confirm the diagnosis, localize the site of perforation, and delineate the esophagus in terms of the presence or absence of associated esophageal pathology (Figs 4 and 5). The preferred contrast agent still is debated. Some prefer meglumine diatrizoate (Gastrografin), a water-soluble contrast medium, because of its relatively innocuous nature if extravasation occurs into the mediastinum or the pleura.[6] Its disadvantages include the following: (1) because of its high osmolality it may produce a severe pneumonitis (a salt-water drowning syndrome) if it is aspirated into the bronchial tree [25] and (2) it may not show extravasation in 5% to 10% of esophageal perforations because of its poor radiologic density. Barium, on the other hand, has superior radiologic density, is isosmotic, and provides excellent mucosal visualization. It suffers from the drawback, however, of producing, at least in experimental animals, severe mediastinitis and granuloma formation when extravasation occurs into the mediastinal tissues.[6]

Hankins and Attar recommend tailoring the type of contrast agent used to the clinical circumstance.[6] In patients with combined esophageal and tracheal injuries or suspicion of an abnormal communication between the esophagus and the tracheobronchial tree, thin barium is the agent of choice. Free perforation into the pleura or mediastinum (the presence of pneumomediastinum or pneumothorax) is demonstrated best by Gastrografin. Once gross extravasation is ruled out, a fluoroscopic study with thin barium is the next step to detect any small perforation that may have been overlooked by the Gastrografin study. DeMeester emphasizes proper positioning of the patient during contrast esophagography.[24] He suggests that contrast progression may be too rapid with the patient in the upright posi-

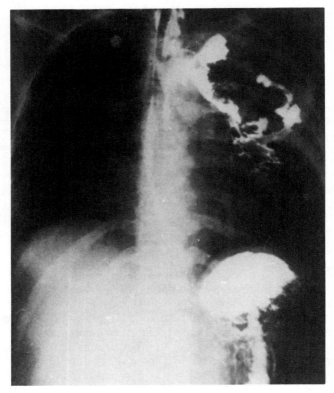

FIG 4.
Delayed recognition of an esophageal perforation. Note the contrast extravasation and pooling in a large abscess in the upper left hemithorax. (From Stirling MC, Orringer MB: Esophageal trauma, in Zuidema GD (ed): *Shackelford's Surgery of the Alimentary Tract,* 3rd ed. Philadelphia, WB Saunders, 1991, p 363. Used by permission.)

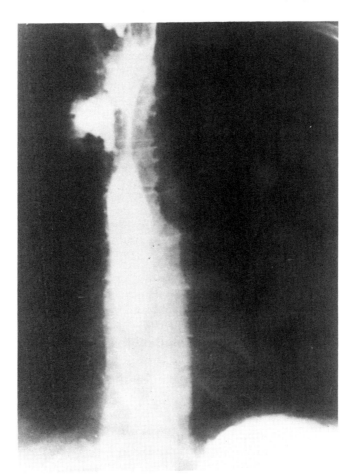

FIG 5.
Esophageal perforation during an emergency endotracheal intubation. Contrast extravasation is seen at the level of the cricopharyngeus muscle. (From Stirling MC, Orringer MB: Esophageal trauma, in Zuidema GD (ed): *Shackelford's Surgery of the Alimentary Tract*, 3rd ed. Philadelphia, WB Saunders, 1991, p 354. Used by permission.)

tion, and recommends that the study be performed in the right or left lateral decubitus position, using multiple-plane radiographs. With these precautions, the incidence of missed injuries by contrast studies may be reduced to less than 10%.[24] Contrast extravasation occurred in 93% of the patients described by Flynn and associates.[13]

Endoscopy

Endoscopy has limited applications when it is used alone. In cases of perforation caused by endoscopic manipulation of the esophagus, its use raises the first suspicion of injury and it is the first diagnostic modality. In cases of blunt or penetrating trauma in which the patient is rushed to the operating room for control of other injuries, intraoperative esophagoscopy may be used to rule out gross esophageal injury. Subtle perforations may be overlooked, especially by flexible endoscopy.[6, 25] It is our practice to perform both intraoperative endoscopy and postoperative contrast studies of the esophagus in such patients. In patients with suspicion of esophageal injury after external trauma, triple endoscopy (laryngoscopy, esophagoscopy, and bronchoscopy) is indicated.[19] Injury to one of these structures should raise the suspicion of injury to the adjacent organs. In their collective review of blunt esophageal trauma, Beal and colleagues noted a 56% incidence of associated injury to the trachea and larynx.[19] The same guidelines are recommended for missile wounds that cross the mediastinum, as well as those that penetrate the cervical region. The sensitivity and specificity of endoscopy in the diagnosis of esophageal injury are unknown, but are related to operator experience. The combination of contrast esophageal studies and endoscopy provides an accurate diagnosis in more than 90% of patients. Pass and associates described rigid esophagoscopy in 11 of their 20 patients.[23] Two false-negative results were obtained, one each in cases of cervical and thoracic perforation. These two injuries were subsequently discovered at operative exploration. Rigid esophagoscopy is considered superior to flexible endoscopy by some, but requires more expertise.[26]

Miscellaneous Diagnostic Methods

Computed tomography may occasionally be of use in the diagnosis of missed perforations and late anastomotic leaks by demonstrating a collection in the neck or thorax. An indium-labeled leukocyte scan may localize an abscess cavity in the neck or mediastinum and prompt a search for a missed esophageal perforation.[19]

Tube thoracostomy for a hydrothorax demonstrating a continuous air leak not in synchrony with respiration may suggest an esophageal injury. Occasionally, an esophageal leak has been confirmed by instilling methylene blue in the proximal esophagus and demonstrating the dye in the chest tube, but the tissue staining this produces may complicate the subsequent operative procedure.

Finally, operative exploration is a useful diagnostic modality.[22] In patients with pressing indications for surgical exploration (i.e., hemorrhage, vascular injury), the esophagus must be inspected in proximity injuries and explored operatively in the region of the penetrating wound. Adjunctive methods at exploration include the intraluminal instillation of saline or dye (methylene blue) with manual compression of the organ to exclude a leak, similar to the procedure performed after an esophagomyotomy. The same end may be achieved by filling the operative field with saline and vigorously injecting air into the esophagus to demonstrate an air leak.[22]

Reevaluation is important to avoid missing delayed perforations. Beal and coworkers reported delayed perforation of the esophagus after the finding of a hematoma on endoscopy or the institution of oral alimentation.[19] Esophageal foreign bodies are known to produce perforation 24 hours after ingestion, probably from a pressure necrosis.[12] The development of new signs, such as unexplained fever or pleural effusion, should raise the suspicion of esophageal perforation, and a complete workup must be repeated.

Treatment of Esophageal Injury

Sawyers has outlined the goals of therapy for esophageal perforation (Table 4).[25] These goals may be met through a wide range of treatment options, both operative and nonoperative. The approach chosen depends on the following factors:

1. Anatomic location of the perforation
2. Interval between the onset of perforation and the initiation of treatment
3. Whether the injury is contained or free
4. Severity of illness of the patient
5. Mechanism of injury
6. Whether the esophagus is normal or there is an associated lesion

Injuries to the Cervical Esophagus

The treatment method used for cervical esophageal perforation depends on the mechanism of injury. Perforation resulting from external trauma is usually treated surgically as part of an exploratory procedure dictated by the presence of cervical subcutaneous emphysema.[19, 22, 23] The diagnosis generally is not delayed. Neck exploration is performed through a left neck incision made along the anterior border of the sternocleidomastoid muscle with medial retraction of the carotid vessels. Adequate mobilization behind the trachea and palpation of the nasogastric tube facilitate identification of the esophagus. The recurrent laryngeal nerve must be protected during the

TABLE 4.
Goals of Treatment of Esophageal Perforation*

1. Stop soilage from the perforation.
2. Restore the integrity of the organ.
3. Eliminate infection from the extravasated esophageal contents.
4. Maintain nutrition of the patient.

dissection and often can be palpated or visualized.[25] The esophageal perforation is identified either by direct visualization or with the help of intraluminal saline or dye. The perforation is repaired in one or two layers. Neither the number of suture layers nor the type of suture material used (absorbable or nonabsorbable) seems to influence the incidence of fistulization after the repair.[25] If the operative exploration is delayed, suturing may be difficult because of extensive inflammation in the area. In either early or delayed operation, wide drainage is the key to success. Closed-suction drains (Jackson-Pratt) are used frequently, and are left in place for 5 to 7 days. Broad-spectrum antibiotics (usually a synthetic penicillin) are instituted. Most surgeons recommend performing a contrast study before removing the drains, because of the common occurrence of fistula without clinical symptoms.[6, 25] Nutritional support may be delivered through a nasogastric tube during this period.

Cervical esophageal fistulas are reported in 10% to 28% of cases after esophageal repair.[27, 28] Factors contributing to this complication include inadequate debridement, esophageal devascularization, tension on the suture line, and associated infection. The potential contribution of an associated tracheostomy to the development of esophageal fistula is discussed later. Adequate drainage, exclusion of distal obstruction, and maintenance of nutritional support are the cornerstones of fistula therapy, and most heal with time.[11, 28]

Nonoperative Treatment of Cervical Esophageal Perforation

Occasionally, some surgeons[25] advocate nonoperative treatment of cervical perforation if the following conditions are met: the perforation is localized, the extravasation "drains back into the esophagus," there is no distal obstruction, and the patient is not septic and has no symptoms related to the thorax.[29] Nonoperative therapy consists of antibiotics and restriction of oral intake. Several authorities emphasize that the leak should be small and the diagnosis made early for nonoperative therapy to be considered.[6, 25, 29] As many as 25% to 50% of such patients, usually with perforation resulting from endoscopy or dilatation, may be treated successfully by this approach.

Injuries of the Thoracic Esophagus

Nonoperative Therapy

A conservative, nonsurgical approach sometimes is advisable for thoracic esophageal perforation in selected patients. The clinical criteria for such an approach are listed in Table 5.

The reported experience with this approach has been small. Lyons and coworkers recorded a survival rate of 91% in a group of 11 patients with spontaneous and instrumental perforation of the esophagus who were treated with gastrostomy, chest tube drainage, and, in some cases, cervical

TABLE 5.
Selection Criteria for Nonoperative Treatment of Esophageal Perforation

Favorable conditions for nonoperative treatment:
1. Perforation localized, no diffuse extravasation of dye
2. Extravasation of dye drains back into esophagus
3. No distal obstruction or disease in esophagus
4. No evidence of systemic sepsis
5. No symptoms related to the thorax

Unfavorable conditions for nonoperative treatment:
1. Diffuse mediastinitis, free perforation
2. Pneumothorax, hydrothorax
3. Obstructing lesions in esophagus
4. Clinical evience of sepsis

---

mediastinotomy.[30] All the lesions were characterized as "free" perforations.

Cameron and colleagues emphasized that the perforation had to be contained for the patient to be eligible for nonoperative therapy.[29] In a group of eight patients with esophageal anastomotic leak (five patients), spontaneous (two patients), or postdilatation (one patient) perforation, they used restricted oral intake, antibiotics, and intravenous hyperalimentation. All the patients survived.

Livingstone supported the concept of nonoperative therapy in patients with achalasia who were treated by pneumatic dilatation.[25] Routine postdilatation contrast esophagograms sometimes demonstrated minor extravasation. If the perforation was contained and the patient had no systemic signs of sepsis, treatment with antibiotic therapy alone was successful.

Flynn and associates treated nonoperatively 8 of 69 patients with esophageal perforation.[13] These patients had the following characteristics: (1) cervical perforation and minimal symptoms (4 patients); (2) thoracic perforation, late diagnosis, contrast leak, and minimal signs of sepsis (2 patients); and (3) poor surgical risk because of advanced age and underlying disease (2 patients). The authors warned that this approach has no role in traumatic perforation of the esophagus because the wounding agent has violated the tissue planes that may have contained the leak.

Indications for Termination of Nonoperative Treatment.—As indicated by Michel and coworkers, surgical intervention is required if the patient worsens on conservative treatment or has a mediastinal abscess or empyema.[31] The presence or development of pneumothorax, pneumoperitoneum, systemic signs of sepsis, or shock are contraindications to a nonoperative approach (see Table 5).[29]

Operative Therapy

Operative repair is the treatment of choice for free thoracic perforation, whether the injury is diagnosed early (<24 hours) or late (>24 hours). The presence of systemic sepsis, pneumothorax, pneumomediastinum, or pneumoperitoneum is an indication for early thoracotomy and repair.

The operative approach consists of thoracotomy on the side of the leak (left thoracotomy for lower esophageal injury and right thoracotomy for upper esophageal injury), exposure of the esophagus, and thorough debridement of all necrotic tissue. The perforation is identified and closed. In cases of penetrating trauma, multiple perforations are common and should be sought diligently. The choice of suture material for closure of the perforation varies between surgeons, as does the preference for a two-layered closure with inner, absorbable and outer, nonabsorbable sutures.[25] Grillo has recommended the use of a pleural flap to cover the suture repair.[32] Other surgeons believe that, with early operation, the pleura is extremely thin and may not add to the suture repair.[25] In this context, perhaps the words of Orloff are worthy of recall[25]: "We all use flaps but I am not sure how much good they do. After I free up a pleural flap that is so thin you can almost see through it and wrap it around the esophagus, I have never been convinced how much good it actually does. Adequate drainage is far more important." Still others suggest using various neighboring structures as a "buttress" to the repair. These have included the diaphragm, intercostal muscle, a vascularized or free graft of pericardium, extracostal chest wall muscle, omentum, or a pedicled jejunal segment.[5, 6, 12] In the lower thoracic area, the gastric fundus has been used as an onlay type of patch by enlarging the esophageal hiatus and bringing the gastric fundus to the perforation. The fundus is sutured around the perforation, which is left unsutured.[25] Some surgeons use the gastric fundus as a "Thal" patch, and still others complete the gastric fundoplication. There is a potential problem of gastroesophageal reflux with gastric flaps that is not entirely prevented by partial or complete gastric wrapping around the lower esophagus.[6] Regardless of the surgical method used, it is extremely important that the area be drained extensively, usually with large-caliber chest tubes placed in the vicinity of the esophageal repair.

Treatment of Delayed Recognition of Esophageal Perforation.—The problems of delayed treatment include extensive mediastinitis, necrosis of the esophageal wall, and difficulty in closing the perforation effectively, even with various buttressing methods (Table 6). Even when repair is technically feasible, subsequent breakdown of the repair is the rule

TABLE 6.
Principles of Therapy for Esophageal Perforation: Late Diagnosis or Anastomotic Leak

1. Wide mediastinal drainage
2. Close with sutures, buttress with pleural or muscle flap
3. Gastrostomy
4. Feeding jejunostomy
5. Consider exclusion procedure
6. Consider esophagectomy and delayed reconstruction
7. Cervical esophagostomy
8. Systemic antibiotics
9. Computed tomography follow-up to diagnose and drain mediastinal collections

rather than the exception. It is in such patients that "exclusion" procedures have been practiced.

Exclusion of the Esophagus.—The rationale for esophageal exclusion is to exclude the repair from the rest of the esophagus and allow it to heal while nutritional support is maintained by the intravenous or enteral route. In 1956, Johnson and associates reported the successful use of this approach in two patients.[33] They diverted the cervical esophagus, transected the gastroesophageal junction, closed both ends, and maintained nutrition by a gastrostomy. The fistula healed and the patients subsequently had restoration of gastrointestinal continuity by jejunal interposition. The decision to perform exclusion or repair depends on the local findings at thoracotomy, as well as the time delay between perforation and operative treatment. In the series of Nesbitt and Sawyers, exclusion procedures generally were reserved for patients with a delay in treatment exceeding 48 hours.[12]

The principles of exclusion procedures are to (1) divert the esophagus from above, (2) prevent gastric reflux from below, and (3) drain the area widely, usually by tube thoracostomy.

Several variations of the esophageal exclusion procedure have been developed.

DIVERSION FROM ABOVE.—Abbott and colleagues used a long T tube with the side arm brought out through the perforation and the chest wall to divert the saliva and achieve a controlled fistula.[17] Urschel and colleagues performed a lateral cervical esophagostomy by making an opening in the cervical esophagus and suturing the opening to the skin.[34] Schwartz and

McQuarrie modified this approach with a muscle bridge between the two loops of the cervical esophagostomy to make the diversion more efficient.[35] Orloff completely divided the cervical esophagus, matured the proximal end as an ostomy, and left the distal end closed.[25] In his experience, the squamous epithelium of the esophagus did not continue to secrete mucus. Others have noted a mucocele of the esophagus in such circumstances. Livingstone suggested creating a modified lateral cervical esophagostomy by suturing a longitudinal opening in the esophagus to the skin.[25] Distal decompression is achieved with a nasogastric tube passed distally. Finally, Greenfield suggested applying a staple line in the cervical esophagus to exclude the perforation.[25]

DIVERSION FROM BELOW.—Urschel and colleagues used a Teflon band to ligate the distal esophagus, which was removed after the perforation healed.[34] Schwartz and McQuarrie used a Silastic band instead of Teflon to reduce adhesion formation.[35]

Recently, Urschel's group modified their original approach by looping the distal esophagus with a Prolene suture that is brought out of the abdomen along with a gastrostomy.[36] After the esophageal perforation healed, the Prolene suture was removed, without laparotomy, restoring esophageal continuity.

Livingstone suggested the use of a heavy chromic catgut suture around the esophagus.[25] Three to 6 weeks after surgery, the sutured area could be dilated open. He also recommended stapling of the distal esophagus as a suitable alternative. The staple line often opened up spontaneously and, if not, could be dilated open by "an interventional radiologist—with a guide wire."

The problem with exclusion-diversion procedures is that most patients require a second operation to restore continuity of the gastrointestinal tract after the fistula has healed. This involves colon or gastric interposition, depending on the surgeon's preference. In a small proportion of patients, the perforation or fistula heals with minimal deformity of the esophagus and the distal diversionary suture or staple line may be dilated to restore normal esophageal continuity.[25] Regardless of the approach used, adequate drainage and a feeding enterostomy are essential for a successful outcome.

The results of exclusion or exclusion-diversion have not been uniformly good. Gouge and associates reviewed the results of 58 cases collected from the literature in 1989.[37] The overall mortality rate was 35%. In an analysis of all causes of esophageal "leaks" (both perforations and anastomotic leaks), Richardson and associates condemned the exclusion procedures.[11] Six of their nine patients who received this treatment died of continued esophageal leak and sepsis. One of the three survivors could not be operated on again for esophageal reconstruction and was left with a permanent feeding jejunostomy. In addition, these authors questioned the physiologic basis for this operation and postulated that the excluded esophagus may enhance the drainage of mucus and bacteria through the perforation. Instead of complete exclusion, these authors preferred primary repair with a muscle buttress initially, reserving cervical esophagostomy for patients with continuing sepsis.

Alternative Approaches to Esophageal Exclusion (Variations of Nonoperative Therapy).—Santos and Frater described a system of "transesophageal irrigation of the mediastinum" as a method of conservative therapy in patients with a delayed diagnosis of spontaneous rupture that led to life-threatening mediastinitis from expulsion of the esophageal contents into the posterior mediastinum.[38] They reported excellent results (7 of 8 patients survived) with a Levin tube placed in the esophagus proximal to the tear, a chest tube placed in proximity to the esophagus, constant irrigation through the Levin tube, and continuous suction to the chest tube, a method that ensured constant mediastinal irrigation.

Another variant of mediastinal irrigation was described by Kanschin and Pogodina, who introduced a transnasal catheter through the esophageal perforation into the periesophageal mediastinal tissues for continuous irrigation.[39] McNamee and associates reported their experience with three cases of instrumental perforation and two cases of esophageal leak after repair.[40] All patients had a periesophageal abscess. The site of perforation was visualized by flexible endoscopy. A flexible guide wire was introduced through the perforation and into the abscess cavity under fluoroscopic guidance. The scope was withdrawn, leaving the guide wire in place. A pharyngotomy was performed with the help of an artery forceps, and a Salem sump tube was withdrawn almost entirely through the oral cavity. The tip of the tube was cut off, and the guide wire was introduced into the sump tube and brought out through its first side hole. Grasping this end, the sump tube was threaded over the guide wire, through the esophagus, and into the abscess. This was followed by minilaparotomy, gastrostomy, and jejunostomy. The cavity was irrigated continuously until postoperative sinograms demonstrated reduction and eventual obliteration of the cavity. All the patients survived. The authors observed that the patients were more comfortable with a pharyngotomy than with a nasogastric tube.

The Role of the Interventional Radiologist.—Maroney and associates described an appealing alternative to surgery in six poor-risk patients with delayed treatment or anastomotic or suture line failure of a perforated esophagus with mediastinitis.[41] In three patients, they placed a guide wire into a mediastinal abscess percutaneously under computed tomographic guidance. A sump tube then was placed over the guide wire and the abscess was drained. In three other patients, they placed a sump tube fluoroscopically through the nose into mediastinal collections using a method similar to that described above (Fig 6). Using serial sinograms, adequate drainage of the abscess cavities was ensured by readjusting the sump tubes as necessary (Fig 7). All six patients survived.

ESOPHAGEAL INTUBATION.—Esophageal tubes (e.g., Celestin tube, Sengstaken-Blakemore tube) have been recommended to "bypass" the perforation, allowing healing to occur in poor-risk patients in whom recognition of the injury was delayed.[6] These anecdotally reported techniques occasionally may prove useful in carefully selected patients.

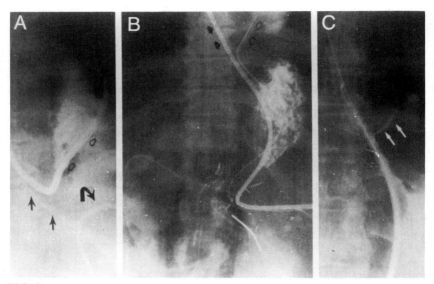

FIG 6.
The role of the interventional radiologist. **A,** a transnasal, transesophageal sump tube *(open arrows)* was placed into a large mediastinal fluid collection. A nasogastric tube with side holes *(straight arrows)* was used to divert esophageal contents. A percutaneous gastrojejunal feeding tube *(curved arrow)* was placed. **B,** a sump tube was placed percutaneously through the gastrostomy site, across the fistula, and into the abscess cavity. A second sump tube was placed into the esophagus through the gastrostomy. **C,** a small residual tract of dye extravasation into the abscess cavity is seen. This gradually closed spontaneously. (From Maroney TP, Ring EJ, Gordon RL, et al: *Radiology* 1989; 170:1055–1057. Used by permission.)

Esophageal Resection.—Emergency resection of the perforated esophagus is the treatment of choice if associated distal obstruction is present. The results of esophagectomy for simple or delayed perforation with or without associated esophageal disease have been poor in most series. In a collective series, Gouge and associates noted a mortality rate of 23% in 26 patients.[37] Based on these data, the authors recommended staged reconstruction (initial resection, followed by reestablishment of continuity when the patient's general status has improved). Richardson and associates also substantiated the high mortality rate with major esophageal resection.[11]

A more optimistic evaluation of emergency esophagectomy for esophageal disruption was recently reported by Orringer and Stirling.[42] A diverse group of 24 patients was presented, including 20 with preexisting esophageal disease (chronic stricture, achalasia, reflux esophagitis, carcinoma, diffuse esophageal spasm, and monilial esophagitis). Forty-five percent of the patients had a delay of more than 3 days before esophagectomy. Alimentary tract continuity was restored in 13 of the 24 patients by esophagogastric anastomosis. In 11 patients, the esophagus was resected, preserving as much of the normal organ as possible. The proximal esophagus then was delivered into the neck, tunneled in front of the clavicle, and the end constructed as an ostomy on the chest wall. There was only one anastomotic leak in the series. Of the 3 patients who died, one had a presumed pulmonary embolism. The authors felt that the risk of esophageal resection in these patients was less than that associated with repair or exclusion procedures. They preferred to avoid exclusion procedures in patients with perforation, because these could keep the source of intrathoracic sepsis active and complicate subsequent reconstruction. They also emphasized that a "safe esophagostomy" was an "end esophagostomy," and that as much of the length of the esophagus as possible should be preserved. The authors went on to suggest that transhiatal esophageal resection was a superior alternative to transthoracic esophagectomy if pleural contamination was minimal. In such patients, thorough irrigation of the pleural cavity through the hiatus and a cervical esophagogastrostomy were recommended. The

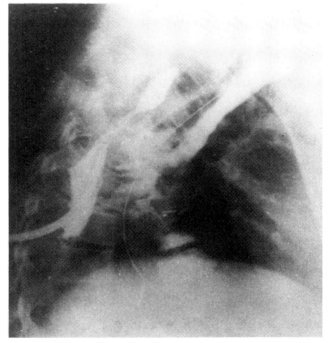

FIG 7.
Percutaneous placement of a sump tube to drain an abscess after esophageal surgery. (From Maroney TP, Ring EJ, Gordon RL, et al: *Radiology* 1989; 170:1055–1057. Used by permission.)

investigators concluded that, "the more critically ill the patient from an intrathoracic esophageal disruption,—the more compelling the argument for esophageal resection." Other, small series have documented a high survival rate with esophageal resection.[24, 43] This represents a significant change in the treatment of perforated esophagus, away from exclusion procedures. Surgeons and their teams must be well versed in esophagectomy for optimal results. As these series have shown, the option of esophageal resection, "as radical as it may seem,"[42] offers promise in carefully selected patients.

Treatment of the Underlying Esophageal Condition or Disease.—If the perforated esophagus is the site of preexisting disease, it generally is agreed that, if at all possible, the underlying pathology should be treated at the time of repair, with or without reconstruction.[6]

Resection is definitely indicated in the following circumstances:

1. Obstructing carcinoma distal to the perforation
2. Extensive, nondilatable stricture of the esophagus distal to the perforation
3. Necrosis of the esophageal wall from extensive ingestion of caustic substances

Resection is not indicated in these circumstances[6, 25]:

1. Unresectable, extensive carcinoma with esophagobronchial fistulas. These patients have such a poor life expectancy that esophageal resection should be avoided and local drainage and antibiotics used.
2. Perforation in achalasia. These patients are best treated by closure of the perforation and careful esophagomyotomy.
3. Perforation during dilatation of a benign stricture. The perforation may be closed and an antireflux procedure considered.
4. Perforation during sclerotherapy. This is a difficult problem because of the patients' poor nutritional and general condition. In addition, the perforation may occur 24 to 72 hours after the sclerotherapy. Orloff recommends a conservative approach.[25] For small leaks, nasogastric intubation and systemic antibiotics may be adequate. Thoracostomy drainage, repeated computed tomography scans, and interventional radiology to establish appropriate thoracostomy drainage are required for larger leaks. For large, free perforations, esophageal exclusion may be necessary. The prognosis is poor in this group of patients.

Results and Prognostic Considerations

The results of various approaches to esophageal perforation have been presented in the section discussing treatment. Survival depends on factors other than the surgeon's approach to the problem. Richardson and associates, in an analysis of 75 patients with esophageal perforation (traumatic,

19 patients; spontaneous, 5 patients; iatrogenic, 32 patients) and anastomotic leaks (19 patients), found the following factors to be important in predicting mortality[11]:

1. Preexisting disease
2. Treatment delay of more than 12 hours
3. Esophageal exclusion and diversion
4. Thoracic site of perforation
5. Anastomotic leak
6. Major esophageal resection
7. Total parenteral nutrition

Hankins and Attar, in an analysis of 64 patients, identified these factors as predictive of mortality[6]:

1. Age
2. Location (cervical perforation was associated with better survival than was thoracic injury)
3. Spontaneous perforation (this produced a higher mortality than did intraluminal or extraluminal injury)
4. Treatment delay of more than 24 hours

In this series, neither the mode of treatment nor the presence of preexisting esophageal disease had a statistically significant influence on mortality. It is apparent from these and other series that spontaneous perforation in a thoracic location associated with a delayed diagnosis has a much poorer prognosis. A survival rate of 92% was reported in one series, however, when primary closure was accomplished within 24 hours.[44] The emphasis, therefore, should be placed on early diagnosis facilitated by a high index of suspicion.

Special Considerations

Combined Tracheoesophageal Injuries

Especially in the setting of trauma, combined tracheoesophageal injuries pose special problems, for several reasons: (1) they are distinctly uncommon and, thus, may lead to treatment errors because of the inexperience of the trauma surgeon; and (2) they produce unique technical problems and may be associated with complex complications in the remote postoperative period.

Feliciano and colleagues brought these injuries to attention in 1985 with a report of an 11-year experience with 23 patients.[27] Combined tracheoesophageal injuries were diagnosed by physical examination in 7 patients. Endoscopy contributed to the diagnosis in 6 patients, and 6 others underwent a combination of these tests, in addition to a barium swallow. Two patients had routine cervical exploration and 2 had resuscitative thoracotomy. Tracheal and esophageal repairs were performed by standard techniques. Five of 6 patients who underwent primary repair of the trachea and esophagus did well without tracheostomy. Many complications were seen in 13 patients with tracheostomy. Of 6 patients who had tracheoesophageal fistulas, 5 had no interposition muscle flap placed between the tracheal and esophageal repairs. Based on their experience, the authors made the following recommendations for improved treatment of combined tracheoesophageal injuries:

1. The addition of tracheostomy to a simple repair of the trachea may actually result in increased infectious morbidity from pneumonia, mediastinal abscess, and wound infection.
2. For extensive esophageal injuries in the cervical area, a cervical esophagostomy (side or end) should be considered at the initial operation (Fig 8). This may prevent subsequent complications such as tracheoesophageal fistula, carotid blowout, and mediastinal abscess.
3. Sternocleidomastoid or strap muscle interposition flaps should be used between tracheal and esophageal repairs, as well as to cover carotid artery repairs (Fig 9).
4. Drainage of combined cervical injuries should be directed anteriorly and through the contralateral neck if a carotid artery injury is present (Fig 10).

The role of tracheostomy in combined tracheoesophageal injuries was examined further by Winter and Wrigelt in a study of 46 penetrating esophageal wounds.[28] Eighteen of the patients had 25 complications, including 4 (9%) esophageal fistulas. Contrary to the advice of Feliciano and colleagues, these authors felt that there was no need for liberal use of cervical esophagostomy because the fistulas were easily controlled with subsequent spontaneous closure.[27] The 4 patients with a fistula had a tracheostomy performed for airway control, either in the emergency department (3 patients) or for a tracheal injury (1 patient). Of all the variables examined, only the presence of shock and tracheostomy were statistically associated with esophageal fistula.

Although these observations do not prove a cause-and-effect relationship between tracheostomy and esophageal fistula, possible mechanisms include contamination of the cervical tissue planes and compression by the tracheostomy tube balloon on the esophageal repair. Security of the airway is important and must be ensured. If this cannot be accomplished by other methods, such as a nasotracheal or orotracheal tube, a tracheostomy may be unavoidable. The performance of tracheostomy must be a deliberate decision, however, and not a "routine" practice.

Thoracoscopy in Esophageal Injuries

With recent advances in video endoscopy, video-assisted thoracic surgery (VATS) has entered the field of esophageal surgery. Reports are forthcom-

Esophageal Injury / 271

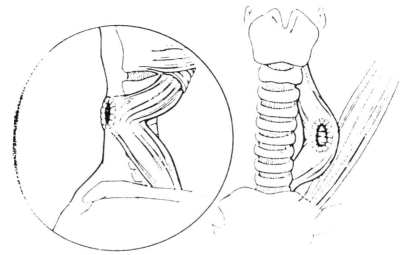

FIG 8.
Construction of a cervical esophagostomy for combined tracheoesophageal injuries. (From Feliciano DV, Bitondo CG, Mattox KL, et al: *Am J Surg* 1985; 150:710–715. Used by permission.)

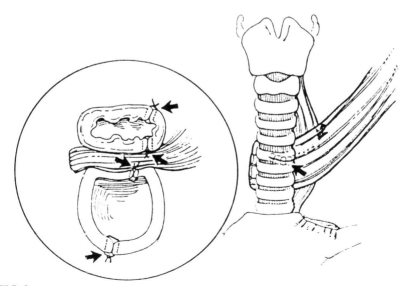

FIG 9.
Sternocleidomastoid or strap muscle flap interposition between tracheal and esophageal repairs helps healing and protects the tracheal suture line in the event of an esophageal leak. (From Feliciano DV, Bitondo CG, Mattox KL, et al: *Am J Surg* 1985; 150:710–715. Used by permission.)

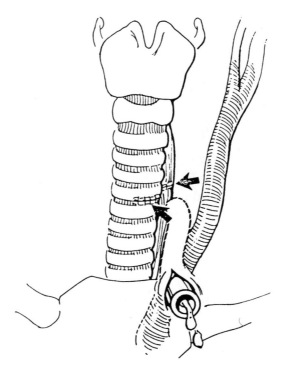

FIG 10.
Drains placed after esophageal repair should be directed anteriorly so that they do not cross over the carotid artery. (From Feliciano DV, Bitondo CG, Mattox KL, et al: *Am J Surg* 1985; 150:710–715. Used by permission.)

ing on the role of thoracoscopy in excising esophageal tumors as well as the organ itself. Thoracoscopic identification and repair of esophageal perforation has been reported.[44] This modality may have the potential to enable earlier, more efficient recognition of esophageal injury.

Summary

The clinical importance of the esophagus in the fields of critical care, and trauma and thoracic surgery lies in the often insidious and unsuspected nature of injury to this organ. Successful therapy depends on early diagnosis, which can be achieved only through heightened awareness. Judicious selection of operative vs. nonoperative therapy, adequate nutritional support, and appropriate antibiotic treatment are the basics of good patient care. Buttressed repair is the preferred operative approach. Drainage must be efficient. Resectional therapy in the presence of concomitant esophageal disease or established mediastinitis, instead of esophageal exclusion, holds promise and requires further evaluation.

References

1. Meade RH: *A History of Thoracic Surgery.* Springfield, Ill, Charles C Thomas, 1961.
2. Frink NW: Spontaneous rupture of the esophagus: Report of case with recovery. *J Thorac Surg* 1947; 16:291.
3. Barrett NR: Report of a case of spontaneous rupture of the esophagus successfully treated by operation. *Br J Surg* 1947; 35:216.
4. Olsen AM, Clagett OT: Spontaneous rupture of the esophagus. *Postgrad Med* 1947; 2:417.
5. Michel L, Grillo HC, Malt RA: Esophageal perforation. *Ann Thorac Surg* 1982; 33:203–210.
6. Hankins JR, Attar S: Esophageal injuries, in Turney SZ, Rodriguez A, Cowley A (eds): *Management of Cardiothoracic Trauma.* Baltimore, Md, Williams & Wilkins, 1990, pp 197–218.
7. Silvis SE, Nebel O, Rogers G, et al: Endoscopic complications: Results of the 1974 American Society of Gastrointestinal Endoscopy. *JAMA* 1976; 235:928–930.
8. Katz D: Morbidity and mortality in standard and flexible gastrointestinal endoscopy. *Gastrointest Endosc* 1969; 15:134–141.
9. Postlethwait RW: Surgery of the esophagus, 2nd ed. East Norwalk, Conn, Appleton-Century-Crofts, 1986, pp 17–19.
10. Goldstein LA, Thompson WR: Esophageal perforations: A 15 year experience. *Am J Surg* 1982; 143:495–503.
11. Richardson JD, Martin LF, Borzotta AP, et al: Unifying concepts in treatment of esophageal leaks. *Am J Surg* 1985; 149:157–162.
12. Nesbitt JC, Sawyers JL: Surgical management of esophageal perforation. *Am Surg* 1987; 53:183–191.
13. Flynn AE, Verrier ED, Way LW, et al: Esophageal perforation. *Arch Surg* 1989; 124:1211–1215.
14. Kinsella TJ, Morse RW, Hertzog AJ: Spontaneous rupture of the esophagus. *J Thorac Surg* 1984; 17:613–631.
15. Mackler SA: Spontaneous rupture of the esophagus: An experimental and clinical study. *Surg Gynecol Obstet* 1952; 95:345–356.
16. Guth AA, Gouge THE, Depan HJ: Blast injury to the thoracic esophagus. *Ann Thorac Surg* 1991; 51:837–839.
17. Abbott OA, Mansour KA, Logan WD, et al: Atraumatic so-called "spontaneous" rupture of the esophagus: A review of 47 personal cases with comments on a new method of surgical therapy. *J Thorac Cardiovasc Surg* 1970; 59:67–83.
18. Skinner DB, Little AG, deMeester TR: Management of esophageal perforation. *Am J Surg* 1980; 139:760–764.
19. Beal SL, Pottmeyer EW, Spisso JM: Esophageal perforation following blunt trauma. *J Trauma* 1988; 28:1425–1432.
20. Hagan WE: Pharyngoesophageal perforations after blunt trauma to the neck. *Otolaryngol Head Neck Surg* 1983; 91:620–626.
21. Oparah SS, Mandal AK: Operative management of penetrating wounds of the chest in civilian practice: Review of indications in 125 consecutive cases. *J Thorac Cardiovasc Surg* 1979; 77:162.
22. Symbas PN, Hatcher CR, Clasis SE: Esophageal gunshot injuries. *Ann Surg* 1980; 191:703–707.

23. Pass LJ, LeNarz LA, Screiber JT, et al: Management of esophageal gunshot wounds. Ann Thorac Surg 1987; 44:253–256.
24. DeMeester TR: The perforation of the esophagus (editorial). Ann Thorac Surg 1986; 42:231–232.
25. Sawyers JL, Greenfield LJ, Livingstone AS, et al: Esophageal perforation. Contemp Surg 1991; 39:91–110.
26. Carter PR: Discussion of companion article. Arch Surg 1989; 124:1215.
27. Feliciano DV, Bitondo CG, Mattox KL, et al: Combined tracheobronchial injuries. Am J Surg 1985; 150:710–715.
28. Winter RP, Wrigelt JA: Cervical esophageal trauma. Arch Surg 1990; 125:849–852.
29. Cameron JL, Kieffer RF, Hendrix TR, et al: Selective nonoperative management of contained intrathoracic esophageal disruption. Ann Thorac Surg 1979; 27:404–408.
30. Lyons WS, Seremetis MC, deGuzman VC, et al: Ruptures and perforations of the esophagus: The case of conservative supportive management. Ann Thorac Surg 1978; 25:346–350.
31. Michel L, Grillo HC, Malt RA: Operative and nonoperative management of esophageal perforations. Ann Surg 1981; 194:57–63.
32. Grillo HC: Esophageal perforation. Surg Rounds 1983; 6:50–71.
33. Johnson J, Schwegman CW, Kirby CK: Esophageal exclusion for persistent fistula following spontaneous rupture of the esophagus. J Thorac Surg 1956; 32:827–832.
34. Urschel HC Jr, Razzuk MA, Wood RE, et al: Improved management of esophageal perforation: Exclusion and diversion in continuity. Ann Surg 1974; 179:587–591.
35. Schwartz ML, McQuarrie DG: Surgical management of esophageal perforation. Surg Gynecol Obstet 1980; 151:668–670.
36. Gouge THE, Depan HJ, Spencer FC: Experience with the Grillo pleural wrap procedure in 18 patients with perforation of the thoracic esophagus. Ann Surg 1989; 209:612–619.
37. Urschel HC JR: Discussion of companion article. Ann Surg 1989; 209:612–619.
38. Santos GH, Frater RWM: Transesophageal irrigation for the treatment of mediastinitis produced by esophageal rupture. J Thorac Cardiovasc Surg 1986; 91:57–62.
39. Santos GH: Spontaneous esophageal rupture (letter). Ann Thoac Surg 1991; 52:1369.
40. McNamee CJ, Meyns B, Pagliero KM: New method for dealing with late-presenting spontaneous esophageal rupture. Ann Thorac Surg 1991; 52:151–153.
41. Maroney TP, Ring EJ, Gordon RL, et al: Role of interventional radiology in the management of major esophageal leaks. Radiology 1989; 170:1055–1057.
42. Orringer MB, Stirling MC: Esophagectomy for esophageal disruption. Ann Thorac Surg 1990; 49:35–43.
43. Attar S, Hankins JR, Sutter CM: Esophageal perforation: A therapeutic challenge. Ann Thorac Surg 1990; 50:45.
44. Nathanson LK, Gotley D, Smithers M, et al: Videothorascopic primary repair of early distal oesophageal perforation. Aust N Z J Surg 1993; 63:399.

Early Fixation of Long-Bone Fractures

Lawrence B. Bone, M.D.

Associate Professor of Orthopaedic Surgery, State University of New York at Buffalo; Director of Musculoskeletal Trauma Service, Erie County Medical Center, Buffalo, New York

Philip M. Stegemann, M.D.

Clinical Assistant Professor of Orthopaedic Surgery, State University of New York at Buffalo, Erie County Medical Center, Buffalo, New York

Historical Perspective

During World War I, the mortality rate for an open fracture of the femur was 80%. With minimal stabilization of the femur using a Thomas splint, the mortality rate dropped to 16%.[1] The reason that mortality was reduced by the use of the Thomas splint initially was not recognized, but has since been attributed to the traction effect of the splint in restoring the length of the bone and reducing the volume of the muscle compartment and, thereby, the amount of blood lost. This simple maneuver saved many lives. It was not until the 1970s, however, that operative stabilization of femur fractures was recognized to reduce morbidity and mortality.

Peltier showed a relationship between the fat emboli syndrome and long-bone fractures in 1957.[2] Not until the mid-1970s, however, did reports from Europe indicate the beneficial effect of further stabilization with internal fixation in the early period after injury in reducing fat emboli syndrome and pulmonary failure. In an early series in 1976, Riska in Helsinki reported a decrease in the incidence of fat emboli syndrome from 22% in the 384 patients treated nonoperatively for long-bone fracture to 4% in the 245 patients treated with early operative stabilization.[3] All patients had multiple injuries and were cared for in the intensive care unit. A prospective study performed by Riska from 1975 to 1978 on 211 patients with multiple injuries and long-bone fractures treated with early internal fixation showed a further decrease in the fat emboli syndrome to 1.4%.[4]

In The Netherlands, Goris also showed a significant decrease in respiratory complications when patients with major trauma and long-bone fractures underwent early stabilization.[5] He retrospectively studied 58 consecutive trauma patients admitted to the University Hospital at Nijmegen between 1977 and 1980. The patients were placed in three groups. Those who underwent early endotracheal intubation for respiratory control and early fracture stabilization had the lowest rates of death, pulmonary failure, and adult respiratory distress syndrome (ARDS), and the lowest rate of late mortality from sepsis.

Early Fracture Fixation

Femur fractures traditionally were treated with skeletal traction until they healed enough for the patient to be stabilized in a spica cast. The balanced skeletal traction, however, forced the patient to remain in a supine position for 6 to 10 weeks. With the development of North American trauma centers and the specialization of orthopaedic traumatologists, earlier stabilization of these injuries was accomplished with either intramedullary rods or plate and screw fixation. During the 1980s, numerous retrospective reviews of early vs. delayed stabilization of long-bone fractures, especially femur fractures, were performed. In 1980, Meek from Vancouver, British Columbia, reviewed the effects of early operative vs. nonoperative treatment of long-bone fractures in patients sustaining blunt trauma.[6] His patients had an average injury severity score (ISS) of 38. Of the 22 patients who underwent early stabilization, 1 died, compared with 14 of the 49 patients who received nonoperative therapy for their femur fractures. This occurred even though the groups appeared to be identical on admission on the basis of several criteria.

A large retrospective study of 132 patients treated at Parkland Memorial Hospital in Dallas, Texas, was performed by Johnson.[7] Included in his study were patients with at least two long-bone fractures or one major long-bone fracture and a spinal or pelvic fracture. The ISS in all cases was at least 18.[8] Among the 132 patients in the study, 511 fractures were identified, for an average of 3.9 fractures per patient. Johnson analyzed two groups of patients: those with early fracture stabilization within the first 24 hours of injury and those with an indefinite delay of at least 48 hours. The mean ISS of the 83 patients with early fracture stabilization was 38.2. Adult Respiratory Distress Syndrome (ARDS) developed in 7% of these patients. Among the group of 49 patients who underwent late stabilization, the mean ISS was 38. ARDS developed in 39% of these patients. A stepwise logistic regression was performed on the data to identify the important factors associated with the presence of ARDS. The dependent variable was the absence or presence of ARDS. The independent variables tested were age, sex, number of injuries, ISS, units of blood transfused during the first week, presence or absence of early fracture stabilization, date of first surgery, and length of operation. In the group of patients with ARDS, the average intensive care unit stay, duration of intubation, and length of hospitalization were longer than in the group without ARDS. The independent variables that contributed significantly to the prediction of ARDS by this process were the ISS and early fracture stabilization. In a group of patients with an ISS of 40 or greater (the more severely injured patients), the effect of early stabilization was even more significant. ARDS developed in 17% of the patients who underwent early fracture stabilization, compared with 75% of those who received late stabilization. Based on these results, Johnson drew the following conclusions: (1) the incidence of ARDS increases with a higher ISS and a delay in fracture stabilization; (2) the more severe are the patient's injuries (i.e., ISS >40), the more significant is fracture stabilization in preventing ARDS; (3) patients with an ISS higher than 40 have an increased mortality rate associated with a delay in fracture stabilization; and (4) major systemic infection is associated with a delay in fracture stabilization, as is ARDS.

Seibel and colleagues reviewed 56 patients with an ISS of 22 or greater associated with a femur or acetabular fracture and at least one other injury.[9] These patients had a total of 446 recognized anatomic injuries, 576 diagnoses, and 516 procedures. They were divided into three groups: (1) those who received immediate stabilization of their fractures and postoperative ventilatory support; (2) those who were given ventilatory support and left in skeletal traction for at least 10 days; and (3) those who remained in skeletal traction for an average of 30 days. When the three groups were compared, a statistically significant increase in acute care days was seen from group 1 to group 3. There also was a statistically significant increase in days of ventilation of 3.4, 9.7, and 21, respectively, for the three groups. In addition, a significant increase in fracture complications was noted with prolonged skeletal traction. Seibel observed a close association between pulmonary failure and sepsis, and the duration of femoral traction. Ten days of femoral traction doubled the period of pulmonary failure and the cost of care, and quadrupled the incidence of fracture complications.

Further documentation of the beneficial effect of early long-bone fracture stabilization was provided in 1990 by Behrman and associates.[10] A retrospective study was performed comparing 121 patients stabilized within the first 48 hours of injury vs. 218 patients stabilized after 48 hours. This study was similar to Johnson's in that more severely injured patients (ISS ≥ 36) obtained a greater benefit from early stabilization, with a decreased incidence of both ARDS and increasing pulmonary shunt. Late fixation resulted in a significantly longer stay in the intensive care unit and a more extended hospitalization.

These retrospective studies corroborated the results of the earlier studies performed in Europe. They were limited by their retrospective nature, however. Therefore, a prospective, randomized study was undertaken between September 1984 and September 1986 by Bone and coworkers from Parkland Memorial Hospital in Dallas, Texas.[11] All patients admitted to the Parkland Memorial Hospital with acute femur fractures were assigned randomly either to early stabilization within 24 hours of injury or to late stabilization after 48 hours. Based on the previous retrospective reviews, 48 hours was the maximum delay that the authors believed would be safe without increasing mortality. The patients were divided into those with an ISS of less than 18 (primarily isolated femur fractures) and those with an ISS of 18 or higher (82 multiply injured patients). The latter group showed the greatest benefit from early stabilization. Forty-five patients were randomized to early fixation and 37 were randomized to fixation after 48 hours. The two groups were identical in terms of ISS (average ISS, 31) and similar in age (27.9 vs. 29.4 years), and had comparable associated injuries. Among the 37 patients who had delayed stabilization of their femur fracture, ARDS developed in 5 (13.5%), compared to only 1 (2%) of the 45 patients who had early stabilization. In addition, 14 of the patients with delayed stabilization had pulmonary complications in the form of pneumonia, pulmonary dysfunction, or fat emboli syndrome. No additional pulmonary complications developed in the group that underwent early fracture stabilization. This increase in the pulmonary failure state increased the time spent using a ventilator, the number of days spent in the intensive care unit, and the overall hospital stay for the delayed treatment group. This was associated with increased costs of more than $13,000 per patient.

This prospective, randomized study clearly shows that long-bone fracture stabilization within 24 hours of injury in the multiply injured patient (i.e., ISS ≥18) has a significant benefit in reducing pulmonary failure. Because 48 hours was the length of delay used in the study, no difference in the mortality rate was observed between the early and delayed treatment groups. The femur fracture was the dependent variable, with all other fractures and serious injuries treated within the first 24 hours.

The results of all these studies indicate that morbidity is increased in patients with multiple injuries when major fracture stabilization is delayed more than 48 hours. Mortality rates appear to be increased with delayed stabilization as well. Johnson pointed out in his retrospective study that the mortality rate was higher in those patients with an ISS of greater than 40 and delay in fracture stabilization.[7] To define better the decreased mortality rate in multiply injured patients who undergo early fracture fixation, Bone performed a multicenter study using data from six trauma centers,[12,13] all of which followed a protocol emphasizing early fracture stabilization in patients with multiple injuries. A group of 676 patients from these trauma centers was compared with a group of 906 patients from the American College of Surgeons' Multitrauma Outcome Study of 1985 and 1986.[14] The criteria for inclusion in both studies were an ISS of at least 18, a minimum age of 16 years, and the presence of at least one of the following fractures: femur, pelvis or acetabulum, both tibias, or one tibia associated with other fractures. Patients had to survive initial resuscitation and be taken to the operating room. Both groups were divided according to age (<50 or >50 years) and ISS (18 to 34, 35 to 45, 46 to 60, or >60). Among patients younger than 50 years who had an ISS of 18 to 34, 350 underwent early fixation, with a 5.1% mortality rate. In the comparable Multitrauma Outcome Study group, there were 570 patients with an 11.8% mortality rate. There were 104 patients with an ISS of 35 to 45 who received early fixation, with an 11.5% mortality rate. In the comparable Multitrauma Outcome Study group, there were 97 patients with a

25.8% mortality rate. The mortality rate was reduced similarly in patients with a higher ISS, but the number of patients in each group was too small to allow comparisons to be made.

Among patients 50 years and older, 137 underwent early stabilization, with an 8% mortality rate. Among the 159 patients of the comparable Multitrauma Outcome Study group, the mortality rate was 26.4% with an ISS of 18 to 34. An even greater increase was present in patients with an ISS of 35 to 45: 31 underwent early fixation and had a mortality rate of 18.4%. The mortality rate among a similar group of 26 patients in the Multitrauma Outcome Study was 42.3%. These data support previous retrospective work by Johnson and Border showing an increased mortality rate in patients with multiple injuries in whom fracture stabilization is not emphasized.

All reports indicate that multiply injured patients with major musculoskeletal injury benefit from early fracture stabilization.

Indications for Early Long-Bone Stabilization

The data presented clearly shows a beneficial rate in reducing morbidity and mortality in the multiply injured patient, i.e., ISS with early fracture stabilization. Long-bone fracture stabilization, especially of the femur, should be performed in all hemodynamically stable patients who are adequately oxygenated and would benefit from the procedure. This includes children, who have been shown to benefit from early fracture stabilization as much as adults. Pediatric patients may be stabilized using intramedullary rods (if the child is large enough), plate fixation, or external fixation.

Some debate has surrounded the use of early fracture stabilization in patients with significant closed head injury. Because the femur fracture is not an immediately life-threatening injury, the safety of a general anesthetic and operative procedure in a patient with increased intracranial pressure is questionable. Hoffman and Goris performed a retrospective study to assess the effect of early fracture stabilization on the outcome of patients with severe head injury (i.e., a Glasgow Coma Scale score of 7 or less).[15-17] In a series of 58 consecutive patients, 15 underwent early fracture stabilization and 43 had a delayed procedure. The brain injuries were similar on computed tomographic scanning in both groups. Mortality was lower in the group that received early stabilization, despite a significantly higher ISS. There were 2 deaths among 15 patients who underwent early stabilization compared with 20 deaths among 43 patients who received late stabilization ($P < .02$).

These results are similar to those obtained by Bone.[12] Glasgow Coma Scale scores, as reported in the emergency department, were used in both the multicenter study and the Multitrauma Outcome Study. Among patients younger than 50 years who had the most serious head injury (i.e., Glasgow Coma Scale score of 8 or less), the mortality rate was 18% in those who underwent early fixation compared to a mortality rate of 38% in the Multitrauma Outcome Study group. The anatomic brain lesions were not identified in this review, somewhat limiting the usefulness of the data. The statistical significance is great enough, however, to suggest that at least no increased mortality is associated with early fracture stabilization in patients with serious head injury.

Recent controversy has arisen over the potentially harmful effect of using reamed intramedullary rods for stabilization of femur fractures in patients with multiple injuries who have pulmonary contusion or multiple rib fractures.[18, 19] Animal studies have shown that reaming of an intact femur produces significant fat emboli into the right ventricle.[20] The effect of this embolization of intramedullary fat is reduced in the fractured femur, however.[21] Animal studies also reveal an increase in vascular permeability accompanying fat embolization.[22] Clinical studies have not supported the hypothesis that there is an increased rate of ARDS or death in patients with chest injuries and femoral fractures who are treated with reamed intramedullary rods.[23] Because of the high incidence of pulmonary failure and ARDS in patients with pulmonary contusion, it is impossible to demonstrate an increase in this rate caused by the use of intramedullary reaming for femur fracture stabilization.[24-26]

Case I.—A 45-year-old man was involved in a head-on motor vehicle accident. He sustained bilateral hemopneumothoraces and bilateral pulmonary contusions (Fig 1). His initial Po_2 was 26 mm Hg on room air (Table 1). He also had a closed head injury, a Glasgow Coma Scale score of 10, and a left midshaft femur fracture (Fig 2). The patient was resuscitated and stabilized. Bilateral chest tubes were placed and he was taken to the operating room for reamed intramedullary stabilization of his left femur (Fig 3) within 2 hours of his injury. A 12-mm intramedullary rod was used after minimal reaming of the femoral canal to 12.5 mm. He tolerated

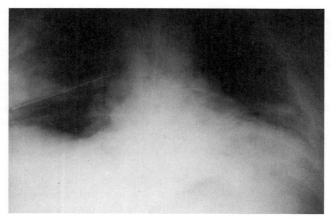

FIG 1.
Radiograph of chest showing bilateral pulmonary contusion with bilateral chest tubes.

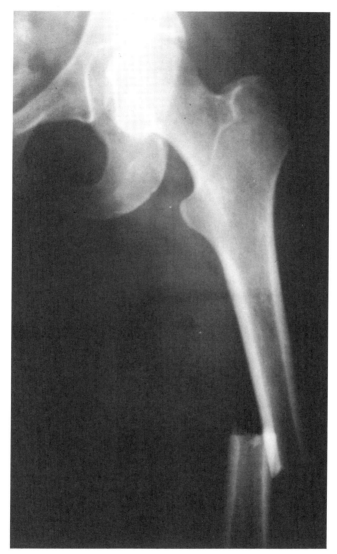

FIG 2.
Radiograph of femur fracture (case I).

this procedure well and was admitted to the intensive care unit for observation with intubation still in place.

By the first postoperative day, his Po_2 had improved to 145 mm Hg on 50% FIO_2 (Table 2). By the fourth postoperative day, he was extubated on a 40% venting mask (Table 3), and significant improvement was seen in the chest radiograph (Fig 4).

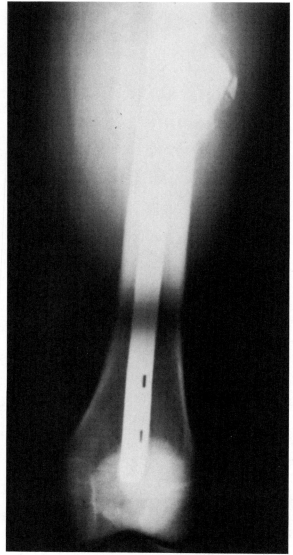

FIG 3.
Radiograph of intramedullary rod for left femur fracture (case I).

Because of his chest injury, it was thought that femur stabilization was essential to avoid skeletal traction in the forced supine position. A small reamed intramedullary rod was placed, reducing the effect of reaming. An unreamed intramedullary rod could have been used or even plate and screw stabilization. It is my opinion that, by stabilizing this patient's femoral fracture rapidly, pulmonary complications

TABLE 1.
Initial Arterial Blood Gases on Room Air: Case 1

Blood Gas	Level
pH	7.31
P_{CO_2}	53
P_{O_2}	26
Bicarbonate	27

TABLE 2.
Postoperative Arterial Blood Gases: Day 1*

Blood Gas	Level
pH	7.34
P_{CO_2}	45
P_{O_2}	145

*Arterial blood gas levels with 50% F_{IO_2}, 5 positive end-expiratory pressure.

TABLE 3.
Postoperative Blood Gases: Day 4*

Blood Gas	Level
pH	7.46
P_{CO_2}	36
P_{O_2}	126

*Patient extubated on the fourth day after injury; 40% mask.

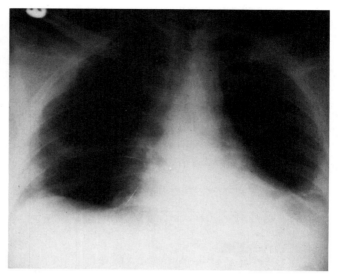

FIG 4.
Radiograph of chest on postoperative day 4 after extubation and removal of chest tubes.

were avoided. The patient recovered rapidly from his pulmonary contusion without further complications.

Contraindications to Early Fracture Stabilization

In patients with multiple injuries who may require several lifesaving operations, continued operative intervention for fracture stabilization must be reassessed. Contraindications to continuing a surgical procedure include hemodynamic instability, hypothermia, or coagulopathy.[27] These patients should remain intubated on a volume cycle ventilator, be resuscitated again, and be warmed and stabilized with the appropriate fluids and blood replacement products. When they are hemodynamically stable, with a normal temperature, adequate clotting factors, and sufficient oxygenation, stabilization of the long-bone fracture should be performed. The longer the delay in fracture stabilization, the greater is the risk of pulmonary failure, multiple organ failure, and death. The patient who has a major pulmonary insult from blunt trauma should be monitored closely for oxygenation during the operative procedure. Although the clinical data do not reveal an increased rate of complications associated with reaming of a fractured femur, they do show fat embolization and the potential risk for further pulmonary compromise. In these patients, an unreamed intramedullary rod or plate stabilization should be considered.

Case II.—A 24-year-old man was involved in a high-speed head-on collision. He was hemodynamically unstable in the emergency department and was taken to the operating room for urgent exploratory laparotomy. He was found to have suffered major blood loss from a lacerated liver. He also had a closed head injury, a Glasgow Coma Scale score of 10, multiple rib fractures (Fig 5), a right femur fracture (Fig 6), an open left tibia fracture (Fig 7), a right tibia fracture, and a sacroiliac dislocation with pelvic fractures (Fig 8). After exploratory laparotomy, during which 12 units of packed erythrocytes and a large volume of crystalloid was administered, the patient was hypothermic and had a coagulopathy. He was not a candidate for continued surgical intervention at that time. The patient remained intubated on a volume cycle ventilator and was taken to the intensive care unit, where he was warmed and hemodynamically stabilized, and his coagulopathy was corrected. Eighteen hours after the initial injury, he was taken back to the operating room for debridement of the open tibia fracture and placement of unreamed intramedullary rods in both the tibia and the right femur (Fig 9). The right tibia was placed in a splint. The patient's pelvic injuries were unstable, but would not prevent him from being mobilized into an upright chest position. Therefore, he was taken back to the intensive care unit, where he was reevaluated over the next 36 hours. His oxygenation improved and he regained hemodynamic stability. The trauma team (the general surgeon, orthopaedic surgeon, and anesthesiologist) believed him to be stable enough to undergo further stabilization of his musculoskeletal system. He was taken back to the operating room 48 hours after his initial orthopaedic surgery and underwent plate fixation of the distal tibia fracture on the right and screw stabilization of the sacroiliac joint (Fig 10).

This case illustrates the necessity of reevaluating a patient with multiple injuries after each stage of treatment. If the patient is stable, complete

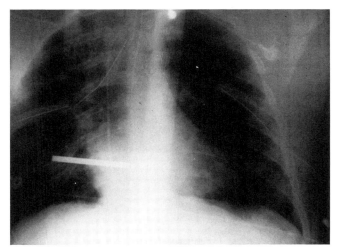

FIG 5.
Radiograph of chest showing pulmonary infiltrate and bilateral chest tubes.

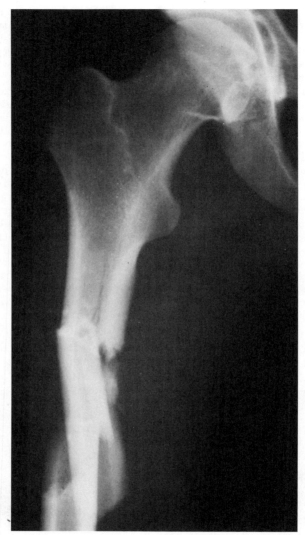

FIG 6.
Radiograph of right femur with comminuted midshaft fracture.

therapy can be accomplished at the first procedure. If the patient is unstable or hypothermic, however, or if a coagulopathy is present, further surgery should be delayed. At the earliest possible time, the patient should undergo long-bone fracture stabilization so that he or she can be mobilized into an upright chest position. A delay of 48 to 72 hours can be used to stabilize the patient again, allow hemodynamics to improve, and enable oxygen transport to resume. At that time, the remainder of the musculo-

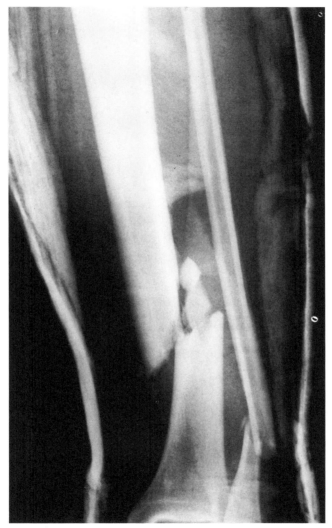

FIG 7.
Grace II open tibia fracture.

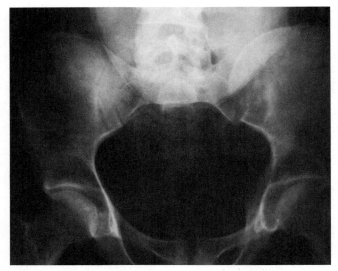

FIG 8.
Anteroposterior radiograph of pelvis showing disrupted left sacroiliac joint.

skeletal injuries can be stabilized. A delay of more than 72 hours, however, places the patient at risk for the development of pneumonia and other septic processes that could delay operative fracture stabilization indefinitely and result in a less than optimal outcome.

Physiologic Response to Early Fracture Stabilization (the Wound and Its Local Consequences)

After an injury, capillary permeability is increased, with entry of plasma into the wound and the development of edema. Concurrently, the edema fluid delivers to the wound all the elements of the plasma, including complement.[28] The presence of devitalized cells activates the complement system and releases C3a and C5a.[28, 29]

The initial phagocytosis that occurs in the wound is by polymorphonuclear cells. These are short-lived cells that give way to activated lymphocytes and monocytes. The macrophage-lymphocyte couplet then releases a variety of substances that have profound effects on both the wound and the systemic body.[28] These substances (e.g., prostaglandin E_2, leukotrienes, complement, leukin-cytokine complex) result from local wound damage and the body's normal physiologic response to injury.[28–31] If excessive production and escape of both macrophage destructive processes and macrophage immune suppressive processes occur, these products can aggregate in the lung and result in pulmonary damage.[32–34]

C5a is the major complement split product that produces cellular invasion of the wound.[28] It is normally confined to the wound. With major

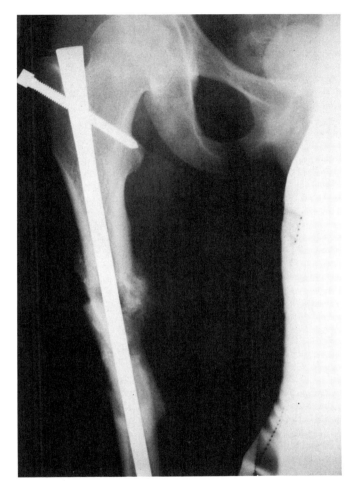

FIG 9.
Radiograph of femur fracture stabilized with an unreamed intramedullary rod.

trauma or sepsis, however, C5a can escape the wound and produce excessive activation of intravascular leukocytes. These can aggregate and travel to the lung.[35] In the lung, these activated leukocytes adhere to the endothelium and cause direct pulmonary damage and vascular leakage. This process is accentuated in man in the forced supine position.[36]

The forced supine position also produces elevation of the diaphragm from the weight of the abdominal viscera (Fig 11). Capillary pressure in the posterior lung is increased by the dependent position, leading to posterior edema.[36] Progressive atelectasis develops because of the patient's inability to cough adequately and breathe deeply, and the resulting retention of secretions. It is the forced supine position causing atelectasis and retained se-

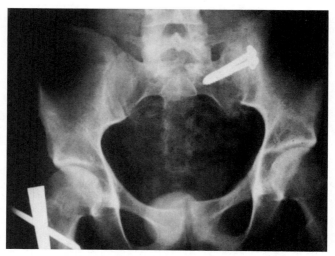

FIG 10.
Pelvic stabilization with screws across the left sacroiliac joint.

cretions combined with the effect on the lung of the destructive processes released from the peripheral wound because of macrophage activation that leads to pulmonary failure.[28, 36]

The exact reason that early fracture stabilization has a beneficial effect on pulmonary function has not been determined. Bone has shown a reduction of C5a levels in rats with femur fractures that are stabilized compared with rats with femur fractures that are not stabilized.[37] The systemic C5a level in the stabilized rats was similar to that of the control rats, whereas it was elevated in the rats with unstabilized femur fractures. This preliminary work supports the hypothesis that early stabilization of long-

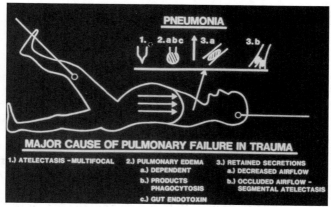

FIG 11.
Diagram of effects of forced supine position.

bone fractures reduces the systemic release of inflammatory mediators from the fracture wound and limits the associated destructive pulmonary processes.

Conclusion

Timely and complete care of patients with multiple injuries, including early fracture stabilization, reduces their morbidity and mortality. Early cardiopulmonary resuscitation with good oxygen transport is vital to survival. Life-threatening hemorrhage requires immediate control, and appropriate early care of head injuries also can reduce mortality.[38, 39] As part of the overall management of a patient with multiple injuries, musculoskeletal stabilization should be performed as early as possible, because stabilizing the traumatic wound, avoiding the forced supine position, and mobilizing the patient into an upright chest position all appear to be critical to achieving the optimum outcome.

References

1. Border J, Bone L, Babikian G, et al: A history of the care of trauma, in Border J, Allgower M, Hansen T, et al (eds): *Blunt Multiple Trauma, Comprehensive Pathophysiology and Care*. New York, Marcel Dekker, 1990.
2. Peltier LF: An appraisal of the problems of fat emboli. *Surg Gynecol Obstet* 1957; 104:313–324.
3. Riska EB, von Bonsdorff H, Hakkinen S, et al: Prevention of fat embolism by early internal fixation of fractures in patients with multiple trauma. *Injury* 1976; 6:110–116.
4. Riska E, Myllynen P: Fat embolism in patients with multiple injuries. *J Trauma* 1982; 22:891–894.
5. Goris RJA, Gimbrere JSF, Van Niekirk JLM, et al: Early osteosynthesis and prophylactic mechanical ventilation in the multitrauma patient. *J Trauma* 1982; 22:895–903.
6. Meek R, Vivoda E, Crichton H: A comparison of mortality in patients with multiple injuries according to type of fracture treatment. *J Bone Joint Surg [Am]* 1981; 63B:456.
7. Johnson KD, Cadambi A, Seibert GB: Incidence of adult respiratory distress syndrome in patients with multiple musculoskeletal injuries: Effect of early operative stabilization of fractures. *J Trauma* 1985; 25:375–384.
8. Baker S, O'Neill B, Haddon W: Injury severity score: A method for describing patients with multiple injuries and evaluating emergency care. *J Trauma* 1974; 14:187–196.
9. Seibel R, LaDuca J, Hassett J, et al: Blunt multiple trauma, femur traction and the pulmonary failure-septic state. *Ann Surg* 1985; 202:283–295.
10. Behrman S, Fabian T, Kudsk K: Improved outcome with femur fractures: Early vs. delayed fixation. *J Trauma* 1990; 30:792–798.
11. Bone LB, Johnson KD, Weigelt J, et al: Early versus delayed stabilization of fractures: A prospective randomized study. *J Bone Joint Surg [Am]* 1989; 71A:336–340.
12. Bone L, McNamara K: Mortality with early total care in the multiply injured

patient with fractures. Presented at the Combined OTA and AAST Meeting, New Orleans, September 1993.
13. Dunham M, Cowley A, Gens D, et al: Methodologic approach for a large functional trauma registry. *Maryland Medical Journal* 1989; 38:227–233.
14. Copes WS, Champion HR, Sacco WJ, et al: The injury severity score revisited. *J Trauma* 1988; 28:69–76.
15. Hoffman P, Goris R: Timing of osteosynthesis of major fractures in patients with severe brain injury. *J Trauma* 1991; 31:261–263.
16. Teasdale G, Jennett B: Assessment of coma and impaired consciousness: A practical scale. *Lancet* 1974; 2:81–83.
17. Jennett B, Teasdale G, Braakman R, et al: Predicting outcomes in individual patients after severe head injury. *Lancet* 1976; 1:1031–1034.
18. Wenda K, Runkel M, Degreif J, et al: Pathogenesis and clinical relevance of bone marrow embolism in medullary nailing. *Injury* 1993; 24:573–581.
19. Pape H, Regel G, Tscherne H, et al: Influence of thoracic truama and primary femoral intramedullary nailing on the incidence of ARDS in multiple trauma patients. *Injury* 1993; 24:S82–S103.
20. Baire P, Minnear F, Med-Malik A: Increased pulmonary vascular permeability after bone marrow injection in sheep. *Am Rev Respir Dis* 1981; 123:648.
21. Manning J, Beek A, Herman C, et al: Fat release after femur nailing in the dog. *J Trauma* 1983; 23:322–326.
22. Sturmer K, Schuchardt W: Neue Aspekte der Gedeekten Markmagelung und des Aufbohrens der Markhohle in Tiereexperiment. *Unfallheilkunde* 1980; 83:341–345.
23. Pape H, Auf 'm' Kolk M, Polfrath T, et al: Primary intramedullary femur fixation in multiple trauma patients with associated lung contusion. *J Trauma* 1993; 34:540–548.
24. Gaillard M, Hewe C, Mandin L, et al: Mortality prognostic factors in chest injury. *J Trauma* 1990; 30:93–95.
25. Fulton R, Peter E: The progressive nature of pulmonary contusion. *Surgery* 1970; 67:499.
26. Johnson J, Cogbill T, Winga E: Determinants of outcome after pulmonary contusion. *J Trauma* 1986; 26:695–697.
27. Phillips T, Contreras D: Timing of operative treatment of fractures in patients who have multiple injuries. *J Bone Joint Surg [Am]* 1990; 72A:784–788.
28. Border JR, Bone LB: Multiple trauma and major extremity wounds: Their immediate management and its consequences. *Adv Surg* 1987; 21:263–292.
29. Burke JF: Events in early inflammation, in Simmons R, Howard R (eds): *Surgical Infectious Disease.* New York, Appleton-Century-Crofts, 1982, pp 235–285.
30. Meakin J, Hobin D, Hunt T: Host defenses, in Simmons R, Howard R (eds): *Surgical Infectious Disease.* New York, Appleton-Century-Crofts, 1982, pp 235–285.
31. Kluger M, Oppenheim T, Powanda M: The physiologic, metabolic and immunologic actions of interleukin 1, in *Progress in Leukocyte Biology,* vol 2. New York, Alan R Liss, 1985, p 47.
32. Beal S, Reed L, Hemiback D, et al: Pulmonary microembolism: A cause of lung injury. *J Surg Res* 1987; 43:303–311.
33. Slotman G, Burchard K, Yellin S, et al: Prostaglandin and complement interaction in clinical acute respiratory failure. *Arch Surg* 1986; 121:271–275.
34. Anner H, Kaufman R, Kobzik L, et al: Pulmonary leukosequestration induced by hind limb ischemia. *Ann Surg* 1987; 206:162–168.

35. Olson L, Moss G, Baukus O, et al: The role of C5 in septic lung injury. *Ann Surg* 1985; 202:771–777.
36. Border J, Rodriguez J, Bone L, et al: Role of immediate surgery in prevention of multiple organ failure, in Deitch E (ed): *Multiple Organ Failure: Pathophysiology and Basic Concepts of Therapy*, New York, Thieme Medical Publishers, 1989, pp 261–274.
37. Bone L, Sultz J, Anders M: Physiologic response to femur fracture stabilization in a rat model. Unpublished data, 1989.
38. Becker DP, Miller JD, Ward JD, et al: The outcome from severe head injury with early diagnosis and intensive management. *J Neurosurg* 1977; 47:491–502.
39. Gennarelli TA, Champion HR, Sacco WJ: Mortality of patients with head injury and extracranial injury treated in trauma centers. *J Trauma* 1989; 29:1193–1202.

Variations on a Theme: Does Enteral Feeding Make a Difference?

J. David Richardson, M.D.

Professor and Vice Chairman, Department of Surgery, University of Louisville, Louisville, Kentucky

The development of effective nutritional support, which began in the late 1960s and continued during the next decade, coincided with a period of great progress in surgery. Advances such as total parenteral nutrition (TPN), effective ventilator management, the entire field of critical care, and more effective antibiotics occurred and allowed for the development and refinement of surgical techniques that previously had only been imagined.

One of the difficulties in evaluating the success of various operations and procedures is determining the impact of individual components of treatment on the success of the whole. Antibiotics, as an example, are often touted as a major contribution to the surgeon's ability to advance surgical technology further and further; however, it is difficult to say that we would cease performing complex procedures if we were limited to only a few reliable antibiotics, rather than being able to choose from the large number that currently are available. One of the common tenets of surgical practice in the United States has been to adopt a standard protocol (often with little or no scientific rationale and little regard for the cost of treatment) and continue to use it under the assumption that it works.

In my opinion, the use of nutritional support has developed in such an environment (i.e., it is difficult to define the role of nutritional support in the well-being of many of our patients). For example, we often do not know what type of feeding is best, when it should be started, or who should receive it, and cannot determine whether it affects ultimate patient outcome.

Sandstrom and associates recently described the effects of TPN on the outcome of 300 general surgical patients who were assigned randomly to receive either TPN or glucose.[1] Patients who were malnourished also were included in the study. Approximately 60% of all patients were able to resume oral intake within 8 or 9 days. No differences were observed between the groups that received TPN and glucose only with respect to mortality or complications. Patients who received 14 days of glucose treatment had a higher mortality rate than did those who were given TPN or short-term glucose therapy. The complication rate also was higher in the group that received long-term glucose therapy. Patients who were not able to resume oral alimentation appeared to need the increased nutritional intake, particularly if complications occurred.

The authors concluded that most patients did not require advanced nutritional support, and that "semi-starvation is not a limiting factor for outcome." If oral alimentation could not be resumed or complications developed, TPN was a necessary adjunct to improve survival and decrease complications. The authors noted that, in terms of "malnutrition," overfeeding was more of a problem than was underfeeding. They indicated that TPN probably was a lifesaving therapy in 20% of the patients who received it, but stated that it was not possible to identify preoperatively which patients would benefit from this adjunct.

Buzby drew similar conclusions when he recently reviewed the randomized clinical trials of TPN for malnourished surgical patients.[2] He recommended the following guidelines for TPN use:

1. Postoperative TPN should be considered when oral or enteral feeding is not anticipated within 7 to 10 days in previously well-nourished patients, and within 5 to 7 days in malnourished patients..
2. Preoperative TPN should be considered for patients who cannot eat, when their operation is delayed 3 to 5 days.
3. Preoperative TPN should be considered in the most severely malnourished patients if their operation can be delayed. Patients with only mild to moderate malnutrition do not require preoperative TPN.

Patients who are without oral nutritional support for a protracted period seem to require adjunctive nutritional support. The "motherhood" nature of this statement is difficult to refute, although the data to support it are woefully lacking. In a similar fashion, it seems intuitively correct to assume that nutrition that can be delivered through the gut is preferable to that provided intravenously. Having admitted to accepting these two premises based more on intuitive processes than on data, I still believe that enteral nutrition has assumed a somewhat "inflated" importance in clinical medicine. In the spirit of critical analysis, a position contrary to many of those espousing the benefits of routine, early enteral feeding is presented. For the purposes of this discussion, the assumption is made that nutrition must ultimately be provided (if oral intake cannot be resumed), lest the patient die of starvation. If feasible, this nutrition should be provided through the gut. The gastrointestinal tract may be used through the stomach or the small intestine, although gastric ileus generally requires jejunal intubation if early enteral feeding is to be used. This discussion examines (1) whether early feeding through the gut has inherent advantages relative to the immune system; (2) whether virtually all critically injured or ill patients should receive early enteral nutrition, as advocated by numerous authors; and (3) whether the early use of enteral feeding makes a difference in overall outcome.

Because the purpose of this discussion is to present a somewhat different opinion regarding enteral nutrition, viewpoints contrary to the often-accepted principle that early enteral nutrition represents proven therapy are emphasized. The contrary positions can be summarized as follows:

1. Much of the scientific rationale favoring enteral feeding is based on the concept that bacterial translocation (BT) is a cause of disease in humans and can be prevented by enteral feeding. In fact, BT has no proven role in disease states in humans, calling into question the rationale for early enteral feeding.

2. Clinical studies demonstrating a beneficial effect may be biased, and certainly oversimplify a complex set of interactions.

3. The disadvantages of enteral feeding have been virtually ignored.

4. Placing a feeding tube in every patient who has a major operation or serious injury is unnecessary, needlessly expensive, and potentially dangerous.

The Case for Early Enteral Feeding

Direct delivery of nutrients into the small intestine is required because of poor gastric emptying in many patients, and this technique eliminates the risk of aspiration associated with direct delivery into the stomach early in the postoperative period. In many critically ill patients, gastric atony persists for several weeks. Fortunately, several methods are available for the provision of direct nutrient delivery to the small intestine. These include the peroral route through nasoenteric tubes and direct delivery through a tube placed into the intestine. A standard tube such as a red rubber catheter, Foley catheter, or T tube can be used, or the needle catheter jejunostomy (NCJ) may be employed. The NCJ was described in 1977 by Delaney and associates[3] and has been perfected and popularized by several authors.[4-7] Problems associated with its early use have largely been overcome, and the catheter can be inserted and maintained with a low complication rate. Recent reports of its use document a technical complication rate of only 1% to 2%; the more common problem of diarrhea requiring medication can be treated easily.[4] Thus, the problem of nutrient delivery can be solved readily in those patients who require celiotomy. In those who do not require an abdominal operation, the use of a nasoenteric tube can aid in providing early nutritional support.

Aside from the caloric value, what are the theoretic advantages of enteral nutrition? Table 1 lists six potential advantages of enteric feeding. Some have been demonstrated in experimental models and others are theoretic considerations. The common theme that has been used by proponents of early enteral feeding is that it enhances immunologic function and, by doing so, lessens the "stress response" or directly decreases infectious complications when comparisons are made between unfed and enterally fed patients. A variety of mechanisms could explain a decreased stress response and immunologic enhancement.[8]

TABLE 1.
Potential Benefits of Enteral Feeding

Maintains secretion of IgA
Promotes hepatic blood flow
Maintains villous height and tight cell cross-links, prevents mucosal atrophy
Prevents bacterial translocation and endotoxemia (in animal models)
Decreased cytokine elucidation may allow for favorable hepatic protein prioritization
Maintains normal insulin levels (allows for better fat utilization)

In humans, secretory IgA is stimulated in Peyer's patches after oral antigenic challenge and is later present in numerous sites, including the gut. In rats, bile appears to contribute most of the IgA to the gut lumen. Studies by Alverdy and associates have shown that rats fed an isocaloric, isonitrogenous formula through the gut or vein have different IgA responses (i.e., animals fed by the gut have a significantly higher level of IgA than do those fed by vein).[9] If this phenomenon occurs in humans, it could be an important advantage of enteral feeding. No studies confirm these observations in humans, however.

An instance in which early enteral nutrition is believed to offer a significant theoretic advantage over intravenous nutrition is in the hepatic prioritization of proteins. The body's normal response to trauma is to increase the acute-phase reactants produced by the liver. This usually occurs at the expense of production of the constitutive proteins. Studies by Peterson and colleagues demonstrated that enteral feeding attenuated the rise in certain acute-phase proteins and increased the level of albumin and retinal-binding protein when compared with animals fed parenterally.[10] Whether this is beneficial to patients is unclear.

The use of enteral feeding promotes hepatic blood flow. This effect could theoretically lead to increased deactivation of toxins produced by the gut or actual bacterial killing by the hepatic reticuloendothelial system.

Most articles favoring early enteral feeding stress the importance of maintaining gut mucosal barrier function and preventing mucosal atrophy. These phenomena are known to occur with starvation or gastrointestinal tract disease. Theoretically, the ability to maintain normal mucosa with tight cellular cross-links prevents BT. Virtually every paper written on the importance of early enteral nutrition stresses the risk of BT without such feeding.

Bacterial Translocation

The phenomenon of BT was described decades ago, but the term itself appears to have been coined by Wolochow and associates in 1966.[11] Introduction of the term also has been attributed to Keller and Engley in 1968.[12] BT is the phenomenon of microorganism migration across the mucosal barrier into the host. Specifically, Deitch has defined BT as the "passage of viable indigenous bacteria from the gastrointestinal tract through the epithelial mucosa to the mesenteric lymph nodes and then organs."[13] Berg described three general mechanisms of BT: (1) increased permeability of the intestinal mucosa after insults such as shock, sepsis, or endotoxin administration; (2) decreased host defenses (e.g., after immunosuppression or starvation); and (3) increased intraluminal bacterial content.[14]

BT is caused by a variety of stresses in experimental animals. These include shock, burns, endotoxemia, radiation injury, and chemotherapy, among others. Associated conditions that appear to augment the process of BT include starvation, parenteral nutrition, immune suppression, and alteration in intestinal bacterial flora. Although BT occurs in a variety of experimental circumstances, many of the models appear to yield results that cannot be directly extrapolated to human disease states; many of the experimental results actually seem contradictory. Even though the prevention of BT is the scientific rationale generally given for the use of early enteral feeding. Deitch and associates showed that protein-free diets, given for as long as 3 weeks, did not cause BT in rats.[15] Starvation for 48 or 72 hours caused no translocation, whereas the addition of endotoxin caused uniform BT. Three weeks of a protein-free diet led to 30% total weight loss, but no BT. These findings are in conflict with reports from Alverdy and associates, who found bacteria in 18 of 27 mesenteric lymph nodes after TPN was given either intravenously or into the gut.[16] None of the 30 nodes sampled after enteral nutrition were positive for bacteria. This corresponded to an increased cecal bacterial content in the TPN group.

The feeding of a high-protein solution orally resulted in BT in another group of experiments, but this could be reversed by adding fiber in the form of cellulose powder.[17] Although endotoxin was used frequently as a cofactor to induce BT, tolerance to its use could be produced by pretreatment with endotoxin.[18] Deitch and coworkers have presented several scenarios in which the translocation of organisms could be responsible for the septic state or multiple organ failure, but the thread between laboratory observations and clinical data is a tenuous one.[13]

To make matters even more confusing for clinicians, there are side issues such as the relationship of glutamine and the gut. Wilmore and colleagues have proposed what is termed "the gut hypothesis," in which they speculate, based on accumulated laboratory evidence, that either systemic or gastrointestinal insults alter gut mucosal permeability.[19] This leads to BT and the "egress of toxins," which results in systemic responses. Wilmore and colleagues stated that "enteral feedings maintain the intestinal mucosa and thus may support gut barrier function during a critical illness." They also described the "gut-glutamine cycle," in which glutamine, which was scavenged from skeletal muscle, was used in the repair of defects in gut permeability. It was noted that, after an extensive small-bowel resection, animals that were fed glutamine-enriched diets had much greater mucosal activity than did control animals. This line of thought has led to recommendations that glutamine-enriched diets be part of enteral feedings to maintain normal gut mucosal barrier functions in stressed surgical patients.

Recently, Deitch's group studied the protective effect of glutamine on BT induced by an elemental diet.[20] One diet contained no glutamine, whereas glutamine constituted 30% of the amino acids in the other. The incidence of BT was 88% in the glutamine-fed group, 75% in the no-glutamine group, and only 13% in the chow-fed group ($P < .05$). These investigators also studied immunologic function and found that the use of glutamine did not prevent immunologic dysfunction. These observations are not reported to imply that glutamine does or does not have merit, but to indicate the difficulty in extrapolating highly contrived laboratory models to human disease states and the questionableness of recommending therapy based on these contradictory observations.

Bacterial Translocation in Surgical Patients

Although much has been made of the importance of BT in experimental models, this process remains difficult to document in surgical patients. Rush and coworkers described 50 patients admitted to a trauma unit.[21] Positive blood cultures were present in 56% when the admission arterial pressure was less than 80 mm Hg. The average admission blood pressure for the 10 patients with positive blood cultures was 45 mm Hg, and 8 of these patients died. Thirteen of the 16 overall deaths occurred in the first 24 hours, including 8 in the emergency department or operating room. Although this does not necessarily negate the value of the observations, it does not lend credence to the association between BT and sepsis or organ failure, which is usually a delayed event occurring several days after injury.

Several clinical studies have attempted to detect BT in injured patients who appear to be at highest risk for this problem. Peitzman and associates studied 29 patients undergoing laparotomy, including 25 with trauma and 4 with surgical problems in the gastrointestinal tract.[22] Mesenteric lymph nodes were cultured and correlated with patient data and clinical outcome. Whereas three fourths of the patients undergoing lymph node biopsy at operation for gastrointestinal disease had positive lymph nodes, none of the 25 injured patients had positive cultures. In addition, none of the patients with positive nodes at the time of gastrointestinal surgery had infectious complications. The injured patients had multiple complications, including infections (7 patients) and the adult respiratory distress syndrome (2 patients), despite the lack of BT. Thus, it would be difficult to argue that this group of patients was not sick enough to manifest BT.

An even more compelling argument against the clinical importance of BT can be made from a review of the work of Moore and colleagues.[23] This group has been a leading proponent of the value of enteral feeding and, therefore, is unlikely to be biased against the theoretic concept of BT. Portal vein catheters were inserted at laparotomy in 20 seriously injured patients. Portal and systemic blood samples were obtained for culture, endotoxin assay, complement, tumor necrosis factor, and other cytokines. Multiple organ failure developed in 30% of the patients. Two of the patients with multiple organ failure had a single positive blood culture, one with a coagulase-negative *Staphylococcus* species and one with *Propionibacterium acnes*. There was no discernible pattern of portal bacteremia, and none of the samples were positive for endotoxin. In the 12 lymph nodes that were sampled, the four positive cultures included *Enterobacter,* enterococcus, α-streptococcus, and a coagulase-negative *Staphylococcus*. None of these patients had multiple organ failure. Thus, these authors could find no convincing data that bacteremia or endotoxemia occurred after major trauma. Likewise, there was no correlation between positive cultures and subsequent multiple organ failure. Follow-up studies did show a high incidence of bacteremia in patients who had blood cultures before exsanguination. Like the work of Rush, it does not appear that these observations are related to typical patients with sepsis and multiple organ failure.

Winchurch and coworkers noted a correlation between the magnitude of injury and the level of circulating endotoxin.[24] There was a slight increase in endotoxin after small burns, whereas injuries over more than 40% of the total body surface area resulted in a 500% increase in endotoxin levels. The peak of endotoxin activity occurred on the third to fourth day after injury. Subsequently, this group reported studies on 76 patients with burns over more than 20% of the body surface.[25] The patients were given polymyxin B to treat the endotoxemia, and levels of endotoxin and interleukin-6 were measured as general markers of the inflammatory response. This group also calculated a sepsis score and measured survival. Treatment with polymyxin B significantly decreased the level of endotoxemia, but did not influence the level of interleukin-6, the sepsis score, or survival. The authors concluded that other factors must be involved in the generation of organ failure.

If BT occurs in humans, it must do so by a mechanism and in a time frame different from that seen in experimental animals. Despite many attempts to detect BT in humans, it does not seem to happen commonly. In addition, positive mesenteric lymph nodes appear to have little relationship to disease states in humans. There is no evidence that BT is *the cause* of any disease process in humans, and there is even less evidence that the use of enteral feeding has any relationship to the prevention of BT. Regardless of how one feels about enteral feeding, current evidence suggests that prevention of BT cannot be used to justify the use of enteral feeding until more confirmatory evidence in humans is available.

Clinical Studies of Enteral Feeding

Several studies have compared enteral feeding to other forms of nutritional support. An outline of the most widely referenced studies is provided in Table 2.[26-36] In the mid-1980s, several studies showed that enteral nutrition could be provided safely. No difference was noted in outcome, from the standpoint of either nutritional parameters or infectious complications.[26, 27] Moore and associates reported on the use of enteral nutrition given through an NCJ and compared the outcome of these patients to the outcome of those receiving no supplemental nutrition (controls).[28] In both instances, nutritional parameters such as albumin and ferritin were the same. There was an increased rate of sepsis in the control group (29% vs. 9% in the enteral feeding group). In the same year (1986), Hadley and colleagues described 45 patients with head injuries who were assigned randomly to receive either TPN or enteral nutrition, and noted no difference in metabolic parameters, infectious complications, or outcome.[29]

Cerra and coworkers studied 66 patients who were hypermetabolic at days 4 to 6 after sepsis and who were assigned randomly to receive either parenteral or enteral nutrition.[30] No differences were noted in the incidence of multiple organ failure or mortality. The researchers concluded that further investigation was needed to elucidate the complex interrelationships between sepsis, organ failure, and the route of administration of nutrition. This study can be criticized, however, because the hypermetabolic state was already under way before supplemental feeding was initiated. Cerra and coworkers had previously suggested that the use of a modified formula might improve patient outcome, but this was not proven to be true in the later study.[37]

Although the first few papers on enteral nutrition described it as a safe and efficacious alternative to TPN, it did not appear to be superior to other types of nutritional support. In particular, no difference was noted in the infection rate of patients fed enterally or parenterally.[26, 27, 29] There have now been several studies using patients assigned randomly to receive parenteral vs. enteral nutrition in which the risk of infection appears to be less with feeding through the gut.[28, 31-34] Thus, there is an implied criticism that failure to use enteral feeding represents substandard care! Referring to a group of high-risk patients from their study, Kudsk and coworkers noted that "failure to administer enteral feeding to this population of patients increased the risk of septic complications by a factor of 6.3."[34] These authors, as well as others, believe that enteral access should be sought at the initial operation, particularly in the high-risk patient.

The first paper that purported to show a beneficial effect of enteral feeding in terms of a decreased infection rate was published by Moore and associates from Denver General Hospital.[28] In this study published in 1986, patients were assigned randomly to receive either enteral nutrition or standard intravenous fluids (not TPN). Septic complications developed in nine patients (29%) in the control group compared with three patients (9%) in the enterally fed group. This difference was statistically significant ($P <$ .05). In the fed group, seven patients had intra-abdominal abscesses and two had pneumonia, whereas in the control group, three patients had abdominal abscesses. This paper has been criticized because the control group did not receive nutritional support, and the authors subsequently completed a study in which patients were assigned randomly to either enteral or parenteral feeding.[31] In the second study, an NCJ was placed in patients with an Abdominal Trauma Index of greater than 15. There was a 3% incidence of sepsis in the enterally fed group, which consisted of one patient with an intra-abdominal abscess. In the TPN-fed group, there were two patients with intra-abdominal abscesses and six patients with pneumonia. In the discussion, the authors presented a diagrammatic representation of their theory of the development of organ failure. They postulated that delayed enteral feeding in combination with shock caused the gut to lose bacteria and endotoxin, which then caused the failure of several end organs, including the kidney and lung. Interestingly, no data were presented to suggest that any of these events happened. In fact, no patient had the adult respiratory distress syndrome or renal impairment, and the author's own previously mentioned clinical study[23] could not confirm loss of bacteria or endotoxin from the gut.

In a related study published in the neurosurgical literature, patients with severe head injuries (Glasgow Coma Scale <10) were randomly assigned to enteral feeding through a nasoenteric tube or to gastric feeding through a tube when bowel sounds resumed.[32] These authors also noted a difference in infectious complications. There was a markedly decreased incidence of infections in the enterally fed group compared with the gastric fed group (20% vs. 100%). The rate of pneumonia was the same, but the gastric fed group had ten patients with "bronchitis," whereas the enterally fed group had only one. Bronchitis was defined as "sputum with 3 to 4+ polymorphonucleocytes with culture positive for pathogenic bacteria" without chest radiograph signs suggestive of pneumonia.

Moore and associates published a meta-analysis in 1992, comparing the results of enteral vs. parenteral nutrition in patients with eight randomized, prospective trials.[33] These trials were conducted to compare the utility of Vivonex total enteral nutrition (TEN) with TPN solutions that were "nutritionally similar" in moderately to severely stressed surgical patients. Two of the eight studies used had previously been published and six were unpublished. The authors chose to focus attention on the incidence of septic complications in the two groups, noting that 24 infections occurred in 19 patients in the TEN group and 46 infections occurred in 39 patients in the TPN group. The incidence of wound infections, abdominal abscesses, and bacteremia was the same. There were three urinary tract infections in the TPN group vs. one in the TEN group. A large difference was noted in the incidence of pneumonia, with six cases occurring in the TEN group and 15 in the TPN group. No catheter sepsis occurred in the enteral group, whereas seven cases occurred in the parenteral group. The overall difference in infectious complications was statistically significant, with the inclu-

TABLE 2.
Outcome With Enteral Feeding*

Author	Ref. No.	Number of Patients	Type of Patient	Type of Study	Outcome	Conclusions
Bower et al.	26	20	Major elective GI operation	TPN vs. TEN	No difference	TEN maintained "adequate nutritional support" at less cost
Adams et al.	27	46	Trauma	TPN vs. TEN	No difference in infections; TEN supplied 73% of caloric needs; 2 TEN patients required abdominal operations	TEN was a "safe" and efficacious choice"
Moore et al.	28	75	Emergency celiotomy with ATI >15	TEN vs. no supplemental nutrition for 5 days	Nutritional parameters exchanged from controls; overall sepsis rate was 29% vs. 9% (no nutrition vs. TEN) and 26% vs. 4% in ATI 15–40; survival was equal	"Suggests early nutrition reduces septic complication"
Hadley et al.	29	45	Neurotrauma; GSC <10	TPN vs. TEN	No difference in metabolic parameters, infectious complications, or outcome	Same as outcome
Cerra et al.	30	66	Hypermetabolic patients; 4 to 6 days after sepsis	TPN vs. TEN	No difference in multiple organ failure or mortality	"Complex relationship between sepsis and route of nutrition; much more investigation required"

Author	Ref	N	Population	Comparison	Results	Conclusion
Moore et al.	31	75	Abdominal trauma; ATI >15	TPN vs. TEN	TEN restored nutritional protein makes better; TEN had 7% infection rate vs. 37% for TPN, 6 cases of pneumonia	"Early feeding via the gut reduces septic complications in the severely stressed patient"
Grahm et al.	32	32	Head injury; GSC <10	Gastric vs. enteral	Enteral feedings were tolerated despite ileus; significant reduction in infectious complications in enteric groups (3 vs. 14); 10 cases of "bronchitis" in gastric group	"Markedly reduced infections"
Moore et al.	33	Meta-analysis; TEN = 118; TPN = 112	"High-risk surgical patients"	TPN vs. TEN	TEN had 18% septic complication vs. 35% in TPN group	TEN patients have "reduced septic morbidity compared to those administered TPN"
Kudsk et al.	34	98	Abdominal trauma; ATI >15	TPN vs. TEN	Sixfold increase in sepsis in TPN; increased incidence of pneumonia and line sepsis	TEN reduces septic complications compared to TPN
Daly et al.	35	85	Upper abdominal malignancies	Standard TEN vs. TEN with arginine, RNA, and omega-3 fatty acids	Improved lymphocyte mitogenesis, decreased infections, and decreased length of stay in supplemental group	Better outcome with supplemental formula
Eyer et al.	36	52	Blunt trauma	Early (24 hrs) vs. late (>72 hrs) enteral feeding	No differences in metabolic responses, infectious complications, or outcome	"Early enteral feeding did not alter patient outcome"

*GI = gastrointestinal; ATI = Abdominal Trauma Index; GSC = Glasgow Coma Scale; TPN = total parenteral nutrition; TEN = total enteral nutrition.

sion or exclusion of patients with catheter sepsis. No data were provided on the organisms causing pneumonia. Despite the preponderance of infections in the TPN group, there was no overall difference in 10- and 30-day outcome when mortality, length of hospital stay, or cost of treatment was compared. No benefit was noted in the group of patients undergoing elective surgery, and all the benefit occurred in the group of trauma patients.

In 1992, Kudsk and associates from Memphis published a paper comparing TEN and TPN, focusing on the "effects of septic morbidity after blunt and penetrating abdominal trauma."[34] They included injured patients who required a laparotomy and the placement of either an NCJ or a red rubber catheter at the surgeon's discretion. The incidence of infections was much higher in the TPN group, especially with regard to pneumonia (6 of 51 TEN patients vs. 14 of 45 TPN patients) and intra-abdominal abscess (1 of 51 TEN patients vs. 6 of 45 TPN patients). The effect was noted particularly in the more severely injured group; no difference was seen in patients with an Injury Severity Score of 20 or less. The authors observed no difference in septic complications in patients with injury to the gastrointestinal tract, but a significant difference in those with injuries to the pancreas and liver who received subsequent nutritional support with TPN. The authors admitted that "enteral feeding was not risk free." One patient had to be operated on again because of a jejunostomy tube obstruction. Abdominal distention requiring reoperation developed in another patient in whom "no pathology was found at operation," but this was not included as a complication. It seems safe to assume that at least 2 of 50 patients underwent repeated operation as a consequence of TEN therapy. Despite the differences in infection rates, there were no differences between the two groups in terms of number of antibiotics used, duration of antibiotic therapy, days using a ventilator, length of hospital stay, or mortality.

In the studies described, benefits related to enteral feeding were noted in patients with major trauma. In addition, most of the studies compared standard enteral formulas to either TPN or no additional nutritional support. Recently, Daly and colleagues demonstrated that enteral nutrition supplemented with arginine, RNA, and omega-3 fatty acids improved outcome in patients undergoing elective abdominal operations when compared with enteral feeding with a standard formula.[35] Not only were the infectious complications reduced, but the length of the hospital stay also was shorter.

Thus, a review of available data on enteral nutrition yields variable results. Several studies have documented the safety of enteral feeding, but no advantage other than possible cost savings. Others have shown that small-bowel feeding is better than gastric feeding, and that infections are reduced in injured patients with enteral feeding compared with TPN, but that a special formula is advantageous in elective situations compared with standard enteral feeding.[35] For a clinician interested in providing proper patient care, these studies raise many questions. Should every patient undergoing a laparotomy have a jejunostomy tube placed for feeding? Should enteral feeding be started immediately? Should a standard formula or an immunologically enhanced formula be used? If the advantages of enteral feeding in regard to sepsis are so obvious, should all critically ill patients have a jejunostomy tube placed on admission, whether they require laparotomy or not? Before attempting to answer these questions definitively, perhaps a more critical examination of the data regarding sepsis and the impact of enteral feeding should be undertaken

Critical Analysis of the Effect of Enteral Feeding on Sepsis

The initial study showing a positive benefit of enteral feeding compared this modality with traditional intravenous fluid therapy with dextrose and water.[28] No difference was seen at day 4 or 7 in the albumin or transferrin levels of the two groups. At day 7, the total lymphocyte count was significantly different, with a mean of 2,054 in patients receiving enteral nutrition compared to 1,482 in those receiving dextrose and water. Nitrogen balance was -11 g at day 7 in the group fed dextrose and water compared with -5 g in the group fed enterally. The major benefit was believed to be the decreased rate of sepsis in the enterally fed group. Nine patients (29%) who received dextrose and water had major infections, compared with only 3 of those fed enterally. This difference in infections, although statistically significant, prompts speculation regarding the reason that septic complications developed in one group rather than the other. In particular, no information is provided about the 10 patients (7 in the dextrose group and 3 in the enteral group) in whom intra-abdominal abscesses developed. What were their specific injuries? This is important information because of the small number of patients involved in the study; the change of 1 patient in either group would affect statistical significance. The method of enteral feeding also was interesting. Twenty of the 32 patients receiving enteral feeding were maintained on an elemental diet for 5 or more days. Nine of the remaining patients were said to have received TPN, although no data were provided on when, why, or how much they received. It is unclear what happened to the other 3 of the 32 patients. It was noted that 12 of 32 patients were intolerant of "full-scale jejunostomy feedings"; presumably, these were the patients who received less than 5 days of enteral feeding. Of note, 5 of the 6 patients with an Abdominal Trauma Index[38] of greater than 40 "could not tolerate being maintained on the elemental diet." Thus, this study described patients who needed the treatment the most, but were unable to tolerate it and so were dropped from further analysis. The authors presented an algorithm in which they recommended the placement of an NCJ in patients with an Abdominal Trauma Index of greater than 15, but the use of TPN was recommended in those with an Abdominal Trauma Index of greater than 40. Of note, an Abdominal Trauma Index of 15 can be obtained by a patient with a "moderate" isolated colon wound.

In the follow-up paper comparing TEN with TPN, 29 and 30 patients were studied, respectively.[31] The differences in infectious complications were noted again, with a higher rate in the TPN group. In this study, the significant difference in intra-abdominal infections that was noted previously was not observed. There was only one intra-abdominal abscess in the TEN group and two in the TPN group. Six patients in the TPN group had pneumonia, however, compared with none in the TEN group. The patients who had pneumonia were an interesting group, and the greater incidence among those who received TPN is unclear. It seems unlikely that malnutrition was the reason, because 3 of the patients had pneumonia within 5 days of injury. In the discussion, the authors postulate that BT was "central" to an understanding of their data. Yet, a review of organisms cultured showed 2 patients with *Staphylococcus aureus* and 1 each with *Streptococcus pneumoniae, Pseudomonas aeruginosa, Serratia marcescens,* and *Citrobacter.* These are unlikely organisms to have translocated from the gut. In fairness, it should be added that there was 1 patient with *Escherichia coli* pneumonia.

In reviewing the risk factors for pneumonia, 2 patients had splenectomy (which may predispose to pneumonia through mechanical factors alone), 1 had a thoracic injury, and 4 were in shock. Although TPN use was the only factor statistically associated with pneumonia, there were other factors that could have been related to this complication.

Grahm and coworkers noted that enteral feeding produced fewer infections compared with gastric feeding with the same formula.[32] This difference resulted entirely from the development of bronchitis in the gastric fed group. Bronchitis is a relatively nonspecific diagnosis, and there is the additional problem of determining the impact of aspiration from gastric feeding on its incidence. Thus, these differences could be explained by mechanical factors in the gastric fed group rather than by immunologic benefits of enteral feeding.

A review of the meta-analysis also raises some questions regarding the clear superiority of enteral feeding.[33] The inclusion criteria permitted the initiation of feedings within 72 hours; when treatment was begun and how long it was administered are not indicated. In the subgroup with penetrating trauma, the randomization produced a TPN group that had a significantly higher Abdominal Trauma Index than did the enteral group (TEN 23.8 mean vs. TPN 30 mean; $P = .02$). In addition, significantly more patients dropped out of the TEN group than the TPN group (26 vs. 10; $P = .001$). Of the 92 TEN patients entered into the study, 16% were classified as treatment failures because of gastrointestinal intolerance. Treatment failures occurred in only 3% of the TPN patients ($P = .001$). The most powerful statistical observations were not related to sepsis, but to the inability to complete treatment in the enterally fed group. The incidence of infection in the TPN group was the result of a higher incidence of pneumonia (15 of 112 vs. 6 of 118 patients) and catheter sepsis (7 of 112 vs. 0 of 118 patients). The diagnosis of pneumonia was a clinical one, left to the individual physicians at the eight participating institutions. No culture data on the causative organisms involved or clinical information on other possible risk factors associated with pneumonia were provided. Of note, this increased rate of infection appeared to have little effect on outcome. There were no differences in the TEN vs. TPN groups with respect to length of hospital stay, cost of treatment, or mortality (10- or 30-day).

The study from the Memphis trauma unit also noted a significant increase in infection in patients randomly assigned to receive TPN.[34] There were increased incidences of intra-abdominal abscess (6 of 45 vs. 1 of 51 patients), pneumonia (14 of 45 vs. 6 of 51 patients), and line sepsis (6 of 45 vs. 1 of 51 patients). No detailed clinical information is provided on the patients with intra-abdominal abscess or pneumonia, and no culture data are provided on the patients with pneumonia. In the most seriously injured patients, there was no significant difference in rate of infection. As noted in other studies, this epidemic of infectious problems seemed to occur in a vacuum, in that no difference in outcome could be detected. There was no difference in days spent in the intensive care unit, days using a ventilator, number of antibiotics used, duration of antibiotic therapy, length of hospital stay, or mortality. Nonetheless, the authors state, "we believe that the current prospective study provides conclusive evidence of the beneficial effect of TEN feeding in injured patients."

These studies indicate several trends that are fairly consistent: (1) there is relatively little difference in the measured metabolic or nutritional parameters between patients fed with TEN or TPN; (2) there is a higher incidence of minor gastrointestinal problems that limits treatment with enteral feeding; (3) infectious problems appear to be more common in the TPN group; and (4) despite septic complications, no study has shown a difference in patient outcome. Length of stay and mortality are consistently the same in these studies. The parameters used to measure infectious morbidity, such as antibiotic use, are unchanged. Kudsk and coworkers argue that this is because the differences in outcome are obscured by the complex nature of the patients being treated.[34] A skeptic would almost certainly agree, and might suggest that this complexity of injured patients probably also is responsible for the differences observed in infections.

Because differences in the rates of infection have been reported by many authors, are there reasons other than immunologic enhancement, BT, or other unproven causes that explain the increased risk of infection in patients receiving TPN? It is important to carefully evaluate other factors, because many of the observed differences are small. Many studies have shown no difference in the infection rate between TPN and enteral feeding. Are the differences observed in some studies real? The difference in the number of intra-abdominal infections has usually been negligible, with sepsis from central venous lines and pneumonia accounting for most of the significant differences. Catheter infections are a problem with TPN, and effective protocols for line management must be enforced to avoid infection. This does not mean that enteral feeding itself offers specific protection through the immune system. It also is well recognized that patients in whom catheter sepsis develops are more prone to other infections, such as bacteremia and pneumonia.[34] Thus, catheter infections may be the initial domino that causes a cascade of multiple infections. In addition, pneumonia is notoriously difficult to diagnose in the clinical setting of trauma and in the postoperative state, in which pulmonary contusion, fluid overload, atelectasis, and other diagnoses also must be considered. Kudsk and colleagues noted in their study that "atelectasis, pulmonary contusion, and pleural effusions were excluded as the source of infiltrates."[34] Yet, it must be questioned how this was done, because it has been difficult to accomplish in a clinical setting. Recent studies have shown that the standard clinical criteria may either underdiagnose or may overdiagnose pneumonia by 25% to 40% when compared with autopsy results.[39] The protected specimen brush technique also frequently yields erroneous results.[40] Given the inherent biases that are often difficult to overcome in any nonblinded clinical study, and the problems inherent in making a diagnosis of pneumonia based on an undefined infiltrate, the difference in reported pneumonia rates must be carefully interpreted. This is particularly true when the need for antibiotic treatment is the same in patients who receive enteral nutrition and those who are given TPN.

What Are the Disadvantages of Nutritional Therapy?

The complications associated with TPN have been well documented since its inception, although their incidence has decreased dramatically. Nonetheless, problems with line placement (including pneumothorax) persist, and catheter sepsis remains a major complication. Hyperosmolar coma and various metabolic derangements occur sporadically as well.

The hazards associated with enteral feeding have not been as well defined. The frequent use of a procedure or technique reduces the incidence of problems; however, a low, but clear, risk of major complications is associated with the use of enteral feeding (Table 3). The risk of aspiration with gastric feeding has been noted. If the small intestine is used, specific problems relating to the tubes or the NCJ must be considered. Included among these are complications such as tube dislodgment, intraperitoneal infusion of nutrients, pneumatosis intestinalis, necrotizing fasciitis, small-bowel perforation, and kinking with secondary bowel obstruction.

The incidence of complications with NCJ is low, but real, in recently reported series. Sarr and Mayo noted no complications requiring reoperation in 83 patients undergoing NCJ.[4] There were two minor complications, and 11 patients required antidiarrheal medications. Adams and associates noted one intestinal leak requiring reoperation in the 23 patients assigned randomly to jejunal feeding; an additional patient given TPN who was changed over to jejunostomy feeding had a small-bowel obstruction.[27] Kudsk and coworkers had 1 patient (2%) who required reoperation because of small-bowel obstruction at the insertion site of the jejunal tube.[34]

Other groups have noted a much higher rate of mechanical problems. The group from Milwaukee described a series of 73 patients who underwent jejunostomy by either a tube or a Roux-en-Y technique (the NCJ was not used).[41] Aspiration was noted to occur in these patients, even though

TABLE 3.
Complications of Enteral Feeding
I. Solution-specific.
   A. Diarrhea 20% to 40%, usually mild and controllable.
   B. Intestinal necrosis occurred with early use of enteral nutrition in shock and low-flow states.
   C. Bloating, abdominal pain, vomiting.
II. Catheter-related.
   A. Needle catheter jejunostomy.
      1. Dislodgment, intraperitoneal feeding.
      2. Pneumatosis intestinalis.
      3. Intramural placement.
   B. Feeding tube.
      1. Dislodgment.
      2. Bowel obstruction.
      3. Volvulus.
      4. Intussusception (balloon-tipped).
      5. Persistent fistula.

this complication is thought to be uncommon with jejunostomy. Complications also included leaks from the tube (8 patients), tube dislodgment (3 patients), peritonitis (3 patients), tube obstruction (3 patients), bowel obstruction (3 patients), and wound infection (2 patients). Seven deaths were believed to result directly from complications of the jejunostomy. Although these results are the worst reported, they do indicate that the procedure is not innocuous, and that it must be performed with care and for the proper indications.

A much more common problem associated with enteral feeding is the development of bloating, cramping, or diarrhea. These complications often can be managed by slowing the infusion rate of the nutrient solution or using antidiarrheal medications. Jones and associates noted that 83% of enterally fed patients had gastrointestinal symptoms, but that "most were manageable with careful monitoring and reassurance by the nutrition staff."[42] The rate of diarrhea usually is 10% to 40%, and bloating or true intolerance also often is a problem, particularly in the critically ill. Our unit has frequently noted the paradox of patients tolerating enteral feeding well when it is not needed, whereas the critically ill, who are purported to need such feeding the most, have the greatest difficulties.

Small-bowel ischemia also has been reported as a consequence of enteral feeding. In one report, five patients died of small-bowel ischemia and infarction after the initiation of jejunal feeding.[43] All were critically ill, and four of the five had hypotension more than 24 hours before intestinal necrosis was detected. Our unit has noted small-bowel necrosis in two patients who were given enteral feeding soon after massive fluid resuscitation from shock. It was our belief that the small-bowel necrosis was caused by a combination of hypoperfusion secondary to shock and the increased mucosal demands necessitated by the tube feedings. It is now our practice to withhold tube feedings until the patient has been resuscitated well for several days.

Virtually any treatment is associated with complications, and the risk-benefit ratio must be estimated before a specific treatment is instituted. Because the overall outcome in most series is the same, the presence of even a single instance of tube complication requiring reoperation may obviate the potential good record of enteral therapy.

The Cost of Nutritional Support: Parenteral vs. Enteral

Numerous studies have attempted to determine the cost of nutritional therapy.[31, 33, 34] Several have concluded that enteral therapy is much less expensive than is TPN. These studies have determined "costs" of therapy by assessing pharmacy charges for TPN vs. the cost of the enteral formulas used. Even if one accepts the concept that "charges" truly reflect "costs" in a hospitalized patient, the cost data previously reported are so simplistic that they deserve further comment.

To determine accurately the cost of a treatment regimen, all components of treatment must be considered. Thus, all the differences in costs incurred with the placement of a jejunostomy tube vs. a central venous catheter must be considered. The nursing time spent regulating enteral and parenteral fluids must be taken into account. How much manpower is expended unclogging the NCJ and how is that "counted" in the costs? Does the significantly increased incidence of diarrhea reported in virtually every series result in higher nursing costs related to the time needed to administer antidiarrheal drugs, assist the patient to the bathroom, and change the bed linen more frequently? What happens to the cost data when one patient requires reoperation for bowel obstruction secondary to a tube complication? To determine the true costs of therapy, a complex time and motion log would need to be kept for many patients and these findings correlated with outcome. None of the studies that claim to have examined costs have done anything but the most simplistic cost analysis, which adds little to our knowledge about the true cost of these therapies.

Does the Method of Nutritional Support Affect Outcome?

Regardless of whether one agrees with the studies showing a higher rate of infection with TPN, none of the reported studies show a difference in outcome. In addition, Eyer and associates from the University of Minnesota studied the effects of initiating enteral feeding early vs. delaying it for more than 3 days.[36] They noted no difference in metabolic parameters, infectious outcome, length of stay in the intensive care unit, or any measurable outcome.

The concept of outcome-based research is difficult to define. It is often impossible to detect what appear to be real differences in treatment because of the statistical "noise" generated by a myriad of complex clinical factors. It could be argued that preventing infection by enteral feeding (if this actually occurs) will eventually make a difference in outcome, even though one cannot be shown at present. The philosophical approach argues that, if "process" measurements are improved, improvement in outcome is likely to follow. This is not a philosophical argument, but a practical issue that will influence huge expenditures of resources. Should every major abdominal operation be completed with the placement of a jejunostomy tube? Should feeding be started in the recovery room, and with what solution? Table 4 provides a partial list of commercially available nutritional products.[44] The fact that more than 40 such products are on the market leads to the following conclusions: (1) no single product is superior enough to dominate the field, and (2) there must be significant financial return to attract the product development and marketing that has already emerged. The field of nutritional therapy needs (1) independently conducted studies (i.e., without commercial sponsorship) to determine whether any type of treatment is indicated, and (2) proof that any of the stress formulas actually improve patient outcome.

Who Should Receive Enteral Support?

Several recommendations have been made regarding the use of enteral nutrition. Sarr and coworkers advocate placing an NCJ for the routine administration of fluids and medication instead of using the intravenous route.[4] Moore[31] and Kudsk[34] have recommended the routine placement of a feeding tube for all patients undergoing laparotomy who have an Abdominal Trauma Index of greater than 15. This results in tube placement in most patients with multiple injuries or moderate colon injuries. We contend that most healthy patients with penetrating trauma need no special nutritional support (either enteral or parenteral) until a delay in the return of gastrointestinal function is demonstrated.

There are, however, several instances in which the routine placement of a jejunostomy tube is indicated, such as esophageal or major esophagogastric operations, or injuries in which a leak may preclude oral alimentation for a considerable period. Patients with pancreaticoduodenal injuries, particularly those who require a resection, are excellent candidates for routine tube placement at the time of operation. In some cases, the tube will not be used (even though it is present) because oral intake is begun within a few days.

Tube placement in patients with blunt trauma who do not require a laparotomy is troublesome. If a patient with a severe head injury needs an abdominal operation, a feeding tube may be added, but the additional operating time required must be balanced against the value of the tube. Our unit relies on a nasoenteric tube placed a few days after injury in most patients, rather than on operative placement of a jejunostomy tube. A percutaneous gastrostomy may be performed later for patients with head injuries, or an open jejunostomy may be performed at the time of tracheostomy if long-term nutritional support is required.

Summary

It is widely accepted that early enteral therapy should be provided for seriously ill patients or those undergoing major operations. Several studies

TABLE 4.
Nutritional Formulas in Clinical Use: Standard Formula*

Formula (calories/mL)		mOsm (g/L)	Protein (%)	Carbohydrates (%)	Fat
Standard					
Tube only					
Isocal	1.06	300	34	50	37
Osmolite	1.06	300	37	55	31
Oral tube					
Ensure	1.06	450	37	55	31
Resource	1.06	450	37	55	31
Calorie-dense					
Medium					
Ensure Plus	1.50	690	55	53	32
Sustacal HC	1.50	650	60	50	34
High					
Magnacal	2.00	590	80	50	36
Isocal HCN	2.00	690	75	40	45
Two-cal HN	2.00	700	84	43	40
Protein-dense					
Low-calorie					
Sustacal	1.00	625	61	55	21
Osmolite HN	1.06	310	44	53	30
Medium-calorie					
Sustacal HC	1.50	650	60	50	34
Ensure Plus	1.50	690	55	53	32
Elemental/semielemental					
Vivonex TEN	1.00	630	38	82	3
Vital HN	1.00	500	42	74	9
Criticare HN	1.06	650	37	83	3

(Continued.)

TABLE 4 (cont.).

Formula (calories/mL)	mOsm	(g/L)	Protein (%)	Carbohydrates (%)	Fat
Short-peptide semielemental					
Peptamen	1.00	260	40	51	33
Reabilan	1.00	350	31	53	35
Milk-based oral					
Meritene	.96	505	58	46	30
Sustagen	1.85	840	111	68	8
Carnation Instant	1.06	677	57	51	27
Fiber-enriched					
Jevity	1.06	310	44	54	30
Enrich	1.10	480	40	55	31
Sustacal with Fiber	1.06	480	46	53	30
Stress/trauma					
Stresstein	1.2	910	70	57	20
Traumacal	1.5	490	83	40	38
Hepatic					
Hepatic-Aid	1.2	560	44	57	28
Travasorb-Hepatic	1.1	600	29	78	12
Renal					
Amin-Aid	1.9	700	19	75	21
Travasorb Renal	1.4	590	23	81	12
Pulmonary					
Pulmocare	1.5	520	63	28	55
Traumacal	1.5	490	83	40	38
Diabetes					
Glucerna	1.0	375	42	33	50
Immunostimulant					
Impact	1.0	375	56	53	25

*Modified from McClave SA, Lowen CC, Snider HL: *Dig Dis Sci* 1991; 37:1153–1161. Used by permission.

have shown enteral therapy to be safe, although it is attended by a 1% to 2% incidence of serious complications and a 10% to 20% incidence of manageable complications. The scientific rationale for this therapy was examined in this chapter, particularly regarding BT. The lack of documentation of BT in the clinical setting was reviewed.

Several recent studies have indicated that enteral nutrition produces fewer infections than does parenteral nutrition, although the data are conflicting. There are several situations in which enteral therapy should be used routinely. A feeding tube always should be placed in patients with major esophageal injuries or reconstructions. Patients with major gastric and pancreaticoduodenal injuries or operations are excellent candidates for the performance of a jejunostomy at the initial operation. In patients with combined multisystem trauma, a feeding tube may be placed with the assurance that it will be used as a source of nutritional support. We usually do not perform jejunostomy in patients with moderate colon wounds, however, even if the Abdominal Trauma Index is 15. Patients who have severe head injuries may be candidates for jejunostomy at the time they undergo other procedures, such as tracheostomy. Generally, we have relied on the use of nasoenteric tubes for patients with head injuries, with excellent results.

References

1. Sandstrom R, Drott C, Hylander A, et al: The effect of postoperative intravenous feeding (TPN) on outcome following major surgery evaluated in a randomized study. Ann Surg 1993; 217:185–189.
2. Buzby GP: Overview of randomized clinical trials of total parenteral nutrition for malnourished surgical patients. World J Surg 1993; 17:173–177.
3. Delaney HM, Carnevale N, Garvey JW, et al: Postoperative nutritional support using needle catheter feeding jejunostomy. Ann Surg 1977; 186:165–170.
4. Sarr MG, Mayo S: Needle catheter jejunostomy: An unappreciated and misunderstood advance in the care of patients after major abdominal operations. Mayo Clin Proc 1988; 63:565–572.
5. Page CP, Ryan JA, Haff RC: Continual catheter administration of an elemental diet. Surg Gynecol Obstet 1976; 142:184–187.
6. Hoover HC, Ryan JA, Anderson EJ, et al: Nutritional benefits of immediate jejunal feeding of an elemental diet. Am J Surg 1980; 139:153–159.
7. McArdle AH, Palmason C, Morency I, et al: A rationale for enteral feeding as the preferable route for hyperalimentation. Surgery 1981; 90:616–623.
8. Lowry SF: The route of feeding influences injury responses. J Trauma 1990; 30:510–515.
9. Alverdy J, Chi HS, Sheldon GF: The effect of parenteral nutrition on gastrointestinal immunity. Ann Surg 1985; 202:681–684.
10. Peterson VM, Moore EE, Jones TN, et al: Total parenteral nutrition versus total parenteral nutrition after major torso injury: Attenuation of hepatic protein reprioritization. Surgery 1988; 104:199–207.
11. Wolochow H, Hildebrand GJ, Lammanna C: Translocation of microorganisms across the intestinal wall of the rat: Effect of microbial size and concentration. J Infect Dis 1966; 16:523–528.
12. Keller R, Engley FB: Fate of the bacteriophage particles introduced into mice by various routes. Proc Soc Exp Biol Med 1968; 18:577.
13. Deitch EA: Bacterial translocation of the gut flora. J Trauma 1990; 30:S184–187.
14. Berg RD: Promotion of the translocation of enteric bacteria from the gastrointestinal tracts of mice by oral treatment with penicillin, clindamycin, or metronidazole. Infect Immun 1981; 33:854–861.
15. Deitch EA, Winterton J, Li M, et al: The gut as a portal of entry for bacteremia. Ann Surg 1987; 205:681–692.
16. Alverdy JC, Aoys E, Moss GS: Total parenteral nutrition promotes bacterial translocation from the gut. Surgery 1988; 104:185–190.
17. Spaeth G, Berg RD, Specian RD, et al: Food without fiber promotes bacterial translocation from the gut. Surgery 1990; 108:240–246.
18. Deitch EA, Specian RD, Berg RD: Induction of early-phase tolerance to endo-

toxin-induced mucosal injury, xanthine oxidase activation, and bacterial translocation by pretreatment with endotoxin. *Circ Shock* 1992; 36:200–212.
19. Wilmore DA, Smith RJ, O'Dwyer ST, et al: The gut: A central organ after surgical stress. *Surgery* 1988; 104:917–923.
20. Dazhong X, Qi L, Thirstrup C, et al: Elemental diet-induced bacterial translocation and immunosuppression is not reversed by glutamine. *J Trauma* 1993; 35:821–824.
21. Rush BF, Sori AJ, Murphy TF, et al: Endotoxemia and bacteremia during hemorrhagic shock. *Ann Surg* 1988; 207:549–554.
22. Peitzman AB, Udekwu AO, Ochoa J, et al: Bacterial translocation in trauma patients. *J Trauma* 1991; 31:1083–1087.
23. Moore FA, Moore EE, Poggetti R, et al: Gut bacterial translocation via the portal vein: A clinical perspective with major torso trauma. *J Trauma* 1991; 31:1083–1087.
24. Winchurch RA, Thepari TN, Munster AM: Endotoxemia in burn patients: Levels of circulating endotoxins are related to burn size. *Surgery* 1987; 102:808–812.
25. Munster AM, Smith-Meek M, Dickerson C, et al: Translocation—incidental phenomenon or true pathology? *Ann Surg* 1993; 218:321–327.
26. Bower RG, Talamini MA, Sax HC, et al: Postoperative enteral versus parenteral nutrition. *Arch Surg* 1986; 121:1040–1045.
27. Adams S, Dellinger EP, Wertz MJ, et al: Enteral versus parenteral nutritional support following laparotomy for trauma: A prospective randomized study. *J Trauma* 1986; 26:882–891.
28. Moore EE, Jones TN: Benefits of immediate jejunostomy feeding after major abdominal trauma: A prospective randomized study. *J Trauma* 1986; 26:874–881.
29. Hadley MN, Grahm TW, Harrington T, et al: Nutritional support and neurotrauma: A critical review of early nutrition in forty-five acute head injured patients. *Neurosurgery* 1986; 19:367–373.
30. Cerra FB, McPherson JP, Konstantinides FN, et al: Enteral nutrition does not prevent multiple organ failure syndrome (MOFS) after sepsis. *Surgery* 1988; 104:727–733.
31. Moore FA, Moore EE, Jones TN, et al: TEN vs TPN following major abdominal trauma—reduced septic morbidity. *J Trauma* 1989; 29:916–923.
32. Grahm TW, Zadrozny DB, Harrington T: The benefits of early jejunal hyperalimentation in the head-injured patient. *Neurosurgery* 1989; 25:729–735.
33. Moore FA, Feliciano DV, Andrassy RJ, et al: Early enteral feeding, compared with parenteral, reduces postoperative septic complications. The results of a meta-analysis. *Ann Surg* 1992; 216:172–183.
34. Kudsk KA, Croce MA, Fabian TC, et al: Enteral versus parenteral feeding— effects on septic morbidity after blunt and penetrating abdominal trauma. *Ann Surg* 1992; 215:107–117.
35. Daly JM, Lieberman MD, Goldfine J, et al: Enteral nutrition with supplemental arginine RNA and omega-3 fatty acids in postoperative patients: Immunologic, metabolic and clinical outcome. *Surgery* 1992; 112:56–67.
36. Eyer SD, Micon LT, Konstantinides NN, et al: Early enteral feeding does not attenuate metabolic response after blunt trauma. *J Trauma* 1993; 34:639–644.
37. Cerra FB, Shronts EP, Konstantinides NN, et al: Enteral feedings in sepsis: A prospective, randomized double-blind trial. *Surgery* 1985; 98:632–639.

38. Moore EE, Dunn EL, Moore JB: Penetrating Abdominal Trauma Index. *J Trauma* 1981; 21:439–445.
39. Andrews CP, Coalson JJ, Smith JD, et al: Diagnosis of nosocomial bacterial pneumonia in acute, diffuse lung injury. *Chest* 1981; 80:254–258.
40. Chastre J, Viau F, Brun P, et al: Prospective evaluation of the protected specimen brush for the diagnosis of respiratory infections in ventilated patients. *Am Rev Respir Dis* 1984; 130:924–929.
41. Adams MB, Seabrook GR, Quebbeman EA, et al: Jejunostomy—a rarely indicated procedure. *Arch Surg* 1986; 121:236–238.
42. Jones TN, Moore FA, Moore EE, et al: Gastrointestinal symptoms attributed to jejunostomy feeding after major abdominal trauma: A critical analysis. *Crit Care Med* 1989; 17:1146–1150.
43. Gaddy MC, Max MH, Schwab CW, et al: Small bowel ischemia: A consequence of feeding jejunostomy? *South Med J* 1986; 79:180–182.
44. McClave SA, Lowen CC, Snider HL: Immunonutrition and enteral hyperalimentation of critically ill patients. *Dig Dis Sci* 1991; 37:1153–1161.

A New Look at Penetrating Carotid Artery Injuries

David V. Feliciano, M.D.

Chief of Surgery, Grady Memorial Hospital; Professor of Surgery, Emory University School of Medicine, Atlanta, Georgia

Carotid artery injuries account for about 5% of the arterial trauma treated in urban trauma centers.[1] Penetrating wounds comprise 95% to 98% of the injuries reported in published series, although the number of reports describing blunt injuries has been rising in recent years.[2-7]

Much has been written about carotid artery trauma over the past 40 years, and there is widespread consensus regarding the appropriate treatment of routine injuries.[8] The treatment of patients with a profound neurologic deficit accompanying the arterial injury, those with delayed recognition of a blunt carotid injury with or without an associated neurologic deficit, and those with an injury above the angle of the mandible, however, remains controversial.

Many retrospective series do not include the wide spectrum of clinical presentations and problems that are seen by trauma surgeons with long experience in the treatment of carotid artery injuries. This review focuses on the following nine clinical scenarios, each of which is illustrated by patients from the author's experience:

1. Cervical hematoma with compromise of the airway
2. Diagnostic evaluation of penetrating wounds in zone I (below the sternal notch)
3. Treatment of penetrating wounds in zone III (above the angle of the mandible)
4. Occlusion of the internal carotid artery in an asymptomatic patient
5. Routine repairs in zone II injuries
6. Treatment of the carotid artery injury with associated stroke or coma
7. Balloon catheter tamponade
8. Treatment of the carotid-jugular fistula
9. Blowout of the carotid artery in the postoperative period

Cervical Hematoma With Compromise of the Airway

Case report.—A 23-year-old man sustained a gunshot wound to the anterior right neck in zone II. On arrival in the emergency department, he was noted to have a large pulsatile hematoma with some deviation of the trachea to the left (Fig 1). Although the patient's voice and airway were intact, an experienced surgical resident noted swelling of the floor of the mouth on the right and displacement of the tongue toward the hard palate. The patient was immediately moved to the operating room, where a rapid intubation over a fiberoptic bronchoscope was performed with little manipulation of the patient's neck. A subsequent lateral repair of an injury to the right common carotid artery was completed in a routine fashion.

Penetrating injuries to the carotid artery often result in lateral defects with contained active bleeding. On occasion, the bleeding may exit the track of the missile externally or enter the trachea or esophagus if either has simultaneously been injured by the missile or knife. Such patients are rarely seen, presumably because they die in the field from exsanguination or asphyxiation. In the patient whose bleeding is "contained," there is often rapid dissection of the acute pulsatile hematoma along the carotid sheath. The expanding cervical hematoma that results leads to deviation of the trachea and elevation of the floor of the mouth, much as in the patient described. The rapid progression of the acute pulsatile hematoma is well known to experienced trauma surgeons, but this information has not been transmitted to junior surgical residents and personnel in emergency medicine, who are the first to see such patients in many trauma centers.

The single greatest priority in the patient with an expanding cervical hematoma is control of the airway. If an operating room is not immediately available, intubation in the emergency department is appropriate, even in

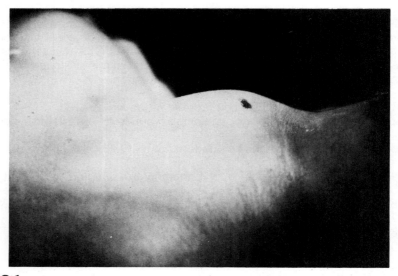

FIG 1.
Large, pulsatile cervical hematoma in a patient with a gunshot wound to the right common carotid artery. (From Brown MF, Graham JM, Feliciano DV, et al: Am J Surg 1982; 144:748–753. Used by permission.)

a patient without obvious airway distress. The choice of sedation (lorazepam vs. midazolam) for the patient about to undergo nasotracheal intubation varies from center to center, as does the choice of a neuromuscular blocking agent (succinylcholine vs. vecuronium) in the patient who is to undergo orotracheal intubation. If the operating room is immediately available, rapid transport followed by intubation by an experienced anesthesiologist is appropriate. If severe deviation or compression of the upper airway is obvious during attempted intubation, conversion to orotracheal intubation over a fiberoptic bronchoscope is ideal. Because any of these maneuvers may fail in the patient with a large hematoma, the surgical team must have a cricothyroidotomy tray immediately available in either the emergency department or the operating room.[9]

To summarize, the ideal approach to control of the airway in such patients should recognize the following:

1. A delay in obtaining an airway may cause hypoxia or even asphyxiation.

2. The agitation and hypertension that result in the hypoxic patient make attempts at intubation difficult without complete paralysis and may precipitate external bleeding or exsanguination into the upper aerodigestive tract.

3. Fiberoptic bronchoscopy under appropriate sedation in the operating room may allow for controlled intubation even when marked tracheal deviation or compression is present.

4. Cricothyroidotomy is indicated if less invasive maneuvers fail or if there is impending asphyxiation, despite the risk of contamination to the subsequent arterial repair.

Diagnostic Evaluation of Penetrating Wounds in Zone I[10, 11]

Case report.—A 34-year-old man sustained a gunshot wound to the right supraclavicular area and arrived in the emergency department with a large hematoma underneath the wound. He was hemodynamically stable, his distal right carotid and upper extremity pulses were intact, and his breath sounds were decreased over the right hemithorax. A right thoracostomy tube was inserted, and 700 mL of blood was evacuated rapidly. Because of the location of the injury, overlapping zone I of the right neck and the right supraclavicular fossa, there was concern regarding the choice of incision around the thoracic inlet. A right retrograde brachial arteriogram performed with a blood pressure cuff inflated to 300 mm Hg on the ipsilateral distal arm (below the arterial puncture) by the surgical team demonstrated a pseudoaneurysm of the right common carotid artery just above the thoracic inlet (Fig 2). After the patient was transferred to the operating room, a median sternotomy with a right anterior oblique cervical extension was performed. Vigorous hemorrhage was noted from small perforations of the right subclavian artery and vein, and from a 50% transection of the right common carotid artery. The patient underwent ligation and division of the left innominate vein for exposure of the vascular injuries, repair of the subclavian artery and vein, and ligation of the right

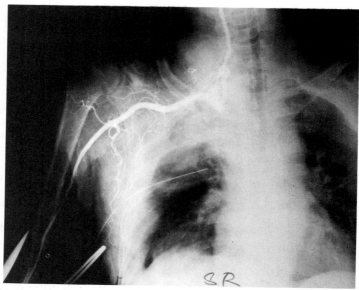

FIG 2.
Right retrograde brachial arteriogram performed by trauma team demonstrated a pseudoaneurysm of the right common carotid artery in this patient with a gunshot wound near zone I.

common carotid artery as blood loss became excessive. The postoperative course was complicated by adult respiratory distress syndrome that was treated with a tracheostomy and ventilator support, but the patient recovered without a neurologic deficit.

In 1968, Monson and colleagues[10] arbitrarily divided the cervical region into zone I (below the sternal notch), zone II ("mid-cervical region" between the sternal notch and the angle of the mandible), and zone III (above the angle of the mandible and below the base of the skull). Roon and Christensen[11] subsequently changed the terminology to "low, middle, and high" cervical zones and altered the definition of a "low" (zone I) wound to one entering below the lower border of the cricoid cartilage. This conflict in the definition of zone I has continued to confuse young surgical house officers and some attending surgeons for the past 15 years. In truth, the original definitions most accurately divide the cervical region into one readily accessible area (zone II) and two somewhat inaccessible areas (zones I and III).

The patient described had an injury near the thoracic inlet (zone I). This bony circle encompasses major vascular structures, the trachea, the esophagus, the thoracic duct, and craniocervical nerves. Because penetrating wounds of the thoracic inlet may involve cervical, mediastinal, pleural, or spinal strictures, localization of the area of injury by radiologic studies in reasonably stable patients allows the trauma team to choose one of the many cervicothoracic incisions that are available to expose this area.[12] Options for therapy in the patient presented included a formal arch aortogram performed in the radiology suite; a rapid, one-shot retrograde brachial arteriogram performed by the trauma team in either the emergency department or the operating room; or a cervicothoracic incision based on the "best guess" by the attending surgeon. The first option is time-consuming in the absence of an in-house team from angiography and the third option is appropriate only for an unstable or exsanguinating patient. The retrograde arteriogram technique involves the placement of an 18-gauge, modified Cournand disposable needle in the brachial or axillary artery proximal to a blood pressure cuff.[13] After the cuff is inflated to 300 mm Hg and the patient's head is turned to the side away from the extremity to be evaluated, 50 mL of angiogram dye is rapidly injected as an assistant stabilizes the position of the needle in the artery. The arteriogram obtained on completion of the injection routinely visualizes the ipsilateral brachial, axillary, subclavian, and carotid arteries, and, on occasion, the vertebral and internal mammary arteries.

Case report.—A 49-year-old man was stabbed in the anterior neck on the right, just above the sternoclavicular junction. He was hemodynamically stable and had normal right carotid and upper extremity pulses, and his chest radiograph was normal. Because the stab wound appeared to pass into zone I, a formal retrograde arch aortogram was performed in the radiology suite. A 5-cm traumatic false aneurysm of the proximal right common carotid artery was noted on the arteriogram (Fig 3). A median sternotomy with a right anterior oblique cervical incision was made, and a lateral repair of a perforation in the right common carotid artery was successfully performed.

Although the role of arteriography in the evaluation of patients with penetrating proximity (to a major artery) wounds of the extremities is in question, the cervicothoracic arteries in the thoracic inlet must be studied in all patients with a proximity wound.[14-16] The risk of tamponade, stroke, compression of aerodigestive structures, or compression of the brachial plexus far outweighs any potential complications of the arteriogram. A retrograde arch aortogram performed through the femoral artery of the average young injured patient carries a complication rate of 2% to 4%, and this is considered to be acceptable in major trauma centers.

The aforementioned patient was stable and had no overt signs of an arterial injury. A patient treatment protocol based on long experience with such injuries prompted a formal radiologic study that allowed for the detection of this occult carotid injury and the use of an appropriate cervicothoracic incision.

Treatment of a Penetrating Wound in Zone III

Case report.—A 24-year-old man sustained a gunshot wound just behind the angle of the right side of the mandible. The patient was hemodynamically stable on arrival in the emergency department, and a small, nonpulsatile hematoma was noted at the entrance site of the missile. Because the wound was close to the internal carotid artery and a hematoma was present ("soft signs"), a selective carotid arteriogram was performed.[16] This revealed a 2-mm intimal defect in the right internal carotid artery at the base of the skull, but no extravasation or interruption of distal flow (Fig 4). Nonoperative therapy was chosen based on the location and size of the defect, as well as the maintenance of cerebral flow. A second carotid arteriogram 10 days later revealed nearly complete healing of the intimal defect.

Excellent data are available from Frykberg and associates,[17] Weaver and coworkers,[18] and others[19] demonstrating that nonocclusive arterial injuries heal in 87% to 95% of patients. These data are particularly clear for arterial lesions such as intimal defects or flaps, narrowing, spasm, or intramural/subintimal hematomas, but less so for lesions with extraluminal blood such as pseudoaneurysms or arteriovenous fistulas. The former lesions are equivalent to those produced during routine arteriographic studies in many patients, and their natural healing is well known.

In the patient described, the small size of the defect and its somewhat inaccessible location in zone III above the angle of the mandible, combined with the maintenance of cerebral flow made the choice of nonoperative

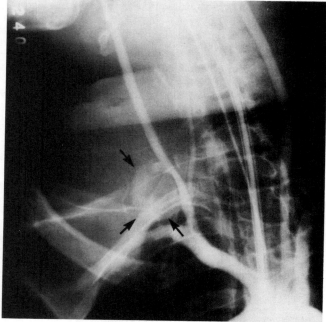

FIG 3.
Unsuspected pseudoaneurysm of the right common carotid artery in a patient with a stab wound passing into zone I. (From Brown MF, Graham JM, Feliciano DV, et al: Am J Surg 1982; 144:748–753. Used by permission.)

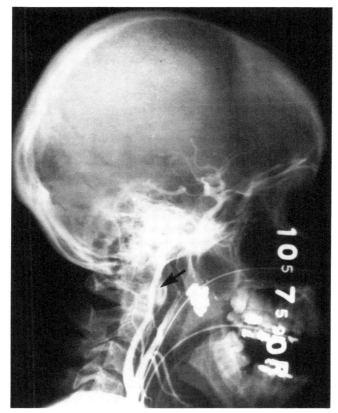

FIG 4.
Nonocclusive defect in the right internal carotid artery in zone III caused by a gunshot wound.

therapy an easy one. The key to nonoperative therapy in patients with injuries to critical cervical, truncal, or proximal extremity arteries is careful follow-up, with a second in-hospital arteriogram mandatory to document healing or worsening of the lesion. Wall lesions often show significant improvement in 7 to 10 days, with complete healing occurring in most patients by 2 to 4 months.[14, 15] Partial healing of the lesion seen on the second in-hospital arteriogram should prompt discharge of the patient, with weekly clinic follow-up and an outpatient arteriogram in 6 to 8 weeks.

Case report.—A 36-year-old woman sustained a gunshot wound over the coronoid process of the right side of the mandible. After an emergency cricothyroidotomy was performed because of marked pharyngeal swelling, a carotid arteriogram revealed significant extravasation of dye around the internal carotid artery at the base of the skull. Through an oblique cervical incision, the right common carotid artery was controlled proximally. The otolaryngology service then performed a "stair-step" right mandibulotomy starting at the mental foramen, and the attachment of the medial pterygoid muscle to the mandible, the posterior belly of the digastric muscle, and the stylohyoid muscle all were divided.[20] Because there was brisk back-bleeding from the distal arterial stump at the base of the skull and no changes on an intraoperative electroencephalogram (EEG) with occlusion of the proximal right internal carotid artery, the proximal and distal portions of the artery around the area of injury were ligated. A preoperative deficit in the right hypoglossal nerve persisted in the postoperative period, but the patient did well, with removal of the Erich arch bars for mandibular fixation during the sixth postoperative week.

Exposure of the distal internal carotid artery near the base of the skull may be performed in a variety of ways. Both neurosurgeons and otolaryngologists have used cervical incisions with preauricular and, sometimes, postauricular extensions to reach the base of the skull during elective procedures. With division of the temporoparotid fascia, identification of the facial nerve, mobilization of the parotid gland, and division of the posterior belly of the digastric muscle, stylohyoid muscle, and stylomandibular ligament, the distal internal carotid artery may be exposed without manipulation of the overlying mandible.[21] An alternate approach involves "drilling out" of the mastoid process and tympanic plate to obtain limited posterior exposure of the distal internal carotid artery.[22]

Trauma surgeons have sought more rapid approaches to high exposures because some patients have active bleeding at the time of presentation. The most rapid technique, which requires only minimal dissection to control hemorrhage at the base of the skull in such patients, involves the passage of a number 3 or 4 Fogarty balloon catheter across the carotid with sequential inflation of the balloon until hemorrhage ceases. In patients without active bleeding, operative techniques for exposure of the distal internal carotid artery have included unilateral or bilateral mandibular subluxation or one of a variety of mandibular osteotomies, much as in the patient described.[23-25]

Fisher and colleagues have comprehensively summarized the evolution of the subluxation techniques used at the Parkland Memorial Hospital in Dallas.[23] The original technique of bilateral mandibular subluxation by full-mouth arch bars with wiring around the teeth took 90 minutes to complete. Over an 8-year period, the oral surgery service developed a technique of unilateral subluxation by wiring around the mandible and across the nose that could be completed in only 10 minutes. A similar 10-minute technique of subluxation using diagonal interdental or Steinmann pin (for edentulous patients) wiring has been described more recently by Dossa and coworkers.[24] Larsen and Smead[25] have subsequently listed some of the disadvantages of the subluxation technique, including the creation of a dislocation rather than a subluxation, and limited improvement in access compared to the osteotomy techniques.[25]

The stair-step mandibulotomy used in the patient described in the case report is one of several horizontal or oblique osteotomies outlined in the literature and illustrated in articles by Dichtel and colleagues[20] and Larsen and Smead.[25] The latter authors have described an alternative approach, namely, a vertical ramus osteotomy that is simple to complete and affords wide exposure of the internal carotid artery at the base of the skull with minimal morbidity to the patient.[25] Particular advantages appear to be the modest risks of intraoral contamination, dysfunction of the temporomandibular joint, and a less than 2% incidence of injury to the inferior alveolar nerve. In the postoperative period, mandibular stability is maintained easily by miniature titanium bone plates.

Case report.—A 23-year-old man sustained a gunshot wound to the left skull base. He was neurologically intact in the emergency department, but had a moderate-sized hematoma overlying the distal left internal carotid artery. A selective left carotid arteriogram demonstrated complete occlusion of the internal carotid artery about 2 cm below the base of the skull. A decision was made to observe the patient, and he was transported to the surgical intensive care unit. As the patient moved himself from the stretcher to the bed, exsanguinating intraoral hemorrhage was noted. This hemorrhage was controlled by packing and manual compression as the patient was moved to the operating room, but several episodes of hypotension occurred. A left anterior oblique cervical incision was made, and proximal control of the left internal carotid artery was obtained. Despite this, vigorous hemorrhage continued to occur from the base of the skull. Rapid dissection along the internal carotid artery revealed a 95% transection about 1 cm below the base of the skull, with hemorrhage from the distal segment causing more hypotensive episodes. With great difficulty, the distal end of the internal carotid artery was oversewn at the base of the skull and the proximal artery was ligated. An EEG was not available in the operating room, so the patient was moved to the surgical intensive care unit. To decrease cerebral edema, the patient was placed in a sitting position, hyperventilated, and given limited intravenous fluids, in addition to 25 g of mannitol. The neurosurgical service was consulted regarding the value of an extracranial-intracranial bypass to restore ipsilateral cerebral flow. They were not willing to perform such a procedure based on the lack of efficacy of these techniques in elderly patients with cerebrovascular disease and on the history of excellent back-bleeding from the intracranial circulation at the time of carotid ligation. The patient awakened in the intensive care unit several hours later and moved all four extremities. About 14 hours after ligation of the carotid artery, the patient rapidly went into a coma and a dilated left pupil developed. An emergency computed tomography scan of the brain revealed severe cerebral edema. All efforts to reverse this problem in the intensive care unit were futile, and the patient died 2 days later without ever regaining consciousness. No autopsy was performed.

Because of difficulty in exposure and control of back-bleeding from the injured internal carotid artery at the base of the skull, ligation may be necessary in the patient who does not have a preoperative neurologic deficit. The development of a new neurologic deficit in the postoperative period is thought to depend on several factors, including hypotensive episodes associated with the injury, the anatomy of the circle of Willis, and secondary cerebral edema.[26]

Excellent historical data from surgical oncologists show that hypotensive episodes during ligation of the carotid artery for neoplasms in the head and neck increase the rate of neurologic sequelae from 28% to 87%.[27] More recent clinical reports have confirmed that intraoperative hypotension has an adverse effect on the outcome of patients with severe head injuries—a clinical scenario that is somewhat analogous to the ischemic hemi-brain that results from carotid ligation.[28] In addition, the anatomic variations in the circle of Willis are well known, and cerebral blood flow studies repeatedly have demonstrated that crossover flow from the contralateral internal carotid artery is not always adequate with ligation of the ipsilateral internal carotid artery.[26, 29, 30] Finally, definitive and effective treatment for severe cerebral edema remains elusive, even in experienced neurosurgical units.

When ligation is performed for injuries of the distal internal carotid artery, an intraoperative or early postoperative EEG may reveal changes suggestive of severe ischemia.[31] In such cases, one consideration is to return the patient to the operating room for an emergency extracranial-intracranial vascular bypass.[31, 32] Although experience with this technique in trauma patients is limited, satisfactory outcomes have been noted in several patients with carotid injuries or ligations and a preoperative neurologic deficit.[32]

In the absence of changes on the EEG, the priorities in patient care are prevention of postoperative hypotension or hypoxia and vigorous treatment of the cerebral edema that is likely to occur. Options for management of the latter problem continue to be intracranial pressure monitoring, sedation or paralysis, intravenous mannitol, drainage of cerebrospinal fluid, and, perhaps, high-dose barbiturates. Based on recent studies, the role of hyperventilation is much less clear in patients without an elevated intracranial pressure.[33]

Occlusion of the Internal Carotid Artery in an Asymptomatic Patient

Case report.—A 35-year-old man sustained a gunshot wound to the left upper neck near the angle of the mandible. He had a normal blood pressure, no palpable hematoma, and no difficulty speaking or swallowing. Because of the proximity of the wound to the internal carotid artery in zone III, a carotid arteriogram was performed. This study demonstrated an occlusion of the internal carotid artery about 2.5 cm above the bifurcation (Fig 5). Because the patient had no neurologic deficit, nonoperative therapy was chosen. After 48 hours of observation, the patient was discharged from the hospital and has continued to do well.

Occlusion of the internal carotid artery in the asymptomatic patient with either penetrating or blunt trauma may lead to delayed neurologic deficits from ischemia, cerebral edema, or emboli. It is impossible to predict which patients will have these complications. The need for operative intervention or anticoagulant therapy was unclear in the patient described above, be-

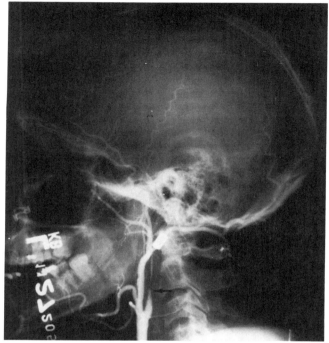

FIG 5.
Gunshot wound with occlusion of the left internal carotid artery in an asymptomatic patient. (From Feliciano DV: *Adv Trauma* 1987; 2:179–206. Used by permission.)

cause he had no neurologic deficits. It is always difficult to improve the condition of a patient who is already doing well, so no attempt at revascularization was considered. The benefits of anticoagulant therapy, including stabilization of the clot, prevention of further thrombosis, and possible prevention of emboli, always must be balanced against the risks of hemorrhage in the brain with a possible ischemic injury. In this asymptomatic patient, the choice was made to avoid anticoagulant therapy. A recent multicenter study on blunt carotid artery injuries did not demonstrate a significant advantage to the use of anticoagulants with blunt carotid thrombosis.[7]

Routine Repairs in Zone II Injuries

Case report.—A 26-year-old woman sustained a close-range gunshot wound to the right cheek resulting in severe facial lacerations and significant hemorrhage, but no neurologic deficit. After an emergency tracheostomy was performed, a right carotid arteriogram demonstrated numerous intimal defects over a 4-cm section of the internal carotid artery. Through an oblique cervical incision, a vein patch arterioplasty was performed to repair the area of perforations (Fig 6). Members of the plastic surgery service then repaired the facial lacerations. The patient's postoperative course was without incident, and she was neurologically intact at the time of hospital discharge.

In the patient with a penetrating wound in zone II and a large anterior cervical hematoma (pulsatile or not), external bleeding, or bleeding into the upper aerodigestive tract, immediate operation is indicated. The patient is placed in the sitting position with the chin and endotracheal tube directed away from the surgeon. All hair around the ipsilateral ear is shaved to allow ready access to both preauricular and postauricular areas, if needed. Skin preparation includes both sides of the neck to the chin anteriorly, around the ipsilateral ear, the entire anterior chest down to the umbilicus, and the anterior thigh on the side of the surgeon. This extensive skin preparation allows for anterior or posterior extension of the incision above the ear lobe, the addition of a median sternotomy for proximal vascular control, and retrieval of the greater saphenous vein for use as an interposition graft.[8]

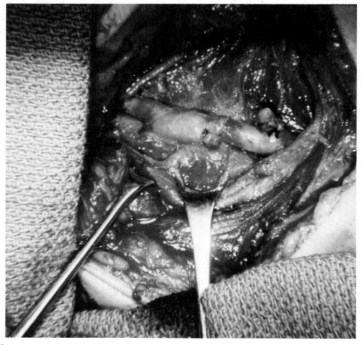

FIG 6.
Vein patch arterioplasty used to repair multiple perforations from a gunshot wound to the internal carotid artery.

The oblique skin incision is made along the anterior border of the sternocleidomastoid muscle, with a length appropriate to attain proximal and distal arterial control around the area of injury. In most zone II injuries, there is room to encircle the proximal common carotid artery above the clavicle before entering the hematoma. If the hematoma fills zone II or active external bleeding is present, a direct approach through the hematoma at the suspected level of injury often is performed by experienced trauma surgeons.

Angled DeBakey vascular clamps are used for vascular control of the common carotid artery. The internal carotid artery is soft and small in young injured patients, and vascular control is usually maintained with Silastic loops or bulldog vascular clamps. At the time of clamping, question often exists regarding the need for a shunt to maintain cerebral flow, much as in elective carotid endarterectomy. It is the policy of many experienced trauma surgeons to avoid the use of a shunt in young, healthy patients who were neurologically intact before operation and have excellent back-bleeding from the cerebral circulation, and in whom repair can be performed within 15 to 20 minutes. If the patient has a preoperative neurologic deficit or multiple episodes of hypotension before vascular control is obtained, the insertion of a rigid Argyle or looped Javid shunt is appropriate.[34, 35] There are no convincing data, however, suggesting that the use of these shunts improves the outcome in young, previously healthy patients who have an expeditious arterial repair.[36]

The choice of repair depends on the size of the defect.[37] Perforations from stab wounds or low-velocity missiles are debrided minimally and closed in a transverse direction with continuous 6–0 polypropylene suture. With loss of tissue from one wall, a vein or prosthetic patch angioplasty is appropriate, as in the patient described. Such patches are difficult to size in collapsed arteries and tedious to sew, but save the time that would be needed to perform a segmental resection and an end-to-end anastomosis or insertion of an interposition graft. An oversized, thin polytetrafluoroethylene (PTFE) patch is the easiest to insert and should not be trimmed until half the defect is closed and flushing is allowed temporarily to "balloon" the patch to an appropriate fit.

Segmental resections are usually performed if through-and-through injuries are present or there is extensive destruction (>50%) of a portion of the wall. The carotid artery is elastic and easily dissected proximally and distally after segmental resection, and an end-to-end anastomosis is readily performed with a two-point (sutures tied 180 degrees apart) fixation technique (Fig 7).

An extensive segmental resection mandates the insertion of an interposition graft. Either a reversed autogenous saphenous vein graft from the ipsilateral thigh or an appropriately sized PTFE graft may be used, although the vein graft is preferred in routine cases because of its long-term patency.[38] If there has been excessive hemorrhage or periods of hypoten-

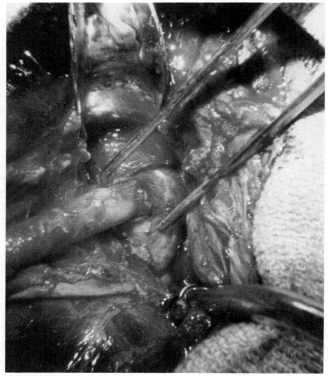

FIG 7.
End-to-end anastomosis of the right common carotid artery just above the bifurcation of the innominate artery was performed through a cervical incision in a patient with a shotgun wound of the anterior neck.

sion, a PTFE graft off the shelf is an appropriate choice (Fig 8). Much as with elective surgery on the carotid artery, thrombosis of an extensive repair or interposition graft often leads to the death of the patient.[39]

Treatment of the Carotid Artery Injury With Associated Stroke or Coma

Case report.—A 23-year-old man sustained a gunshot wound to the left neck. He was noted to have a large pulsatile hematoma under the entrance site of the missile and a Glasgow Coma Scale score of 5. Despite rapid repair of a transected left internal carotid artery, the patient remained in a coma postoperatively and was transferred to a chronic care facility.

The controversy surrounding repair vs. ligation in patients with preoperative neurologic deficits is at least 75 years old.[40] Much of the current debate started in 1970 when Cohen and associates described 8 patients (from a total group of 86) with neurologic deficits in combination with injuries to the carotid artery.[41] After repair of the carotid artery, these researchers noted that "the neurologic deficit in two of these patients reverted to normal, three patients died of progressive cerebral vascular damage, two had an increase in neurologic deficit, and one patient's neurologic condition remained unchanged." One of the conclusions reached in this paper was that "ligation may be the procedure of choice in a number of patients who have impairment of neurologic function."[41]

In 1973, Bradley reviewed a 10-year experience with penetrating injuries to the carotid artery at Grady Memorial Hospital.[42] In a group of ten normotensive patients who had preoperative neurologic deficits, "six died from cerebral causes, and only two appeared to benefit from vascular repair." Results in the subgroup of five patients with preoperative hemiplegia or quadriplegia were especially dismal, with all dying in the early postoperative period. Bradley noted that postmortem examination in two of these five patients demonstrated hemorrhagic infarction of the revascularized lobe. He concluded that "ligation might be considered in this group of patients," and suggested that prospective studies were needed to resolve the controversy.

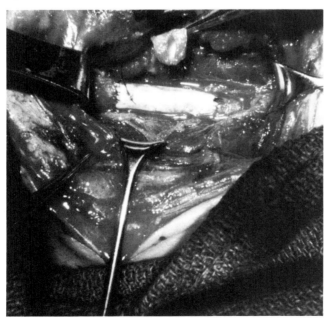

FIG 8.
Eight-mm PTFE graft used to repair a transection of the right common carotid artery from a gunshot wound. Note the resected artery specimen in the forceps. (From Brown MF, Graham JM, Feliciano DV, et al: *Am J Surg* 1982; 144:748–753. Used by permission.)

Subsequent reports describing patients with penetrating wounds have favored attempts at repair, with the caveat that comatose patients do poorly with either repair or ligation.[18, 26, 34-37, 39, 43-47] The literature review of penetrating carotid injuries performed by Liekweg and Greenfield in 1978 is one of the most comprehensive summaries available.[43] Among a group of 40 patients with neurologic deficits *exclusive of coma,* 34 underwent revascularization and 6 had ligation. A favorable outcome occurred in 85% of the patients who underwent revascularization vs. 50% of those who received ligation ($P < .05$). In a report from Brown and coworkers, 22 patients were admitted with neurologic deficits short of coma.[26] Of the 3 patients who were treated with ligation, 2 subsequently died. Revascularization was performed in the remaining 19 patients, and 14 had no deficit at hospital discharge or "their deficit was significantly decreased." Robbs and coworkers subsequently described 15 patients with "localizing neurological signs without coma."[45] Among the 14 patients who underwent reconstruction of either the common or the internal carotid artery, 7 had improvement or complete clearing of the deficit and 6 were left with a permanent hemiparesis.

Liekweg and Greenfield also described a group of 23 patients *with coma,* 15 of whom underwent revascularization and 8 of whom had ligation.[43] A favorable outcome was noted in only 27% and 25% of patients, respectively. Based on their review, these investigators recommended ligation of the carotid artery only in comatose patients without prograde flow or patients in whom repair is technically impossible. Brown and colleagues also described 16 patients admitted with coma.[26] Six of 9 patients who underwent revascularization had partial or total clearing of the preoperative neurologic deficit, and 3 died. Among the 7 patients who had ligation, 5 died and 2 improved. Finally, Robbs and coworkers described 7 patients with coma and localizing neurologic signs.[45] Four patients underwent reconstruction, with 3 recovering completely and 1 left with a permanent hemiplegia. In the group of 3 patients who underwent ligation, 2 died and 1 had a permanent hemiparesis.

Based on the available data, the best chance for recovery of a patient with a neurologic deficit short of coma resulting from a penetrating wound occurring just before arrival in the emergency department is revascularization. Comatose patients should also undergo immediate reconstruction, particularly if hypotension has made the preoperative neurologic examination difficult to interpret. Improvement or clearing of the deficit can be expected in 27% to 66% of comatose patients, with the patient's cerebrovascular anatomy, the surgeon's speed in reestablishing cerebral blood flow, and the quality of postoperative critical care all presumably affecting the final result.

Balloon Catheter Tamponade

Case report.—An 18-year-old man sustained a gunshot wound to the base of the skull at the level of the first cervical vertebra on the left (Fig 9). There was

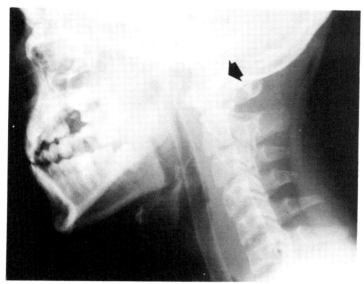

FIG 9.
Gunshot wound to the base of the skull that damaged the left internal carotid artery.

diffuse hemorrhage from behind the mandible, and the patient was rushed to the operating room. The left common and internal carotid arteries were exposed through an oblique cervical incision. Clamping of the internal carotid artery slowed the hemorrhage, but did not cause it to stop. An internal carotid arteriotomy was made, and a number 4 Fogarty balloon catheter was passed to the presumed area of injury at the base of the skull (Fig 10). With inflation of the balloon, all hemorrhage ceased. The oblique cervical incision was closed around the Fogarty catheter, and the patient was moved to the surgical intensive care unit. On the third postoperative day, the patient was returned to the operating room. The incision was partially reopened, the Fogarty balloon was deflated, the catheter was removed, the arteriotomy site was closed, and the patient was observed in the operating room for 15 minutes. During 2 more days of observation in the hospital, the patient remained neurologically intact and then was discharged.

Case report.—A 22-year-old man sustained a stab wound to the high left lateral neck anterior and inferior to the ear. His blood pressure was not palpable on arrival in the emergency department. A left anterolateral thoracotomy, cross-clamping of the descending thoracic aorta, and internal cardiac massage were performed. With the return of cardiac activity, vigorous arterial bleeding was noted to be coming from the site of the stab wound. The patient was rushed to the operating room, where an oblique left anterior cervical incision was performed. Because of the extensive hemorrhage, a number 8 Fogarty balloon catheter was inserted into the site of the stab wound and advanced until resistance was encountered. At this point, the balloon was inflated and all hemorrhage ceased. A dry gauze roll was packed into the depths of the stab wound track around the Fogarty balloon catheter to

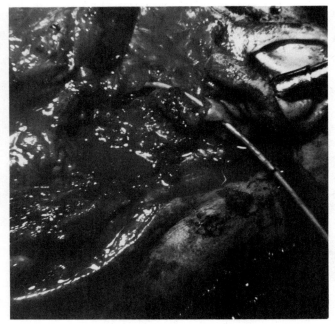

FIG 10.
A transcarotid number 4 Fogarty balloon catheter was used to control hemorrhage at the base of the skull. The balloon catheter was removed on the third postoperative day. (Same patient as in Figure 9.)

hold it in place (Fig 11). The thoracotomy incision then was closed after ligation of the left internal mammary artery. After 3 days of observation in the intensive care unit, the patient was returned to the operating room for removal of the pack and the balloon catheter. He had no neurologic deficits at the time of hospital discharge.

Balloon catheter tamponade has been used for the past 35 years for operative control of hemorrhage from inaccessible or fragile vascular structures, or from the heart.[31] Although the technique is rarely indicated, it is lifesaving in properly selected patients.

The decision to insert balloon catheters in the two patients described was based on the presence of exsanguinating hemorrhage and the inaccessible location of the source. By the time the oral surgery service would have been able to come to the operating room to perform a vertical ramus osteotomy or subluxation of the temporomandibular joint with wiring, both patients would have died of hemorrhage. In the first patient, proximal control of the internal carotid artery through an anterior oblique cervical incision resulted in some slowing of the bleeding. This was presumptive evidence that the distal internal carotid artery was the source of hemorrhage. When a decision is made to pass a balloon catheter through a carotid arteriotomy, a number 3 or 4 Fogarty catheter is used. The catheter is advanced and the balloon is inflated when the suspected area of injury is reached. It may be necessary to deflate the balloon and move it proximally or distally and then inflate it again to find the ideal site at which to control hemorrhage. After hemorrhage is controlled, the surgical team may choose to leave the balloon in place for several days or to proceed with further operative dissection for formal repair (or ligation) of the injured area in the distal internal carotid artery. If balloon catheter tamponade is determined to be the treatment of choice, the balloon may be filled with radiopaque dye for visualization on postoperative radiographs. The catheter also should be sutured to the arteriotomy site and to the skin incision to prevent dislodgment.

Balloon occlusion is equivalent to ligation of the internal carotid artery, and consideration once again should be given to performing a postoperative EEG and monitoring intracranial pressure. With obvious signs of ischemia on the EEG and an unwillingness to attempt repair of the occluded distal internal carotid artery, an extracranial-intracranial vascular bypass is

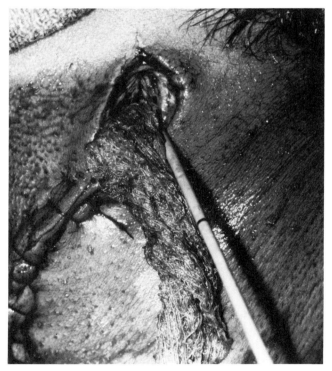

FIG 11.
A number 8 Fogarty balloon catheter was passed directly into the track of a stab wound until bleeding at the base of the skull was controlled. The balloon catheter was removed on the third postoperative day.

indicated. If increased intracranial pressure rather than ischemia results, all the previously described techniques for control are used. In the asymptomatic patient, a return to the operating room is indicated in 48 to 72 hours for deflation of the balloon, removal of the catheter, and closure of the arteriotomy site. It is probably safe to remove the catheter through the skin incision and to apply pressure over the arteriotomy site as an alternative approach.

If hemorrhage from the missile or knife track cannot be controlled by external pressure and there is not enough time to obtain proximal control of the internal carotid artery (as in the second patient described), a larger Fogarty balloon catheter (number 8) or even a Foley catheter with a 5-mL or 30-mL balloon may be inserted directly into the wound. Again, sequential inflation of the balloon should be performed until hemorrhage is controlled. Although the exact position of the balloon can be determined only by performing a postoperative arteriogram, an exsanguinating wound at the base of the skull is presumed to arise from a defect in the distal internal carotid artery. For this reason, the previously mentioned monitoring and precautions are maintained in the surgical intensive care unit after the balloon has been inserted. In recent years, the balloon has been deflated and the catheter removed through the skin incision in the intensive care unit 48 to 72 hours after the original operation. Recurrent bleeding after removal of the balloon catheter for tamponade has not occurred in the author's experience.[31]

Carotid-Jugular Fistula

Case report.—A 26-year-old woman sustained a gunshot wound to the right side of the face at the angle of the mandible. A palpable thrill and audible bruit were present over the right anterior neck, and a carotid arteriogram demonstrated a carotid artery false aneurysm and an associated carotid-jugular arteriovenous fistula (Figs 12 and 13). Through an oblique right anterior cervical incision, proximal control of the carotid artery and jugular veins was obtained. The fistula was then manually detached, bleeding was controlled by compression, and distal control of both vessels was applied. A lateral repair of the internal jugular vein was completed with continuous 5–0 polypropylene suture. The defect in the distal internal carotid artery was of modest size and was repaired with continuous 6–0 polypropylene suture. The patient was neurologically intact at the time of hospital discharge.

Although it is rare, an untreated carotid-jugular fistula decreases arterial flow to the ipsilateral hemisphere, reduces systemic vascular resistance, and leads to increases in the heart rate, stroke volume, and plasma volume. Severe congestive heart failure may result if the fistula is not closed.[48]

Operative division of the fistula and repair of the carotid artery and jugular vein are the preferred treatments because cerebral flow is preserved and the hyperdynamic state is cured.[48, 49] Although balloon or coil occlu-

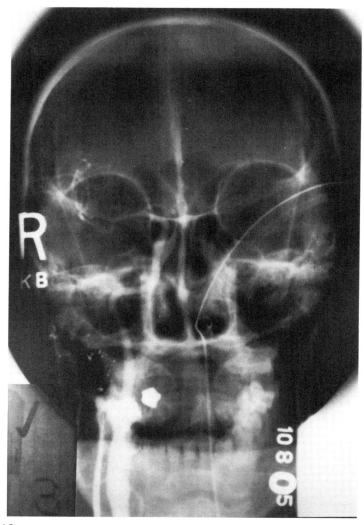

FIG 12.
Anterior view of a right internal carotid artery-internal jugular vein fistula resulting from a gunshot wound to the right side of the face.

sion of the arterial side of the fistula is curative, much as with high vertebral-jugular arteriovenous fistulas, the need to interrupt ipsilateral cerebral flow in the patient without a neurologic deficit or risk of exsanguination is not appealing. If the fistula is located high in the neck, preoperative or intraoperative placement of a balloon catheter into the internal carotid artery proximally should be considered. With passage of the balloon distally and

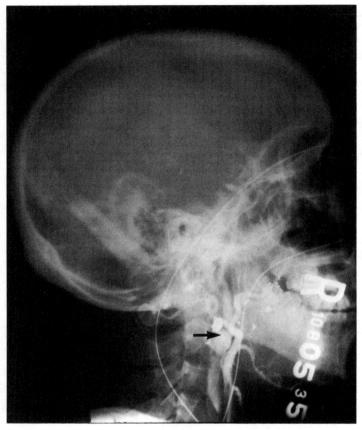

FIG 13.
Lateral view of a right internal carotid artery-internal jugular vein fistula resulting from a gunshot wound to the right side of the face. (Same patient as in Figure 12.)

inflation at the site of the fistula, the distended jugular vein is less engorged and easier to dissect. Ligation of the internal jugular vein after detachment of the fistula is acceptable.

Blowout of the Carotid Artery in the Postoperative Period[50]

Case report.—A 26-year-old man sustained a gunshot wound to the right neck with obvious penetration of the platysma muscle. A moderate-sized hematoma was present, and the patient was taken directly to the operating room. Lateral injuries to the trachea and esophagus were primarily repaired, although the esophageal injury was extensive. The right common carotid artery had a small contusion, but was otherwise intact. After the insertion of a Penrose drain between the esophagus and the carotid artery, the incision was closed. In the early postoperative period, a purulent wound infection developed and was treated conservatively. On the fifth postoperative day, arterial bleeding was noted to be coming from the Penrose drain and the patient was returned to the operating room. A second right cervical exploration demonstrated total dissolution of the wall of the common carotid artery near the Penrose drain and a foul-smelling wound infection, but no obvious leak from the esophageal repair. The site of the blowout in the right common carotid artery was resected, and both arterial ends around the resection were ligated. Pneumonia and meningitis developed, and the patient died of a right cerebral infarction 3 days later.

There are certain technical maneuvers that may be helpful to protect the normal or repaired carotid artery in patients with significant cervical contamination from isolated or combined tracheoesophageal injuries.[50] In the patient with a combined tracheoesophageal injury, there is a significant risk of fistula formation with possible secondary injury to the carotid artery because the repairs in the two structures are frequently in close proximity (i.e, posterior trachea-anterior esophagus). In such a patient, the sternal head of the sternocleidomastoid muscle should be detached and placed between the adjacent repairs. If a Penrose drain is to be used for drainage in the postoperative period, it should be directed anteriorly and *not* pass over the uninjured carotid artery (Fig 14). On the rare occasion when injury to both the carotid artery and either of the aerodigestive structures is present, the sternal head of the sternocleidomastoid muscle should once again be

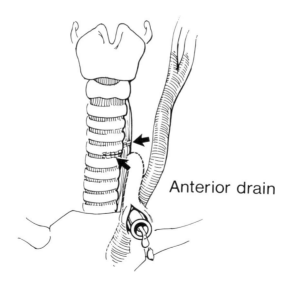

©Baylor College of Medicine 1985

FIG 14.
Drains for esophageal or tracheoesophageal injuries should be directed anteriorly and not pass over the carotid artery. (From Feliciano DV, Bitondo CG, Mattox KL, et al: *Am J Surg* 1985; 150:710–715. Used by permission.)

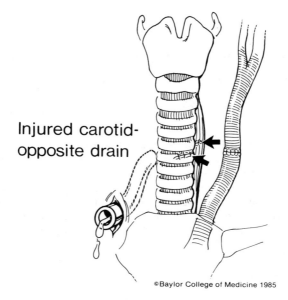

FIG 15.
In the presence of an ipsilateral carotid artery injury, drains for esophageal or combined tracheoesophageal injuries should be established through the side of the neck opposite the injury. (From Feliciano DV, Bitondo CG, Mattox KL, et al: *Am J Surg* 1985; 150:710–715. Used by permission.)

detached and placed between the tracheal or esophageal repair and the carotid repair. In addition, drainage of an esophageal repair or a combined tracheoesophageal repair should be established through the side of the neck opposite the carotid repair (Fig 15). This technique may eliminate a carotid-esophageal fistula resulting from a leak in the esophageal repair.[51]

References

1. Feliciano DV, Bitondo CG, Mattox KL, et al: Civilian trauma in the 1980s. A 1-year experience with 456 vascular and cardiac injuries. *Ann Surg* 1984; 199:717–724.
2. Welling RE, Saul TG, Tew JM Jr, et al: Management of blunt injury to the internal carotid artery. *J Trauma* 1987; 27:1221–1226.
3. Reddy K, Furer M, West M, et al: Carotid artery dissection secondary to seatbelt trauma: Case report. *J Trauma* 1990; 30:630–633.
4. Davis JW, Holbrook TL, Hoyt DB, et al: Blunt carotid artery dissection: Incidence, associated injuries, screening, and treatment. *J Trauma* 1990; 30:1514–1517.
5. Lee C, Woodring JH, Walsh JW: Carotid and vertebral artery injury in survivors of atlanto-occipital dislocation: Case reports and literature review. *J Trauma* 1991; 31:401–407.
6. Hebra A, Robison JG, Elliott BM: Traumatic aneurysm associated with fi-

brointimal proliferation of the common carotid artery following blunt trauma: Case report. *J Trauma* 1993; 34:297–299.
7. Cogbill TH, Moore EE, Jurkovich GJ, et al: The spectrum of blunt injury to the carotid artery: A multicenter experience. Presented at the 24th Annual Meeting of the Western Trauma Association, Crested Butte, Colorado, February-March 1994.
8. Feliciano DV: Vascular injuries, in Maull KI, Cleveland HC, Strauch GO, et al (ed): *Advances in Trauma*, vol 2. St Louis, Mosby, 1987, pp 177–206.
9. Advanced Trauma Life Support Subcommittee: Airway and ventilatory management, in *Advanced Trauma Life Support Subcommittee, Committee on Trauma: Advanced Trauma Life Support Program for Physicians, 1993 Instructor Manual*. Chicago, American College of Surgeons, 1993, pp 47–59.
10. Monson DO, Saletta JD, Freeark RJ: Carotid vertebral trauma. *J Trauma* 1969; 9:987–999.
11. Roon AJ, Christensen N: Evaluation and treatment of penetrating cervical injuries. *J Trauma* 1979; 19:391–397.
12. Feliciano DV, Mattox KL, Graham JM, et al: Hazards and pitfalls of thoracic inlet injury. *Current Concepts in Trauma Care* 1979; 2:5–7.
13. O'Gorman RB, Feliciano DV: Arteriography performed in the emergency center. *Am J Surg* 1986; 152:323–325.
14. Dennis JW, Frykberg ER, Crump JM, et al: New perspectives on the management of penetrating trauma in proximity to major limb arteries. *J Vasc Surg* 1990; 11:84–93.
15. Frykberg ER, Dennis JW, Bishop K, et al: The reliability of physical examination in the evaluation of penetrating extremity trauma for vascular injury: Results at one year. *J Trauma* 1991; 31:502–511.
16. Sclafani SJA, Panetta T, Goldstein AS, et al: The management of arterial injuries caused by penetration of zone III of the neck. *J Trauma* 1985; 25:871–881.
17. Frykberg ER, Vines FS, Alexander RH: The natural history of clinically occult arterial injuries: A prospective evaluation. *J Trauma* 1989; 29:577–583.
18. Weaver FA, Yellin AE, Wagner WH, et al: The role of arterial reconstruction in penetrating carotid injuries. *Arch Surg* 1988; 123:1106–1111.
19. Wigle RL, Moran JM: Spontaneous healing of a traumatic thoracic aortic tear: Case report. *J Trauma* 1991; 31:280–283.
20. Dichtel WJ, Miller RH, Feliciano DV, et al: Lateral mandibulotomy: A technique of exposure for penetrating injuries of the internal carotid artery at the base of the skull. *Laryngoscope* 1984; 94:1140–1144.
21. Sundt TM Jr (ed): *Occlusive Cerebrovascular Disease. Diagnosis and Surgical Management*. Philadelphia, WB Saunders, 1987.
22. Pellegrini RV, Manzetti GW, DiMarco RF, et al: The direct surgical management of lesions of the high internal carotid artery. *J Cardiovasc Surg (Torino)* 1984; 25:29–35.
23. Fisher DF, Clagett GP, Parker JI, et al: Mandibular subluxation for high carotid exposure. *J Vasc Surg* 1984; 1:727–733.
24. Dossa C, Shepard AD, Wolford DG, et al: Distal internal carotid exposure: A simplified technique for temporary mandibular subluxation. *J Vasc Surg* 1990; 12:319–325.
25. Larsen PE, Smead WL: Vertical ramus osteotomy for improved exposure of the distal internal carotid artery: A new technique. *J Vasc Surg* 1992; 15:226–231.

26. Brown MF, Graham JM, Feliciano DV, et al: Carotid artery injuries. Am J Surg 1982; 144:747–753.
27. Moore O, Baker HW: Carotid artery ligation in surgery of the head and neck. Cancer 1955; 8:712–716.
28. Pietropaoli JA, Rogers FB, Shackford SR, et al: The deleterious effects of intraoperative hypotension on outcome in patients with severe head injuries. J Trauma 1992; 33:403–407.
29. Sundt TM, Sharbrough FW, Piepgras DG, et al: Correlation of cerebral blood flow and electroencephalographic changes during carotid endarterectomy. With results of surgery and hemodynamics of cerebral ischemia. Mayo Clin Proc 1981; 56:533–543.
30. Roberts B, Hardesty WH, Holling HE, et al: Studies on extracranial cerebral blood flow. Surgery 1964; 56:826–833.
31. Feliciano DV, Burch JM, Mattox KL, et al: Balloon catheter tamponade in cardiovascular wounds. Am J Surg 1990; 169:583–587.
32. Gewertz BL, Samson DS, Ditmore QM, et al: Management of penetrating injuries of the internal carotid artery at the base of the skull utilizing extracranial-intracranial bypass. J Trauma 1980; 20:365–369.
33. Muizelaar JP, Marmarou A, Ward JD, et al: Adverse effects of prolonged hyperventilation in patients with severe head injury: A randomized clinical trial. J Neurosurg 1991; 75:731–739.
34. Padberg FT Jr, Hobson RW II, Yeager RA, et al: Penetrating carotid arterial trauma. Am Surg 1984; 50:277–282.
35. Pearce WH, Whitehall TA: Carotid and vertebral arterial injuries. Surg Clin North Am 1988; 68:705–723.
36. Demetriades D, Skalkides J, Sofianos C, et al: Carotid artery injuries: Experience with 124 cases. J Trauma 1989; 29:91–94.
37. Meyer JP, Walsh J, Barrett J, et al: Analysis of 18 recent cases of penetrating injuries to the common and internal carotid arteries. Am J Surg 1988; 156:96–99.
38. Feliciano DV, Mattox KL, Graham JM, et al: Five-year experience with PTFE grafts in vascular wounds. J Trauma 1985; 25:71–82.
39. Fabian TC, George SM Jr, Croce MA, et al: Carotid artery trauma: Management based on mechanism of injury. J Trauma 1990; 30:953–963.
40. Makins GH: Gunshot Injuries to the Blood Vessels. Bristol, England, John Wright & Sons, 1919.
41. Cohen A, Brief D, Mathewson C Jr: Carotid artery injuries. An analysis of eighty-five cases. Am J Surg 1970; 120:210–214.
42. Bradley EL III: Management of penetrating carotid injuries: An alternative approach. J Trauma 1973; 13:248–253.
43. Liekweg WG Jr, Greenfield LJ: Management of penetrating carotid arterial injury. Ann Surg 1978; 188:587–592.
44. Ledgerwood AM, Mullins RJ, Lucas CE: Primary repair vs ligation for carotid artery injuries. Arch Surg 1980; 115:488–493.
45. Robbs JV, Human RR, Rajaruthnam P, et al: Neurological deficit and injuries involving the neck arteries. Br J Surg 1983; 70:220–222.
46. Karlin RM, Marks C: Extracranial carotid artery injury. Current surgical management. Am J Surg 1983; 146:225–227.
47. Richardson R, Obeid FN, Richardson JD, et al: Neurologic consequences of cerebrovascular injury. J Trauma 1992; 32:755–760.
48. Kakkar S, Angelini P, Leachman R, et al: Successful closure of post-traumatic

carotid-jugular arteriovenous fistula complicated by congestive heart failure and cerebrovasclar insufficiency. *Cardiovas Dis* 1979; 6:457–462.
49. Meier DE, Ammons DH, Estrera AS: Missile embolus to the lung associated with a carotid-jugular arteriovenous fistula. *J Trauma* 1981; 21:1048–1049.
50. Feliciano DV, Bitondo CG, Mattox KL, et al: Combined tracheoesophageal injuries. *Am J Surg* 1985; 150:710–715.
51. Levine EA, Alverdy JD: Carotid-esophageal fistula following a penetrating neck injury: Case report. *J Trauma* 1990; 30:1588–1590.

Index

A

Abdomen
  CT, 89
    in children, 178
  injuries, in children, 178–179
Absorbable suture: in bladder repair after pelvic fracture, 219
Acetabular fractures, 222–223
N-Acetylcysteine: for immunologic blockade, 157
Acquired immunodeficiency syndrome: *Candida* infections in, 231
Adenosine triphosphate
  levels after hypoxia and ischemia, 143
  -MgCl$_2$ for immunologic stimulation, 148
AIDS: *Candida* infections in, 231
Air
  mediastinal, on plain radiograph after esophageal injury, 255
  rewarmers, convective, 59–60
Airway
  in children, 174–175
  compromise and cervical hematoma after penetrating carotid artery injury, 319–321
  esophageal gastric tube, 6
  esophageal obturator, 6
  management, prehospital, 5–6
  pharyngeal tracheal lumen, 6
  rewarming in hypothermia, 62
Aluminum space blankets: in hypothermia, 61
Amino acids: branched chain, for immunologic stimulation, 148
Anastomosis: end-to-end, after penetrating carotid artery injury, 332
Anatomy
  pelvis, 200
  surgical, of esophagus, 245–248
Angiography of hypogastric vessels after pelvic fracture
  showing hemorrhage, 210
  showing occlusion after placement of coils and Gelfoam, 211
Antiarrhythmics: in hypothermia, 50–51
Antibodies
  interleukin-6, for immunologic blockade, 153–154
  monoclonal, for immunologic blockade, 152, 156

Anticandidal function, polymorphonuclear neutrophil (*see* Polymorphonuclear neutrophil, anticandidal function)
Anticoagulant therapy: in extracorporeal cardiopulmonary support, 118, 120
Antiendotoxin strategies: of immunologic blockade, 151–152
Antigen titers: *Candida*, 228–240
Anti-inflammatory drugs: nonsteroidal, for immunologic blockade, 155–156
Antioxidants: for immunologic stimulation, 149
Antiproteases: for immunologic blockade, 157
Antiserum: to mutant J5 *Escherichia coli*, 151
Antishock garment, pneumatic (*see* Pneumatic antishock garment)
Anti-tumor necrosis factor: for immunologic blockade, 153
Aortic
  laceration complicating laparoscopy, 93
  rupture, traumatic, extracorporeal cardiopulmonary support during repair of, 109–111
Aprotinin: during extracorporeal cardiopulmonary support, 118
Arginine: for immunologic stimulation, 148
Arteriography: in penetrating carotid artery injuries, 323
Arterioplasty: vein patch, after gunshot wound to carotid artery, 330
Arteriovenous rewarming, continuous, after hypothermia, 65–68
  depiction, 67
Artery
  carotid (*see* Carotid artery)
  embolization after pelvic fracture, 209–211
  hypogastric, ligation after pelvic fracture, 207
  pelvic, injury in pelvic fracture, 209–211
  supply of esophagus, 247
Atlantoaxial rotation injuries, 25–26
Axis fracture, 27–28
Azygous vein: esophagus relationship to, 247

B

Backboard: prehospital use, 9
Bacterial translocation
  enteral feeding and, 299–301
  immunosuppression and, 141

347

Bacterial translocation *(cont.)*
  in surgical patients, and enteral feeding, 300–301
Bactericidal/permeability increasing protein: for immunologic blockade, 152
Balloon catheter tamponade: in penetrating carotid artery injuries, 334–338
Barium: in contrast studies of esophageal injury, 255–256
Barotrauma: pulmonary, in mechanically ventilated patients, 101
Beds: specialty, for immobilization of spine, 21
Biologic response modifiers: for immunologic stimulation, 146–148
Biomechanical etiology: of lower cervical spine injuries, 29
Bladder rupture due to pelvic fracture, 217–219
  extraperitoneal, cystogram of, 218
  intraperitoneal, cystogram of, 218
Blankets for rewarming after hypothermia
  aluminum space, 61
  cotton hospital, 60
  convective warm air, 59–60
  fluid-circulating heating, 58–59
Blast injury: esophageal, 250–251
Bleeding complications: of extracorporeal cardiopulmonary support, 120–122
Bloating: and enteral feeding, 311
Blood
  effects of hypothermia on, 54–55
  flow
    hepatic, and enteral feeding, 298
    hepatic, effect of mechanical ventilation on, 101
    path through extracorporeal circuit, 116
    renal, effect of mechanical ventilation on, 101
    splanchnic, effect of hypothermia on, 53
  gases
    after early fixation of femur fracture in chest-injured patient, 283
    hypothermia and, 51–52
  products, warming, in hypothermia, 63–64
  pumps, servo-regulated, in extracorporeal cardiopulmonary support, historical perspective, 104
Blowout: of carotid artery in postoperative period, 340–342
Board: spinal, prehospital use of, 9
Bone, long, fracture *(see* Fracture, long-bone)
Bowel: small, ischemia, and enteral feeding, 311–312

Brace: two- or four-point sternal occipital mandibular immobilization, 22
Bradykinin inhibitors: for immunologic blockade, 154
Branched chain amino acids: for immunologic stimulation, 148
Breathing
  in children, 175–176
  liquid, 123
Bretylium: in hypothermia, 51
Bronchorrhea: cold, 51
Build-A-Board, 10
Burns: immune dysfunction after, 139
Bypass
  cardiopulmonary
    in hypothermia treatment, 65
    partial *(See also* Extracorporeal, cardiopulmonary support)
    partial, discussion of term, 105
    partial, protocol for rapid rewarming with, 109
    roller pump in extracorporeal blood rewarming, 68–69
  extracranial-intracranial, after penetrating carotid artery injuries, 328
  heart-lung *(see* cardiopulmonary *above)*

C

Calcium
  channel blockers for immunologic blockade, 154
  levels in hypothermia, 54
Cancer patients: *Candida* infections in, 231
Candida
  antigen titers, 228–240
  infections, 227–243
    detection methods, 228–229
Cannulation: in extracorporeal cardiopulmonary support, 115–116
Caps: protective surgical, 85–86
Carbon dioxide
  clearance monitoring during extracorporeal cardiopulmonary support, 115
  removal, extracorporeal *(see* Extracorporeal, carbon dioxide removal)
Carcinoma: esophagus, causing esophagus rupture, 251
Cardiac *(see* Heart)
Cardiogenic shock: extracorporeal cardiopulmonary support in, 112
Cardiopulmonary
  bypass *(see* Bypass, cardiopulmonary)
  resuscitation *(see* Resuscitation, cardiopulmonary)

support, extracorporeal (see
    Extracorporeal, cardiopulmonary
    support)
Cardiovascular effects: of hypothermia,
    49–51
Care
  follow-up, of children after treatment in
    adult trauma center, 187–188
  prehospital, 1–14
    conclusions, 10–11
  psychosocial, for children after treatment
    in adult trauma center, 187–188
Carotid artery
  blowout, postoperative, 340–342
  common, pseudoaneurysm (see
    Pseudoaneurysm of common
    carotid artery)
  injury, penetrating, 319–345
    anastomosis in, end-to-end, 332
    arterioplasty for, vein patch, 330
    carotid-jugular fistula due to,
      338–340
    cervical hematoma with compromise
      of airway due to, 319–321
    coma associated, treatment, 332–334
    drain placement in, 340–342
    nonocclusive defect due to, 325
    occlusion of internal carotid artery in
      asymptomatic patient after,
      328–329
    stroke associated, treatment, 332–334
    tamponade in, balloon catheter,
      334–338
    zone I, diagnostic evaluation,
      321–323
    zone II, routine repairs, 329–332
    zone III, treatment, 323–328
  internal, occlusion in asymptomatic
    patient after penetrating carotid
    artery injury, 328–329
  -jugular vein fistula due to penetrating
    carotid artery injury, 338–340
  ligation after penetrating injuries, 328
Cart
  extracorporeal cardiopulmonary support,
    114
  pediatric trauma, components of, 185
Cast: Minerva, for atlantoaxial rotation
    injuries, 26
Catecholamines: and immunosuppression,
    141
Catheter
  Foley, in pelvic fracture patient, 217,
    219
  jejunostomy, needle, 297
  tamponade, balloon, in penetrating
    carotid artery injuries, 334–338

Cell(s)
  -mediated immunity, 137
  suppressor, in immunosuppression, 142
  T, changes after trauma, 138
Central nervous system effects: of
    hypothermia, 52–53
Cerebral edema: after penetrating carotid
    artery injury, 328
Cervical
  collar (see Collar, cervical)
  hematoma with compromise of airway
    after penetrating carotid artery
    injury, 319–321
  Immobilizer Device, prehospital use, 9
  orthosis (see Orthosis, cervical)
  spine (see Spine, cervical)
Chemotaxis: polymorphonuclear
  neutrophil, effect of 8-kd peptide
    on, 142
Chemotherapy: cancer, and Candida
    infections, 231
Chest injuries and reamed intramedullary
    rod fixation of femur fracture, 280
  blood gases after, 283
Children
  (See also Pediatric trauma)
  abdominal injuries in, 178–179
  airway in, 174–175
  atlantoaxial rotation injuries in, 25
  breathing in, 175–176
  circulation in, 176–178
  disability in, 178
  fixation of long-bone fractures in, early,
    279
  head injury in, 174
  laparoscopy in, 93–94
  newborn, complications of ECMO in,
    121
  occipital-atlantal injuries in, 23
  Revised Trauma Score in, 194
  rib fracture in, 174
  vital signs in, normal, 177
Chylothorax: thoracoscopy in, 95
Circulation: in children, 176–178
Circulatory support, extracorporeal (see
    Extracorporeal, cardiopulmonary
    support)
CO_2 (see Carbon dioxide)
Coagulation: effects of hypothermia on,
    54–55
Coils: steel, in embolization of hypogastric
    vessels after pelvic fracture, 210,
    211
Cold bronchorrhea, 51
Collar, cervical
  for C1 fractures, 25
  hard, for atlantoaxial rotation injuries, 26

Collar, cervical (cont.)
  in-hospital use, 22
  prehospital use, 9
  temporary, 20, 21
Colony-stimulating factor
  granulocyte-macrophage, and Candida infections, 232
  for immunologic stimulation, 147–148
Colostomy: after open pelvic fractures, 214, 215
Coma: treatment of penetrating carotid artery injury associated with, 332–334
Combitube: esophageal tracheal, 6
Compartment syndrome: pneumatic antishock garment-associated, 8
Complement activation: during extracorporeal cardiopulmonary support, 122
Compression pelvic fracture (see Fracture, pelvic, compression)
Computed tomography (see Tomography, computed)
Computer-generated guideline sheet printout: for equipment requirements and drug doses for resuscitation of children, 186
Conduction, 55
  system, cardiac, effect of hypothermia on, 50
Contrast studies: in esophageal injury, 255–257
Contusion: pulmonary, radiograph of, 280
Convection, 57
Convective air rewarmers, 59–60
Coquille, 10
Corticosteroids
  for immunologic blockade, 155
  serum, effect of hypothermia on, 54
Cost: of parenteral vs. enteral nutritional support, 312
Cotton hospital vs. convective air blankets: for rewarming after hypothermia, 60
CPR (see Resuscitation, cardiopulmonary)
Cramping: and enteral feeding, 311
Craniocervical injury: Power's ratio for identification, 24
Crepitation: in esophageal injury, 253–254
CT (see Tomography, computed)
C3b receptor expression: decrease after hemorrhage, 138
Cystogram of bladder rupture due to pelvic fracture
  extraperitoneal, 218
  intraperitoneal, 218
Cytokines
  effect on anticandidal function of polymorphonuclear neutrophils, 235, 236
  for immunologic stimulation, 147

D

Decision tree: for triage of pediatric patient, 192–195
Decortication: thoracoscopic, 95
Demographics: pediatric trauma, 170–173
Diaphragmatic
  herniation, pneumatic antishock garment-associated, 8
  injuries
    laparoscopy in, 91
    thoracoscopy in, 94–95
Diarrhea: and enteral feeding, 311
Diathermy: in hypothermia, 61–62
Dilatation: causing esophageal injury, 249
Disability: in children, 178
Dislocation: facet, treatment, 30–31
Drain placement
  after esophageal repair, 270, 272, 341, 342
  after tracheoesophageal repair, 341, 342
Drugs
  antiarrhythmic, in hypothermia, 50–51
  anti-inflammatory, nonsteroidal, for immunologic blockade, 155–156
  doses for resuscitation of children, computer-generated guideline sheet printout for, 186
  inotropic, in hypothermia, 50–51
Dyspnea: in esophageal injury, 253
Dysrhythmias: and hypothermia, 50

E

E5: for immunologic blockade, 152
$ECCO_2R$ (see Extracorporeal, carbon dioxide removal with low-frequency positive-pressure ventilation)
ECMO (see Extracorporeal, membrane oxygenation)
Edema
  cerebral, after penetrating carotid artery injury, 328
  pulmonary
    hypothermia and, 51
    pneumatic antishock garment-associated, 8
Eicosanoids: effect of anti-inflammatory drugs on, 155–156
Elderly, hypothermia in
  fluid-circulating heating blankets for, 59
  pulmonary edema and, 51
Electrocautery: in thoracic cavity, 95

Electroencephalogram: in hypothermia, 53
Electrolytes: effect of hypothermia on, 54
Embolism
  fat
    after pelvic fracture, 221
    early fixation of long-bone fractures and, 275
    gas, systemic, due to mechanical ventilation, 101
    pulmonary, after pelvic fracture, 221
Embolization
  arterial, after pelvic fracture, 209–211
  gas, complicating laparoscopy, 92
Emergency room: laparoscopy in, 92
Emphysema
  pulmonary interstitial, in adult respiratory distress syndrome, 101
  subcutaneous, in esophageal injury, 253
End-expiratory pressure: positive, complications of, 100–101
Endocrine effects of hypothermia, 54
Endorphins: and immunosuppression, 141
Endoscopy
  in esophageal injury diagnosis, 257–258
  esophageal injury due to, 249
Endothelium: immunologic blockade strategies targeting, 156–157
Endotoxin
  immunologic blockade for eradication of, 150–151
  neutralizing protein for immunologic blockade, 152
  pretreatment, enteral feeding, and bacterial translocation, 299
Endotracheal intubation (see Intubation, endotracheal)
Enteral feeding (see Nutrition, enteral)
Equipment
  for extracorporeal cardiopulmonary support, 113–115
  requirements for resuscitation of children, computer-generated guideline sheet printout for, 186
Escherichia coli: mutant J5, antiserum to, 151
Esophagectomy: for esophageal disruption, 266–268
Esophagitis: causing esophageal perforation, 251
Esophagography: contrast, in esophageal injuries, 255–257
Esophagoscopy: rigid, in esophageal injuries, 258
Esophagostomy: cervical, for combined tracheoesophageal injuries, 270, 271
Esophagus
  anatomy, surgical, 245–248

  arterial supply and relationship to azygos vein, 247
  cervical
    fistula after esophageal repair, 260
    injury, treatment, 259–260
    injury, treatment, nonoperative, 260
  disease, preexisting, esophageal perforation in, 251
    treatment of disease, 268
  divisions, classic, and relationship to vertebral levels, 246
  gastric tube airway, 6
  injury, 245–274
    blast, 250–251
    blunt, 251–252
    diagnosis, 252–259
    dilatation causing, 249
    drain placement for, 341, 342
    endoscopy causing, 249
    endoscopy in, 257–258
    etiology, 248–252
    etiology, classification of, 248
    external trauma causing, 251–252
    foreign bodies causing, 250
    iatrogenic operative, 251
    intraluminal force causing, 249–251
    penetrating, 252
    radiography in, 254–259
    radiography in, contrast studies, 255–257
    radiography in, plain, 254–255
    signs, clinical, 253–254
    summary, 272
    symptoms, clinical, 253–254
    thoracoscopy in, 270, 272
    treatment, 259–268
    treatment, drain placement after, 272
    treatment, prognostic considerations after, 268–269
    treatment, results, 268–269
  intubation in esophageal injury, 265
  obturator airway, 6
  perforation (see rupture below)
  relationship to azygous vein, 247
  resection in thoracic esophageal injury, 266–268
  rupture
    in preexisting esophageal disease, 251
    spontaneous, 251
  thoracic, injuries, treatment, 260–268
    esophageal resection in, 266–268
    exclusion of esophagus, 263–265
    nonoperative, 260–262
    nonoperative, indications for termination of, 262
    nonoperative, selection criteria for, 261
    operative, 262–268

Esophagus *(cont.)*
  role of interventional radiologist in, 265–266
  treatment of delayed recognition of esophageal perforation, 262–263
  treatment of underlying esophageal condition or disease in, 268
  tracheal combitude, 6
  tracheoesophageal injuries, combined *(see* Tracheoesophageal injuries, combined)
Evaporation, 57
Extracorporeal
  blood rewarming, cardiopulmonary bypass roller pump in, 68–69
  carbon dioxide removal, partial
    (See also Extracorporeal, cardiopulmonary support)
    discussion of term, 104–105
  carbon dioxide removal with low-frequency positive-pressure ventilation
    (See also Extracorporeal, cardiopulmonary support)
    discussion of term, 104
    historical perspective, 103
  cardiopulmonary support, 99–133
    after CPR failure, 111
    anticoagulant therapy in, 118, 120
    during aortic rupture repair, 109–111
    applications, 106–108
    as bridge to transplantation, 112–113
    cannulation in, 115–116
    in cardiac failure, 112
    in cardiogenic shock, 112
    cart, 114
    complications, 120–122
    contraindications, 107
    equipment for, 113–115
    future, 122–123
    historical perspective, 100–104
    indications for, nonpulmonary, 108–113
    modalities, relative ranges of, 105
    nomenclature, 104–106
    patient selection criteria, 106–108
    pressure monitoring in, 116
    in respiratory failure due to diffuse acute lung disease, 106–107
    in respiratory failure due to status asthmaticus, 107–108
    for rewarming after hypothermia, 108–109
    "sweep gas" in, 115
    technical variations, 117
    technique, 113–115
    ventilator management before and during, 117–118, 119
  circulatory support *(see* Extracorporeal, cardiopulmonary support)
  life support
    (See also Extracorporeal, cardiopulmonary support)
    discussion of term, 105
  lung assistance
    (See also Extracorporeal, cardiopulmonary support)
    discussion of term, 105
  lung support
    (See also Extracorporeal, cardiopulmonary support)
    discussion of term, 105
  membrane oxygenation
    (See also Extracorporeal, cardiopulmonary support)
    discussion of term, 104
    historical perspective, 102
    in newborn, complications of, 121
Extracranial-intracranial bypass: after penetrating carotid artery injuries, 328
Eyewear: protective surgical, 86

F

Facet dislocation: treatment, 30–31
Fat emboli *(see* Embolism, fat)
Fatty acids: N-3 polyunsaturated, for immunologic stimulation, 149
Fc receptor expression, decrease after hemorrhage, 138
Feeding
  enteral *(see* Nutrition, enteral)
  jejunostomy, laparoscopic, 91
Femur fracture *(see* Fracture, femur)
Ferno-Kendrick Extrication Device, 9
Fever: in esophageal injury, 253
Fiber: enteral feeding and bacterial translocation, 299
Fibrin glue: in chylothorax, 95
Fibronectin levels: decreased after hemorrhage, 138
Filter: vena caval, after pelvic fracture, 221
Fistula
  carotid-jugular, due to penetrating carotid artery injury, 338–340
  esophageal, cervical, after esophageal repair, 260
Fixation
  early, of long-bone fractures, 275–293
  in chest-injured patient, blood gases after, 283
  conclusion, 291

contraindications, 284–288
historical perspective, 275–276
indications, 279–284
physiologic response to, 288–291
internal, of type III hangman's fracture, 28
of pelvic fractures, 207–209
CT-guided percutaneous screw, 209
Fixator: external, for pelvic fracture, 208
Flap: sternocleidomastoid or strap muscle interposition, for combined tracheoesophageal injuries, 270, 271
Flexicare bed, 21
Fluid
-circulating heating blankets, 58–59
intravenous, warm, in hypothermia, 63–65
replacement, prehospital, 7
warmer, countercurrent, schematic of, 66
Foley catheter: in pelvic fracture patient, 217, 219
Footwear: protective surgical, 86
Forced supine position: diagram of effects of, 290
Foreign bodies: causing esophageal injury, 250
Formulas: nutritional, 314–315
Fracture
acetabular, 222–223
femur
(See also Fixation, early, of long-bone fractures)
comminuted midshaft, radiograph, 286
radiograph, 280
rod for, intramedullary (see Rod, intramedullary, for femur fracture)
hangman's, 27–28
long-bone
early fixation (see Fixation, early, of long-bone fractures)
pneumatic antishock garment use in, 8
occipital condyles, 22–23
odontoid, 26–27
pelvic, 199–225
classification, 200–204
complications, 219–222
compression, anteroposterior, 201, 203
compression, lateral, 201, 202
concomitant injuries, 204–205
fixator for, external, 208
hemorrhage in, 205–213
hemorrhage in, evaluation of, 212
hypogastric vessels after (see Angiography of hypogastric vessels after pelvic fracture)

incidence, 199–200
neurologic injury with, 219
open, soft tissue injury in, 213–214
orthopedic considerations, 223
pneumatic antishock garment use in, prehospital, 8
rectal injury with, 214–215
respiratory failure after, 219–221
sepsis after, 222
summary, 223
thrombosis after, 221
urinary tract injury with, 216–219
urinary tract injury with, evaluation, 220
vaginal injuries with, 215–216
vertical shear, 201, 204
rib, in children, 174
sacral, 219
spine
C1, 24–25
lumbar, worsening after pneumatic antishock garment use, 8
tibia, grade II open, 287
Fusion, surgical
for C1 fractures, 25
for facet dislocation, reduced unilateral, 31
for occipital-atlantal injuries, 24
for odontoid fractures, 26, 27
for spine injuries, lower cervical, 29–30

G

Garment, pneumatic antishock (see Pneumatic antishock garment)
Gas
blood (see Blood, gases)
embolism, systemic, due to mechanical ventilation, 101
embolization complicating laparoscopy, 92
"sweep," in extracorporeal cardiopulmonary support, 115
Gasless laparoscopy, 93
Gastric distension: in children, 176
Gastritis: erosive, prophylaxis against, 145
Gastrografin: in contrast studies of esophageal injury, 255, 256
Gastrointestinal
effects of hypothermia, 53
hemorrhage during pediatric ECMO, 121
tract and immunosuppression, 141
Gelfoam
in embolization of hypogastric vessels after pelvic fracture, 210, 211
Gianturco coils: in embolization of hypogastric vessels after pelvic fracture, 210, 211

Gloves: protective surgical, 84
Glucocorticoids
  for immunologic blockade, 155
  immunosuppression and, 141
Glue: fibrin, in chylothorax, 95
Glutamine
  enteral feeding and bacterial translocation, 299–300
  for immunologic stimulation, 149
Gott shunt: in aortic repair, 110
Gowns: protective surgical, 84–85
Graft: PTFE, after penetrating carotid artery injury, 331–332, 333
Granulocyte-macrophage colony-stimulating factor
  Candida infections and, 232
  for immunologic stimulation, 148
Grillo pleural wrap: for thoracic esophageal injury, 262
Growth factor
  insulin-like, for immunologic stimulation, 148
  transforming growth factor beta, increase after hemorrhage, 140
Gunshot wound
  carotid artery
    arterioplasty for, vein patch, 330
    hematoma after, cervical, 320
    nonocclusive defect due to, 325
    occlusion of internal carotid in asymptomatic patient after, 329
    pseudoaneurysm after, 322
    PTFE graft for, 333
  esophageal, 252, 253

H

HA-1A: for immunologic blockade, 152
Halo device
  for atlantoaxial rotation injuries, 26
  for cervical spine injuries, penetrating, 33
  for C1 fractures, 25
  for facet dislocation, reduced unilateral, 31
  for hangman's fracture, 28
  in-hospital use, 22
  for occipital-atlantal injuries, 23–24
  for occipital condyle fractures, 23
  for odontoid fractures, 26, 27
  temporary, 21
Halter: head, for atlantoaxial rotation injuries, 25
Hangman's fracture, 27–28
Head
  halter for atlantoaxial rotation injuries, 25
  injury
    in children, 174, 178
    early fixation of long-bone fractures and, 279–280
Heart
  failure, extracorporeal cardiopulmonary support in, 112
  output, effect of mechanical ventilation on, 101
Heat
  loss mechanisms, 55–57
  transfer
    mechanisms, 55–57
    rate, approximate, with rewarming methods, 69
Heating blankets: fluid-circulating, 58–59
Hematologic complications: nonhemorrhagic, after extracorporeal cardiopulmonary support, 121
Hematoma
  cervical, with compromise of airway after penetrating carotid artery injury, 319–321
  pelvic, after pelvic fracture, management, 207
Hemicorpectomy: after pelvic fracture, 207
Hemipelvectomy: after pelvic fracture, 207
Hemodynamic instability: after extracorporeal cardiopulmonary support, 122
Hemolysis: after microwaved warm blood use, 64
Hemorrhage
  immune dysfunction after, 139
  in pelvic fracture, 205–213
    evaluation, 212
    open, with soft tissue injury, 213–214
Heparin
  after pelvic fracture, 221
  during extracorporeal cardiopulmonary support, 118
  surface bonding technology in extracorporeal cardiopulmonary support, historical perspective, 103–104
Hepatic
  blood flow (*see* Blood, flow, hepatic)
  dysfunction in hypothermia, 53
Hepatitis B virus: protective surgical wear against, 82
Herniation: diaphragmatic, pneumatic antishock garment-associated, 8
HIV: protective surgical wear against, 83
HLA-DR receptor expression: decrease after trauma, 138
Hormones: stress, and immunosuppression, 141

Host
  barriers, 135–136
  defenses, normal, 135–138
    preservation for immunomodulation, 144–145
Human immunodeficiency virus: protective surgical wear against, 83
Humoral-mediated immunity, 136–137
Hypercapnia permissive, 101
Hyperoncotic solutions: prehospital, 7
Hypertonic solutions: prehospital, 7
Hypogastric
  artery ligation after pelvic fracture, 207
  vessels, angiography of (see Angiography of hypogastric vessels)
Hypoglycemia: and hypothermia, 54
Hypotension
  pneumatic antishock garment-associated, 8
  in septic shock patients, effect on nitric oxide inhibitors on, 157
Hypothermia, 39–79
  approaches to, practical, 39–79
  blood effects of, 54–55
  cardiovascular effects of, 49–51
  central nervous system effects of, 52–53
  classification, 39
  definitions, 39–41
  detrimental effects of, 49–55
  endocrine effects of, 54
  gastrointestinal effects of, 53
  induced, 47–49
  mortality of, 43
  oxygen consumption and, 45–46
  physiologic responses to, 40
  renal effects of, 53
  respiratory system effects of, 51–52
  rewarming for (see Rewarming)
  summary, 69
  in trauma victim, 41–43
  treatment, 57–69
Hypoxia: and immunosuppression, 143

I

Ibuprofen: for immunologic blockade, 155
Iloprost: during extracorporeal cardiopulmonary support, 120
Imaging
  indium-labeled leukocyte, in esophageal injury, 258
  magnetic resonance, in cervical spine injuries, 20
Immersion: warm water, for hypothermia, 60–61
Immobilization, cervical spine
  beds for, 21
  collars for (see Collars, cervical)
  halo for (see Halo device)
  prehospital, 8–10
  temporary, 20–21
  traction for (see Traction)
Immune
  dysfunction after trauma, 138–140
  system mediators, 137–138
Immunity
  cell-mediated, 137
  humoral-mediated, 136–137
Immunization: for immunologic stimulation, 146
Immunodeficiency
  syndrome, acquired, Candida infections in, 231
  virus, human, surgical protective wear against, 83
Immunoglobulin A secretion: and enteral feeding, 298
Immunologic
  blockade, 150–157
    antiendotoxin strategies, 151–152
    antiproteases for, 157
    anti-tumor necrosis factor strategies, 153
    bradykinin inhibitors for, 154
    for eradication of sepsis or endotoxin, 150–151
    interleukin-1 receptor antagonist for, 153
    interleukin-6 antibodies for, 153–154
    leukocyte receptor antagonist for, 156
    mediator inhibition, 152–154
    nitric oxide inhibition for, 157
    nonspecific agents for, 154–156
    nonsteroidal anti-inflammatory agents for, 155–156
    oxygen radical scavengers for, 156–157
    pentoxifylline for, 156
    platelet activator factor antagonists for, 154
    steroids for, 154–155
    strategies targeting neutrophil and endothelium, 156–157
  stimulation, 146–150
    adenosine triphosphate-MgCl$_2$ for, 148
    biologic response modifiers for, 146–148
    immunization for, 146
    metabolic support for, 148
    nutritional pharmacotherapy for, 148–150
Immunomodulation, 135–167
  preservation of normal defenses for, 144–145

Immunomodulation *(cont.)*
  summary, 157–158
Immunosuppression
  bacterial translocation and, 141
  gastrointestinal tract and, 141
  hypoxia and, 143
  ischemia and, 143
  mechanisms after trauma, 140–143
  mediators, 141–142
  nutritional deficiency and, 143
  stress hormones and, 141
  suppressor cells in, 142
  suppressor factors in, 142
  tissue injury and, 140–141
Indium-labeled leukocyte scan: in esophageal injury, 258
Indomethacin: for immunologic blockade, 155
Inflammatory
  mediators, activation during extracorporeal cardiopulmonary support, 122
  response, systemic, and sepsis, 143–144
Inotropic drugs: in hypothermia, 50–51
Instruments: pediatric laparoscopic, 93
Insulin
  effects of hypothermia on, 54
  -like growth factor for immunologic stimulation, 148
Interferon-gamma
  Candida infections and, 232
  for immunologic stimulation, 147
  level depression after trauma, 138, 140
Interleukin
  -1
    for immunologic stimulation, 147
    level depression after trauma, 138, 140
    receptor antagonist for immunologic blockade, 153
  -2
    for immunologic stimulation, 147
    level depression after trauma, 138, 139
  -3 production decrease after trauma, 139
  -6
    antibodies for immunologic blockade, 153–154
    decrease after trauma, 139
    increase after hemorrhage, 140
  -8 and *Candida* infections, 232
Intracranial
  -extracranial bypass after penetrating carotid artery injuries, 328
  hemorrhage as complication of ECMO in newborn, 121
Intraluminal
  force causing esophageal injury, 249–251
  tubes causing esophageal injury, 250
Intravenous
  access for treatment of shock, in children, 176–177
  fluids, warm, in hypothermia, 63–65
  line placement, field, 7
Intubation
  endotracheal
    in children, 175
    esophageal perforation during, 257
    prehospital, 5–6
  esophageal, in esophageal injury, 265
Irrigation: of mediastinum, transesophageal, after thoracic esophageal injury, 265
Ischemia
  bowel, small, and enteral feeding, 311–312
  immunosuppression and, 143

J

Jejunostomy
  laparoscopic feeding, 91
  needle catheter, 297
Joint, sacroiliac (*see* Sacroiliac joint)
Jugular vein-carotid artery fistula: due to penetrating carotid artery injury, 338–340

K

Kidney (*see* Renal)

L

Laceration: aortic, complicating laparoscopy, 93
Laparoscopy
  complications, 92–93
  gasless, 93
  history, 90–91
  pediatric, 93–94
  review, 90
  technique, 92
Lavage
  peritoneal, 89
    diagnostic, after pelvic fracture, 206
    heated, in hypothermia, 62–63
  pleural, for rewarming in hypothermia, 62–63
Leukocyte
  activation during extracorporeal cardiopulmonary support, 122
  polymorphonuclear (*see* Polymorphonuclear neutrophil)
  receptor antagonist for immunologic blockade, 156

scan, indium-labeled, in esophageal
    injury, 258
Levamisole: for immunologic stimulation,
    147
LFPPV-ECCO$_2$R (see Extracorporeal,
    carbon dioxide removal with
    low-frequency positive-pressure
    ventilation)
Lidocaine: in hypothermia, 51
Life support
  basic vs. advanced prehospital, 3–5
  extracorporeal
    (See also Extracorporeal,
      cardiopulmonary support)
    discussion of term, 105
Ligation
  carotid artery, after penetrating injuries,
    328
  hypogastric artery, after pelvic fracture,
    207
  staple, of thoracic duct for chylothorax,
    95
Line placement: intravenous field, 7
Liquid breathing, 123
Liver (see Hepatic)
Low-frequency positive-pressure ventilation
    with extracorporeal CO$_2$ removal
    (see Extracorporeal, carbon dioxide
    removal with low-frequency
    positive-pressure ventilation)
Lumbar fracture: worsening after
    pneumatic antishock garment use,
    8
Lung
  (See also Pulmonary)
  assistance, extracorporeal
    (See also Extracorporeal,
      cardiopulmonary support)
    discussion of term, 105
  disease, diffuse acute, causing respiratory
    failure, extracorporeal
    cardiopulmonary support in,
    106–107
  heart-lung bypass (see Bypass,
    cardiopulmonary)
  membrane, in extracorporeal
    cardiopulmonary support, historical
    perspective, 103
  support, extracorporeal
    (See also Extracorporeal,
      cardiopulmonary support)
    discussion of term, 105
  transplantation, extracorporeal
    cardiopulmonary support as bridge
    to, 112–113
Lymphocyte function changes: after
    trauma, 138–140

M

Macrophage (see Granulocyte-macrophage
    colony-stimulating factor)
Magnetic resonance imaging: in cervical
    spine injuries, 20
Mandibular
  osteotomy for high carotid exposure,
    326
  subluxation for high carotid exposure,
    326
Mandibulotomy: stair-step, after penetrating
    carotid artery injury, 326
Manipulation
  for cervical spine dislocations,
    unreduced, 31
  for facet dislocation, 30–31
Masks: protective surgical, 85–86
Mediastinal
  air on plain radiograph after esophageal
    injury, 255
  hemorrhage during pediatric ECMO, 121
  irrigation, transesophageal, after thoracic
    esophageal injury, 265
Meglumine diatrizoate: in contrast studies
    of esophageal injury, 255, 256
Membrane
  lung in extracorporeal cardiopulmonary
    support, historical perspective, 103
  oxygenation, extracorporeal (see
    Extracorporeal, membrane
    oxygenation)
Metabolic support: for immunologic
    stimulation, 148
Metabolism: and temperature, 46–47
Microwave warming: of intravenous fluids,
    64
Minerva cast: for atlantoaxial rotation
    injuries, 26
Minimally invasive surgery, 89–97
  summary, 96
Monoclonal antibodies: for immunologic
    blockade, 152, 156
Monitoring
  carbon dioxide clearance, during
    extracorporeal cardiopulmonary
    support, 115
  pressure, in extracorporeal
    cardiopulmonary support, 116
Mortality
  of hypothermia, 43
  of pelvic fracture, 200
  rates
    from pediatric and adult trauma
      centers, 100
    in trauma victims, and core body
      temperature, 41

MRI: in cervical spine injuries, 20
Mucus production: and hypothermia, 51
Muscle interposition flap:
    sternocleidomastoid or strap, for combined tracheoesophageal injuries, 270, 271

N

Nafamostat: during extracorporeal cardiopulmonary support, 118, 120
Necrosis
    pancreatic, due to hypothermia, 53
    tumor necrosis factor (*see* Tumor necrosis factor)
Needle catheter jejunostomy, 297
Nervous system: central, effects of hypothermia on, 52–53
Neurologic injury: due to pelvic fracture, 219
Neutrophil
    immunologic blockade strategies targeting, 156–157
    polymorphonuclear (*see* Polymorphonuclear neutrophil)
Newborn: ECMO in, complications of, 121
Nitric oxide
    extracorporeal life support and, 123
    for immunologic stimulation, 148
    inhibition for immunologic blockade, 157
Nonsteroidal anti-inflammatory drugs: for immunologic blockade, 155–156
Nonunion: of odontoid fractures, 26
Nosocomial pneumonia: after pelvic fracture, 221
Nucleotides: dietary, for immunologic stimulation, 149
Nutritional
    deficiency and immunosuppression, 143
    pharmacotherapy for immunologic stimulation, 148–150
    support
        cost, 312
        disadvantages, 310–312
        immunomodulation and, 146
        method, and outcome, 312–313
Nutrition
    enteral, 295–318
        bacterial translocation and, 299–301
        bacterial translocation and, in surgical patients, 300–301
        benefits, potential, 298
        clinical studies, 302–307
        complications, 311
        cost, 312
        early, case for, 297–298
        effect on sepsis, 307–310
    outcome, 304–305
    patient selection, 313–314
    summary, 314
    formulas, 314–315
    parenteral
        cost, 312
        total, 295–296

O

Occipital
    -atlantal injuries, 23–24
    cervical fusion in occipital-atlantal injuries, 24
    condyle fractures, 22–23
Occlusion: internal carotid artery, in asymptomatic patient after penetrating carotid artery injury, 328–329
Odontoid fractures, 26–27
Operating room temperature: and hypothermia, 60
Opsonic activity: diminished after hemorrhage, 138
Orthopedic considerations: in pelvic fractures, 223
Orthosis, cervical
    for cervical spine injuries, lower, 30
    flexion injuries, 28
    for hangman's fracture, 28
    for odontoid fracture, 26
Osteomyelitis: after cervical spine gunshot wounds, 33
Osteotomy
    mandibular, for high carotid exposure, 326
    ramus, vertical, for high carotid exposure, 327
Overhead radiant warmers: in hypothermia, 61
Oxygen
    consumption and hypothermia, 45–46
    radical scavengers for immunologic blockade, 156–157
    supplementation in acute respiratory failure, complications of, 100–101
Oxygenation, extracorporeal membrane (*see* Extracorporeal, membrane oxygenation)

P

Pain: in esophageal injury, 253
Pancreas necrosis: due to hypothermia, 53
Pancreatitis: acute, after hypothermia, 53
Parenteral nutrition (*see* Nutrition, parenteral)
Pathogens: protective surgical wear against, 82–83

PECO₂R
 (*See also* Extracorporeal, cardiopulmonary support)
 discussion of term, 104
Pediatric trauma
 (*See also* Children)
 cart, components of, 185
 center
  ideal, 179–180
  personnel involved in resuscitation of trauma patient at, 180
  problem with, 179–180
  standards for, 179
 decision tree for triage, 192–195
 demographics, 170–173
 injury types, 170–173
 physiologic differences of injured child, 173–174
 printout of computer-generated guideline sheet for equipment requirements and drug doses for resuscitation, 186
 score, 195
 special aspects, 173–179
 treatment in adult trauma center, 169–198
  commitment, 181–183
  composition of pediatric trauma team, 183–184
  conclusion, 196
  evaluation of program, 188–192
  facilities, 184–186
  follow-up care/rehabilitation/ psychosocial care, 187–188
  scope, 181–183
PEEP: complications of, 100–101
Pelvic
 anatomy, 200
 artery injury in pelvic fracture, 209–211
 fracture (*see* Fracture, pelvic)
 hematoma after pelvic fracture, management, 207
 stabilization with screws across sacroiliac joint, 290
Penrose drain: and blowout of carotid artery in postoperative period, 340–342
Pentoxifylline: for immunologic blockade, 156
Peptide
 8-kd, effect on polymorphonuclear neutrophil chemotaxis, 142
 suppressive active, 142
Peritoneal lavage (*see* Lavage, peritoneal)
Personnel: involved in resuscitation of child at pediatric trauma center, 180
Phagocytic defects: after hemorrhage, 138

Pharmacotherapy: nutritional, for immunologic stimulation, 148–150
Pharyngeal tracheal lumen airway, 6
Philadelphia collar
 in-hospital use, 22
 prehospital use, 9
 for spinal injuries, penetrating cervical, 33
 temporary, 21
Phosphodiesterase inhibitors: for immunologic blockade, 156
Physiologic
 differences of injured child, 173–174
 response
  to fracture stabilization, early, 288–291
  to hypothermia, 40
Platelet(s)
 activator factor antagonists for immunologic blockade, 154
 effect of hypothermia on, 55
 during extracorporeal cardiopulmonary support, 121–122
Pleural
 lavage for rewarming in hypothermia, 62–63
 wrap, Grillo, for thoracic esophageal injury, 262
Pneumatic antishock garment
 after pelvic fracture, 207
 prehospital use, 8
Pneumonia
 enteral feeding and, 309–310
 nosocomial, after pelvic fracture, 221
Pneumothorax
 recurrent, thoracoscopy in, 95
 tension, complicating laparoscopy, 92
Polyethylene cervical collar, 21
Polymorphonuclear neutrophil
 anticandidal function, 233–239
  effect of cytokines on, 235, 236
  effect of supernatants on, 237, 238–239
  study, patient demographics for, 234
 Candida infections and, 231–239
 chemotaxis, effect of 8-kd peptide on, 142
 dysfunction after trauma, 140
Polytetrafluoroethylene graft: after penetrating carotid artery injury, 331–332, 333
Polyunsaturated fatty acids: N3-, for immunologic stimulation, 149
Position: forced supine, diagram of effects of, 290
Positive end-expiratory pressure: complications of, 100–101

Positive-pressure ventilation, low-frequency, with extracorporeal CO_2 removal (see Extracorporeal, carbon dioxide removal with low-frequency positive-pressure ventilation)
Potassium levels: in hypothermia, 54
Power's ratio: for identifying craniocervical injury, 24
Pregnancy: pelvic fracture in, 215
Prehospital
 airway management, 5–6
 care, 1–14
  conclusions, 10–11
  immobilization, 8–10
  intravenous line placement, 7
  life support, basic vs. advanced, 3–5
  pneumatic antishock garment use, 8
  time factor, 2–3
Pressure
 monitoring in extracorporeal cardiopulmonary support, 116
 positive end-expiratory, complications of, 100–101
Prevention: of trauma, 1–2
Printout: of computer-generated guideline sheet for equipment requirements and drug doses for resuscitation of children, 186
Procainamide: in hypothermia, 51
Prostacyclin: during extracorporeal cardiopulmonary support, 120
Prostaglandin E_2
 immunosuppression and, 142
 level increase after trauma, 138
Protective surgical wear, 81–88
 against hepatitis B virus, 82–83
 against HIV, 83
 against pathogens, 82–83
 against tuberculosis, 82
 caps, 85–86
 conclusion, 86–87
 development, 84–86
 eyewear, 86
 footwear, 86
 gloves, 84
 gowns, 84–85
 masks, 85–86
 role, 84–86
Protein
 bactericidal/permeability increasing, for immunologic blockade, 152
 endotoxin neutralizing, for immunologic blockade, 152
Pseudoaneurysm of common carotid artery
 after gunshot wound, 322
 after stab wound, 324

Psychosocial care: for children after treatment in adult trauma center, 187–188
PTFE graft: after penetrating carotid artery injury, 331–332, 333
Pulmonary
 (See also Lung)
 barotrauma in mechanically ventilated patients, 101
 cardiopulmonary (see Cardiopulmonary)
 contusion, radiograph of, 280
 edema (see Edema, pulmonary)
 embolism after pelvic fracture, 221
 emphysema, interstitial, in adult respiratory distress syndrome, 101
 infiltrate, radiograph of, 285
Pump
 blood, servo-regulated, in extracorporeal cardiopulmonary support, historical perspective, 104
 roller, cardiopulmonary bypass, in extracorporeal blood rewarming, 68–69

R

Radiant warmers: overhead, in hypothermia, 61
Radiation, 56
 therapy in cancer, and *Candida* infections, 231
Radical scavengers: oxygen, for immunologic blockade, 156–157
Radiography
 in atlantoaxial rotation injuries, 25
 contrast studies in esophageal injury, 255–257
 criteria for instability of cervical spine, 30
 in esophageal injury, 254–259
 of femur fracture, 280
  comminuted midshaft, 286
 in hangman's fracture, 27
 in occipital-atlantal injuries, 23
 in odontoid fractures, 26
 plain, in esophageal injury, 254–255
 of pulmonary contusion, 280
 of pulmonary infiltrate, 285
 of rod for femur fracture, intramedullary, 282
  unreamed, 289
 of sacroiliac joint disruption, 288
 in spinal fractures, C1, 25
 in spinal injuries, cervical, 16
  initial evaluation, 18–20
 of tibia fracture, grade II open, 287
Radiologist: interventional, role in thoracic esophageal injury, 265–266

Ramus osteotomy: vertical, for high carotid exposure, 327
Rectal injury: with pelvic fracture, 214–215
Reduction
  closed, of facet dislocation, 31
  open, of type III hangman's fracture, 28
Reeves Sleeve, 9–10
Rehabilitation: of children after treatment in adult trauma center, 187–188
Renal
  blood flow, effect of mechanical ventilation on, 101
  effects of hypothermia, 53
Respiratory
  complications and early fixation of long-bone fractures, 275–276
  distress syndrome, adult
    after pelvic fracture, 220
    emergence after development of advanced ventilatory support, 101
    ventilatory support and, historical perspective, 100–101
  failure
    acute, and ventilatory support, historical perspective, 100–101
    after pelvic fracture, 219–221
    diffuse acute lung disease causing, extracorporeal cardiopulmonary support in, 106–107
    status asthmaticus causing, extracorporeal cardiopulmonary support in, 107–108
  system effects of hypothermia, 51–52
Resuscitation
  cardiopulmonary
    failure, extracorporeal cardiopulmonary support after, 111
    in hypothermic cardiac arrest, 50
  of pediatric patient
    at pediatric trauma center, personnel involved in, 180
    printout of computer-generated guideline sheet for, 186
Retinal hemorrhage: after pediatric ECMO, 121
Revised Trauma Score: in children, 194
Rewarmers: convective air, 59–60
Rewarming after hypothermia
  active core, 62–69
  airway, 62
  cardiopulmonary bypass for, partial, 109
  cardiopulmonary support for, extracorporeal, 108–109
  continuous arteriovenous, 65–68
    depiction, 67
  external
    active, 58–62
    passive, 57–58
  methods, approximate rate of heat transfer with, 69
Rib fracture: in children, 174
RNAs: dietary, for immunologic stimulation, 149
Rod, intramedullary, for femur frature reamed
  in chest injured patient, 280
  radiograph of, 282
  unreamed, radiograph of, 289
Roller pump: cardiopulmonary bypass, in extracorporeal blood rewarming, 68–69
Rotorest bed, 21
Rupture
  aorta, traumatic, repair, extracorporeal cardiopulmonary support during, 109–111
  bladder (see Bladder, rupture)
  esophagus (see Esophagus, rupture)

S

Sacral fractures, 219
Sacroiliac joint disruption
  radiograph, 288
  screw stabilization, 290
Screw
  percutaneous, CT-guided, in pelvic fracture, 209
  stabilization of sacroiliac joint, 290
Sengstaken-Blakemore tube: causing esophageal injury, 250
Sepsis
  after pelvic fracture, 222
  effect of enteral feeding on, 307–310
  immunologic blockade for eradication of, 150–151
  systemic inflammatory response and, 143–144
Sex distribution: of adult vs. pediatric trauma, 171
Shock
  cardiogenic, extracorporeal cardiopulmonary support in, 112
  in children, 176–178
Shunt: Gott, in aortic repair, 110
Soft tissue injury: in open pelvic fracture, 213–214
Space blankets: aluminum, in hypothermia, 61
Spine
  board, long, prehospital use, 9
  cervical
    fractures of C1, 24–25

Spine (cont.)
    immobilization (see Immobilization, cervical spine)
    injuries, 15–38
    injuries, clinical risk factors, 16–18
    injuries, patterns and treatment, 22–23
    injuries, penetrating, 33
    injuries, radiographic evaluation, initial, 18–20
    instability, radiographic and clinical criteria, 30
    lower, injuries, 28–32
    lower, injuries, biomechanical etiology, 29
    lumbar, fracture, worsening after pneumatic antishock garment use, 8
Splanchnic blood flow: effect of hypothermia on, 53
Spondylolisthesis: of axis, traumatic, 27–28
Staple ligation: of thoracic duct for chylothorax, 95
Status asthmaticus: causing respiratory failure, extracorporeal cardiopulmonary support in, 107–108
Steel coils: in embolization of hypogastric vessels after pelvic fracture, 210, 211
Sternal occipital mandibular immobilization braces: two- or four-point, 22
Sternocleidomastoid muscle interposition flap: for combined tracheoesophageal injuries, 270, 271
Steroids: for immunologic blockade, 154–155
Stiffneck collar: prehospital use, 9
Strap muscle interposition flap: for combined tracheoesophageal injuries, 270, 271
Stress hormones: and immunosuppression, 141
Stroke: treatment of penetrating carotid artery injury associated with, 332–334
Stryker frame, 21
Subcutaneous emphysema: in esophageal injury, 253
Subluxation: mandibular, for high carotid exposure, 326
Sucralfate: as prophylaxis against erosive gastritis, 145
Sump tube: in treatment of esophageal injury, 265, 266, 267
Supernatants: effect on anticandidal function of polymorphonuclear neutrophils, 237, 238–239

Supine position: forced, diagram of effects of, 290
Suppressive active peptide, 142
Suppressor
    cells in immunosuppression, 142
    factors in immunosuppression, 142
Surgery, minimally invasive, 89–97
    summary, 96
Surgical wear, protective (see Protective surgical wear)
Suture: absorbable, in bladder repair after pelvic fracture, 219
"Sweep gas": in extracorporeal cardiopulmonary support, 115

T

Tamponade: balloon catheter, in penetrating carotid artery injuries, 334–338
T cell changes: after trauma, 138
Temperature
    core body, correlation between mortality rate and, 41
    metabolism and, 46–47
    operating room, and hypothermia, 60
Thermal homeostasis: in children, 174
Thermoregulation, 43–44
Thoracic duct: fibrin glue or staple ligation for chylothorax, 95
Thoracoscopy, 94–95
    in esophageal injuries, 270, 272
Thrombosis: causing pelvic fracture, 221
Thrombotic complications: of hypothermia, 54
Thromboxane
    A_2 receptor antagonists for immunologic blockade, 155
    synthetase inhibitors for immunologic blockade, 155
Thymopentin: for immunologic stimulation, 147
Tibia fracture: grade II open, 287
Tissue
    injury and immunosuppression, 140–141
    soft, injury in open pelvic fracture, 213–214
Tomography
    computed
        abdominal, 89
        abdominal, in children, 178
        in atlantoaxial rotation injuries, 25
        in esophageal injury, 258
        -guided percutaneous screw fixation of pelvic fracture, 209
        in hangman's fracture, 27

in head injury, in children, 178
of hemorrhage after pelvic fracture, 205
in occipital condyle fractures, 23
in odontoid fractures, 26
in spinal fractures, C1, 25
in spinal injuries, cervical, 18, 19–20
in spinal injuries, cervical, penetrating, 33
in hangman's fracture, 27
in occipital condyle fractures, 23
in odontoid fractures, 26
in spinal fractures, C1, 25
thin-section, in cervical spine injuries, 18, 19
Tracheoesophageal injuries, combined, 269–270
drain placement for, 341, 342
esophagostomy for, cervical, 271
flap for, sternocleidomastoid or strap muscle interposition, 271
Tracheostomy: in combined tracheoesophageal injuries, 270
Traction
for atlantoaxial rotation injuries, 25
for facet dislocation, unilateral, 30, 31
for hangman's fracture, 28
in-hospital use, 22
for odontoid fractures, 27
Tranexamic acid: during extracorporeal cardiopulmonary support, 120
Transesophageal irrigation: of mediastinum after thoracic esophageal injury, 265
Transforming growth factor beta: increase after hemorrhage, 140
Transplantation
lung, extracorporeal cardiopulmonary support as bridge to, 112–113
solid organ, *Candida* infections after, 231
Transport of patient: and convective heat loss, 56
Triage: of pediatric patient, decision tree for, 192–195
TRISS
methodology from multiple trauma outcome study, 189
Z-scores and mortality rates from pediatric and adult trauma centers, 190
Tube
intraluminal, causing esophageal injury, 250
sump, in treatment of esophageal injury, 265, 266, 267
Tuberculosis: protective surgical wear against, 82

Tumor necrosis factor
Candida infections and, 232
for immunologic blockade, 153
for immunologic stimulation, 147
level increase after hemorrhage, 140

U

Ultrasound
in abdominal trauma, 89
diathermy in hypothermia, 61
of hemorrhage after pelvic fracture, 205–206
Uracil: for immunologic stimulation, 149
Ureter injury: complicating laparoscopy, 93
Urethral injuries: due to pelvic fracture, 216–217
Urethrography: retrograde, of urethral injury due to pelvic fracture, 216–217
Urinary
output, effect on mechanical ventilation on, 101
tract injury due to pelvic fracture, 216–219
evaluation, 220

V

Vaccine: hepatitis B, 83
Vaginal injuries: due to pelvic fracture, 215–216
Vein
(*See also* Intravenous)
azygous, esophagus relationship to, 247
jugular vein-carotid artery fistula due to penetrating carotid artery injury, 338–340
patch arterioplasty after gunshot wound to carotid artery, 330
Vena caval filter: after pelvic fracture, 221
Ventilation
mechanical
complications, 101
for respiratory failure after pelvic fracture, 219–221
positive-pressure, low-frequency, with extracorporeal CO_2 removal (*see* Extracorporeal, carbon dioxide removal with low-frequency positive-pressure ventilation)
Ventilator management: before and during extracorporeal cardiopulmonary support, 117–118, 119
Ventilatory support: and acute respiratory failure, historical perspective, 100–101

Vertebral levels: esophagus relationship to, 246
Vessels
  cardiovascular effects of hypothermia, 49–51
  hypogastric (*see* Angiography of hypogastric vessels)
Virus
  hepatitis B, protective surgical wear against, 82
  immunodeficiency, human, protective surgical wear against, 83
Vital signs: normal, in children, 177
Vitamins A, C, and E: for immunologic stimulation, 149
Volutrauma, 100

W

Warm water immersion: for hypothermia, 60–61
Warmers
  fluid, countercurrent, 66
  overhead radiant, in hypothermia, 61
Warming
  (*See also* Rewarming)
  of blood products in hypothermia, 63–64
Water immersion: warm, for hypothermia, 60–61